INDEPENDENT NURSING INTERVENTIONS

Second Edition

INDEPENDENT NURSING INTERVENTIONS

Second Edition

Mariah Snyder, Ph.D., RN, FAAN
Professor
School of Nursing
University of Minnesota
Minneapolis, MN

Delmar Publishers Inc.®

NOTICE TO THE READER

This book is dedicated to my parents, Agnes and Peter Snyder

Cover design by Anne M. Pompeo

Delmar Staff:
    Executive Editor: David Gordon
    Developmental Editor: Denise Black Gold
    Project Editor: Carol Micheli
    Production Coordinator: Sandra Woods
    Design Coordinator: Karen Kunz Kemp

For information, address:
Delmar Publishers, Inc.
Two Computer Drive West, Box 15-015
Albany, NY 12212

Printed in the United States of America
published simultaneously in Canada
by Nelson Canada
a division of The Thomson Corporation

10 9 8 7 6 5 4 3 2 1

Library of Congress Cataloging-in-Publication Data

Independent nursing interventions / [edited] by Mariah Snyder. — 2nd
   ed.
      p. cm.
    Includes bibliographical references and index.
    ISBN 0-8273-4845-2 (textbook)
    1. Nursing. 2. Nurse and patient. I. Snyder, Mariah.
    [DNLM: 1. Nursing Process. 2. Therapeutic—nurses' instruction.
WY 100 I38]
RT41.I53   1992
610.73—dc20
DNLM/DLC
for Library of Congress   91-16545
                                      CIP

CONTENTS

SECTION 5   SOCIAL INTERVENTIONS

SECTION 6   RESEARCH

PREFACE

The first edition of *Independent Nursing Interventions* grew out of the need for a text for a graduate nursing course that I taught, Nursing Intervention Models. At that time no text existed that contained the numerous interventions that students were using in working with patients. Students in this course and in graduate nursing courses in many other schools/colleges of nursing have found the text helpful in examining interventions to use with patient populations and in conducting clinical research studies. It has been heartening to see the enthusiasm for the text expressed by nurses around the world.

Since the book was published in 1985, considerably more research on many of the interventions in the first edition has been conducted. Therefore, to maximize the usefulness of the text, content on the 23 interventions presented in the first edition was updated and findings from recent research incorporated. Discussions with students and colleagues during the ensuing years have led to the identification of numerous other independent nursing interventions. A number of these have been included in this revision, thus adding to the completeness of the text. However, the interventions included are not meant to be an exhaustive list of independent nursing interventions. For example, teaching, a very important nursing intervention, is not presented because an adequate description would require more space than was feasible for this text. Also, several excellent texts on patient teaching exist.

Many of the chapters have been authored by nurses who have considerable experience with particular interventions. This adds to the richness of the content.

During the years since the first edition, considerably more discussion of independent nursing interventions has occurred in nursing. This has prompted an expansion of the discussion of independent nursing interventions, including possible classification systems and the relationship of independent nursing interventions and nursing diagnoses. The intent of these chapters is to stimulate thinking and discussion of these areas rather than presenting "the answers." Providing patient care is very complex; chapters on moral and ethical issues related to use of independent nursing interventions and clinical decision-making are included to assist nurses with the broad perspectives needed in selecting and using interventions.

Findings from research studies, particularly nursing research studies, are incorporated into each chapter. However, research is lacking for a number of the interventions and considerably more research needs to be conducted on the use of all of the interventions. A final section on research has been added. The chapter provides an overview of clinical research and presents some strategies that may be useful for the development of a more scientific basis for the use of specific independent nursing interventions.

I view this book as a continuing effort by nurses to identify the scope of nursing practice and to communicate to other health professions and the public the essential role that nurses play in the provision of quality health care to diverse patient populations. Undergraduate and graduate nursing students and nurses in clinical settings will find the book to be a ready reference as they consider possible strategies that can be used to achieve patient outcomes. Each chapter defines the intervention, provides the scientific basis for the effects of the intervention, describes how the intervention may be used, identifies populations with whom the intervention has been used, and identifies parameters that can be used in measuring the effectiveness of the intervention. An extensive reference list gives guidance to persons wishing additional information about the intervention.

It is hoped that the readers will share in the excitement the author, contributors, and students have experienced in the use of the text and in the further development of it. It is the editor's desire that the text will prompt nurses to further develop and test the interventions presented and to identify additional nursing interventions.

The author and contributors wish to thank their families and friends for the immense support and encouragement given during the development of this revised edition. Special thanks are extended to the many students who have provided input on particular interventions.

Mariah Snyder, PhD, RN, FAAN
December, 1990

CONTRIBUTORS

Patricia Crisham PhD, RN
Associate Professor
School of Nursing
University of Minnesota
Minneapolis, MN

Miriam Cameron, MS, RN
Doctoral Candidate
School of Nursing
University of Minnesota
Minneapolis, MN

Sheila Corcoran-Perry PhD, RN
Associate Professor
School of Nursing
University of Minnesota
Minneapolis, MN

Ellen Egan PhD, RN, FAAN
Associate Professor
School of Nursing
University of Minnesota
Minneapolis, MN

Marilyne Gustafson PhD, RN
Assistant Professor
School of Nursing
University of Minnesota
Minneapolis, MN

Michaelene Mirr PhD, RN
Associate Professor
School of Nursing
University of Wisconsin-Eau Claire
Eau Claire, WI

Susan Moch PhD, RN
Associate Professor
School of Nursing
University of Wisconsin-Eau Claire
Eau Claire, WI

Margot Nelson MS, RN
Doctoral Candidate
School of Nursing
University of Minnesota
Minneapolis, MN

Muriel Ryden PhD, RN
Associate Professor
School of Nursing
University of Minnesota
Minneapolis, MN

Carol Schaefer BS, RN
Director of Nursing
Rutledge Home
Chippewa Falls, WI

Kathleen Sodergren MS, RN
Assistant Professor
School of Nursing
University of Minnesota
Minneapolis, MN

Lois Taft MS, RN
Doctoral Student
Rush School of Nursing
Chicago, IL

SECTION 1

OVERVIEW

CHAPTER 1

INDEPENDENT NURSING INTERVENTIONS

Nursing, the Finest Art (Donahue, 1989), an illustrated history of nursing, contains many scenes of nurses "caring." Images of nursing that are captured in Donahue's book are ones that are often mentioned by persons when describing nursing. A nurse's hand placed on a fevered brow and a nurse holding the hand of a wounded soldier are two of the paintings included. More recently, the image of a nurse with a stethoscope around her/his neck working amidst intravenous tubings, monitors, and ventilators has evolved. In each, the patient is the focus of attention.

Nursing has often been described as being an art and a science. Peplau (1988) elaborated on this depiction of nursing as it applies to nursing practice. Art forms comprise three elements: medium, process, and product. The use of self, the nurse as the medium, is key to the art of nursing. Peplau (1988) stated:

> The nurse as medium, as an instrument for change, as a catalyst to animate other persons, uses sensitivity, intuition, imagination, resourcefulness, versatility, and innovation. The art of nursing, its aesthetic aspect, is crucially dependent on the presentation of self of the nurse, specifically as a concerned, caring, compassionate, competent person. [p. 10]

The process aspect of art includes the application of skill, such as in doing treatments, making the environment attractive, or providing comfort measures, and in using health care technology. Nurses employ a vast number of modalities in providing care. The expertness of the nurse in the execution of these modalities is an art form. To achieve the stage of being truly artistic, the nurse's judgment regarding a particular situation is critical. What would be best for this patient in this situation? The nurse's past experience and knowledge contribute to the process being artful. Product, the third component of art, is similar to outcomes. Some are readily measurable—decreased stress or improved functioning—whereas other products are more elusive—new insights or changed perceptions. Peplau noted that nurses who have an intense need to measure all possible outcomes of care may become frustrated when patients do not reveal their innermost responses to nursing actions.

Peplau (1988) defined the major components of nursing practice science as problems, method, theory application, planning, intervention, and process. The nursing process is a chief component of nursing practice; it provides a means for an investigative approach to practice. Nurses collect much data during their assessment of patients; these data serve as a basis for planning care and determining the effectiveness of interventions selected. Facts, objective measurements, and verified evidence are needed for nurses to be able to make scientific judgments. Thus, science is an integral part of nursing practice. According to Peplau, "the art of nursing can inform and nourish nursing science and vice versa" (p. 14). Art focuses on the individual being served whereas science looks for more universal applications. Both are critical to the study and use of nursing interventions.

What is it that nurses do and which of these activities, if any, are done autonomously? How can nursing describe its role in the health care field to others, especially policy makers and legislators? What impact does nursing care have on health outcomes? What is the scientific basis for nursing interventions? These are critical questions in the current health care system. This chapter will explore nursing, nursing interventions, and reasons why it is imperative that nurses give attention to the strategies they use in providing care.

Definition

Defining nursing and its scope of practice has received considerable attention. Numerous definitions of nursing have been proposed. Nightingale (1936) defined nursing as having charge of the personal health of a person; the aim of care is to put the patient in the best possible condition so that nature can act upon him or her. Virginia Henderson (1966) viewed nursing as:

> Assisting the individual, sick or well, in the performance of those activities contributing to health or its recovery (or to a peaceful death) that he would perform unaided if he had the necessary strength, will, or knowledge. And to do this in such a way as to help him gain independence as rapidly as possible. [p.15]

More recently, the American Nurses' Association (1980) defined nursing as "The diagnosis and treatment of human responses to actual or potential health problems" (p. 9). This definition focuses on the persons' responses to illness and to the prevention of problems. Benoliel and colleagues (cited in Taylor, 1989) defined nursing practice as the actions and interventions of nurses in relation to health/illness phenomena and includes the achievement of therapeutic goals as dictated by the chosen substantive problem.

Each of these definitions contains words relating to nurses intervening. Nightingale uses the terms "taking charge" and "to put" which suggest activities in which the nurse is to engage. The first word in Henderson's definition is "assist"; this conveys that the nurse performs activities that will help the person achieve his/her level of optimum functioning. "Treatment" in the ANA definition indicates that nurses are involved in care activities that will assist persons in gaining or retaining their health. Benoliel and colleagues are the only ones to actually use the term "intervention." However, all of the definitions cited indicate that the nurse determines the nature of the interventions needed and carries out these actions in an autonomous manner.

NURSING INTERVENTIONS

Nurses engage in a wide variety of activities: assessing, monitoring, and evaluating; diagnosing; planning, coordinating, and managing care; developing policies and standards of care; and intervening. It is this latter activity, the "doing," that is often thought of as composing nursing. All of the above activities are important; this book will focus only on the intervening activities of nurses.

Interventions often have been classified as being independent or dependent. The latter being those actions nurses use in carrying out orders written by other disciplines, primarily physicians. Martha Rogers (1970) proposed using the term "collaborative" rather than dependent in describing this category of interventions as nurses are responsible for all of their actions. Others prefer to use the term interdependent for labeling interventions used to carry out orders written by other professions.

Nursing practice acts in most states have been revised to allow nurses to intervene independently without orders from physicians. The Minnesota Nursing Practice Act (1974) states:

> The practice of professional nursing includes both independent functions and delegated medical functions, which may be performed in collaboration with other health team members, or may be delegated by the professional nurse to other health team personnel. Independent nursing functions may be performed autonomously. [Sec. 148, 171]

What are independent nursing interventions? Numerous terms have been used interchangeably with the term intervention: nursing measures, treatments, modalities, techniques, and therapies are some of these terms. Watson (1988) preferred using the term "caring processes" rather than interventions to denote activities performed by nurses. Gordon (1987) defined independent nursing interventions as actions taken by nurses to help patients move from their present state of health to the one specified in the outcome. This author defines independent nursing interventions as actions performed by a nurse that will help achieve a patient outcome that falls within the realm of nursing. It is important, therefore, for nurses to have an understanding of what constitutes nursing.

In *Nursing: A Social Policy Statement* (ANA, 1980), a number of areas were identified as being within nursing's purview:

1. Self-care limitations
2. Impaired functioning in areas such as rest, sleep, ventilation, circulation, activity, nutrition, elimination, skin, or sexuality.
3. Pain and discomfort.
4. Emotional problems related to illness and treatment, life-threatening events, or daily experiences such as anxiety, loss, loneliness, or grief.
5. Distortion of symbolic functions that are reflected in interpersonal and intellectual processes such as hallucinations.
6. Deficiencies in decision making and ability to make personal choices.
7. Self-image changes required by health status.
8. Dysfunctional perceptual orientations to health.
9. Strains related to life processes, such as birth, growth and development, and death.
10. Problematic affiliative relationships. [p.10]

The authors of the document emphasized that they do not see the above list as exhaustive, but rather as a beginning in the development of the scope of practice concerns.

Nursing diagnoses are another means by which nursing delineates its scope of practice. Nursing diagnoses specify actual and potential health problems for which nurses plan interventions. These will be discussed further in Chapter 3.

What are interventions that fall within the realm of nursing that nurses can use in achieving patient outcomes? The interventions that are found in the subsequent chapters of this book are a beginning effort to delineate these and propose them for use in clinical practice. A perusal of the Table of Contents will reveal that many of the interventions included in this book are ones that also are used by other professions. Biofeedback is used by nurses, physicians, clinical psychologists, physical therapists, and social workers. One may ask, "What makes it an independent nursing intervention?" If the problem for which it is being used falls within the scope of nursing, then the intervention is appropriately classified as being a nursing intervention. Considerably more research is needed for many of the interventions included before they can be prescribed with certainty for particular patient populations. It is hoped that their inclusion may prompt nurses to initiate research studies.

Reasons for Reluctance

Many nurses are reluctant to intervene without physicians' orders. Despite efforts to move beyond the handmaiden image, many nurses feel that it is easier and safer to function in a dependent fashion. However, a great need exists for nurses to make the assessments necessary to arrive at nursing diagnoses and then to select appropriate independent nursing interventions. Progress is being made. The increasing number of practicing nurses who are prepared at the master's level is resulting in nurses evidencing more autonomy in the intervention realm.

A number of reasons exist for nurses being reluctant to function autonomously and to use independent nursing interventions. Some may relate to nursing being primarily a female profession. Others are related to the use of the medical model for nursing.

Curricula devote considerable time to the teaching of nursing skills. The majority of these are included in the beginning nursing courses; texts for these courses contain few independent nursing interventions. Many of the independent nursing interventions that will be presented in this text are viewed as "extras" that can be carried out if time permits. Nursing students are thus engrained with the idea that the skills emphasized constitute the essence of nursing. If nursing students were exposed early in their education to problems falling within the scope of nursing and the independent nursing interventions to be used in achieving the patient outcomes related to these problems, they would become imbued with the essence of nursing. A factor hindering this change is that agencies place a major emphasis on the expertise the nurse has in performing these skills.

A clearer distinction among the components of the nursing process is needed. Assessing the status of the patient and ongoing monitoring of the status are important aspects of care. However, these activities are part of the assessment or evaluation phases of the nursing process and are not actions that fall within the intervening phase. These actions will not achieve a patient outcome. If a patient outcome is to maintain the blood pressure within a specific range, taking the blood pressure every four hours will not achieve that outcome. Teaching the patient relaxation interventions or using strategies that would help the patient change his/her diet would lead to the possible achievement of the outcome. Assessing and evaluating functions, such as taking the blood pressure or checking for reddened areas of skin, are frequently listed under the intervention column of care plans. The reasons why nurses persist in specifying these as interventions are not evident.

Although the number of nursing research studies has increased exponentially in the past 10 years, studies on nursing interventions have comprised a small segment of the nursing research that has been published. Walker (1986) examined the 1981 issues of four nursing research journals to determine the number of published research articles on nursing interventions. She found that less than 10% of the articles (9 out of 104 articles) tested nursing interventions. This author reviewed the 1986 issues of these journals and found that the percentage had not increased. It is encouraging to see the increased number of research studies that are being published in nursing specialty journals. Conducting intervention studies is time consuming and costly. However, more intervention studies are needed to provide a more scientific basis for nursing practice.

Factors Influencing Progress

Although one would wish to see more progress in the delineation of, research on, and use of independent nursing interventions, there are a number of factors that are hastening the trend toward wider use of the interventions. These include the increasing emphasis from reimbursement agencies on the measurement of outcomes, the increasing emphasis on the concept of caring within nursing, and the striving for autonomy by nurses. Each of these will be discussed as it relates to independent nursing interventions.

A number of legislative and policy bodies are placing increased emphasis on the evaluation of care outcomes. The newly created federal Agency for Health Care Policy and Research (AHCPR) supports research on the quality, delivery, and costs of health services. Nursing is integrally involved in this agency. The Medical Treatment Effectiveness Program (MEDTEP) of AHCPR is examining medical, surgical, nursing, and pharmacological outcomes of treatments. Nursing leaders have stated that collaboration is needed in developing guidelines for these outcomes in which a holistic perspective that considers all modalities for intervening is used. Evaluating the effectiveness of independent nursing interventions is critical to this process.

Because alternative interventions to achieve a patient goal may be available, decisions on which one is best to use need to be made. Traditionally, nursing has prescribed one method for handling a situation. Procedure manuals are a prime example of this approach. Fundamental nursing texts usually present only one way to handle a situation. Nurses need to become more attuned to the many possibilities that exist and the decision analysis that is needed to identify the intervention that is most appropriate for a specific situation. Methods to use for decision analysis are presented in Chapter 4.

An important component of decision analysis is considering the ethical implications of particular interventions. Does the intervention have possible risks? What are the long-term effects of the intervention? Does the nurse have adequate knowledge about the intervention? Chapter 5 provides a model for nurses to use in considering the ethical implications of a particular course of action.

Nursing is giving renewed attention to the concept of caring. Watson, Benner, and Leininger have been leaders in the placement of caring as the core of nursing. Watson (1988) believes that the caring function of nursing is threatened by technology, the high-intensity pace of management, and the manipulation of people that is needed to meet the demands of organizations and government. Mayerhoff (1971) notes that caring is more than good intentions. It requires knowing the person's powers and limitations, the person's needs, and what is conducive to growth. Caring also requires that the caregiver be aware of his/her own powers and limitations. Independent nursing interventions, such as those included in this book, are ones that will allow a nurse to intervene in a caring manner.

One reason many nurses seek advanced education is to enable them to function in a more autonomous fashion. Changes in federal and state legislation are providing reimbursement to nurses for services rendered. As nurses function in these more autonomous roles, they diagnose problems that fall within the domain of nursing and prescribe and use independent nursing interventions to achieve outcomes. Psychiatric mental health nurses are one group who have functioned in an autonomous manner for many years; a review of their journals indicates a significant use of independent nursing interventions. Another speciality in which independent nursing interventions are extensively used is in gerontological nursing. The number of elderly is increasing and, thus, there will be a greater demand for nurses to diagnose and treat health concerns of the elderly. Cunningham (1989) urges nurses to put creativity into practice. Use of independent nursing interventions fosters creativity.

Nurses have been using independent nursing interventions, but little attention has been given to identifying and describing these activities. Peplau (1988) noted that science consists of systematized knowledge. Identifying, classifying, conducting research, and using nursing interventions will advance both the art and science of nursing.

REFERENCES

American Nurses' Association. (1980). *Nursing: A social policy statement.* Kansas City, MO: American Nurses' Association.

Cunningham, M. (1989). Putting creativity into practice. *Oncology Nursing Forum* 16:499–505.

Donahue, M.P. (1989). *Nursing, the finest art.* St. Louis: C.V. Mosby.

Gordon, M. (1987). *Nursing diagnoses.* New York: McGraw Hill.

Henderson, V. (1966). *The nature of nursing.* New York: Macmillan.

Mayerhoff, M. (1971). *On caring.* New York: Harper & Row.

Minnesota Nursing Practice Act. (1974). From *Laws relating to registered nurses, nursing grants-in-aid, and licensed practical nurses, Minnesota statutes.* St. Paul: State of Minnesota.

Nightingale, F. (1936). *Notes on nursing*. New York: Appleton Century.

Peplau, H.E. (1988). The art and science of nursing: Similarities, differences, and relations. *Nursing Science Quarterly* 1:8–14.

Rogers, M.E. (1970). *An introduction to the theoretical basis of nursing*. Philadelphia: F.A. Davis.

Taylor, D. (1989). Interventions. Pp. 31–36 in *Classification systems for describing nursing practice*. Kansas City, MO: American Nurses' Association.

Walker, L. (1986). Nursing diagnoses and nursing interventions: New tools to define nursing's unique role. *Nursing and Health Care* 7:323–326.

Watson, J. (1988). *Nursing: Human science and human care—a theory of nursing*. New York: National League for Nursing.

CHAPTER 2

CLASSIFICATION OF NURSING INTERVENTIONS

Since the delineation of independent nursing interventions is in its infancy, some may feel that it is premature to consider possible classification systems for nursing interventions. The profession has, however, begun to give attention to classifying nursing interventions. In 1986 the American Nurses' Association (ANA, 1989) approved a number of policies related to the development of classification systems in nursing. The Association agreed to facilitate the development of classification systems for nursing practice which includes nursing interventions.

Peplau (1988) noted that science comprises systematized knowledge. She stated:

> Classification of the basic phenomena of a given field provides a systematic arrangement that, among other purposes, serves as a building block for research and education of novices in a given science. [p. 13]

A classification system serves as a common language for members of the profession and for the profession to use in communicating with the public.

A major factor necessitating attention to developing a classification system at this time is the rapid computerization within the health care field. The introduction to *Classification Systems for Describing Nursing Practice* (ANA, 1989) states:

> Nursing must be able to name itself and to describe what it does in order to function effectively in a world where computerized information is used to establish everything from diagnosis related groups (DRGs) to cardiac output. Until nurses can name what they do and assign a computer number to that name, we may be neither reimbursed nor recognized as a profession with unique skills and knowledge. [p. 3]

There is a need, therefore, to identify and describe nursing interventions so that nursing can be competitive with other health professions in securing reimbursement for care provided.

The Nursing Minimal Data Set (NMDS) comprises 16 elements (Table 2.1). One of these elements is nursing interventions. It is difficult to envision what will be placed within the intervention category at this time as nursing has no common nomenclature for describing interventions. This became very clear to this author when reviewing nursing literature related to relaxation interventions. The interventions included in articles obtained from a literature search on relaxation were very diverse. Nurses conducting research on relaxation interventions use the term "relaxation" to cover a wide variety of techniques; thus, confusion exists on what was done. Also, this hampers persons from comparing results across studies. This diversity extended even to a very specific intervention, progressive muscle relaxation. Such diversity is found not only in relation to relaxation but exists with interventions such as exercise, movement therapies, imagery,

Table 2.1
Elements of the Nursing Minimum Data Set

Nursing Care Elements
1. Nursing Diagnosis
2. Nursing Intervention
3. Nursing Outcome
4. Intensity of Nursing Care

Patient or Client Demographic Elements
5. Personal Identification
6. Date of Birth
7. Sex
8. Race and Ethnicity
9. Residence

Service Elements
10. Unique Facility or Service Agency Number
11. Unique Health Record Number of Patient or Client
12. Unique Number of Principal Registered Nurse Provider
13. Episode Admission or Encounter Number
14. Discharge or Termination Date
15. Disposition of Patient or Client
16. Expected Payer for Most of This Bill (Anticipated Financial Guarantor for Services)

From H. Werley & C. Zorn. (1989). The Nursing Minimum Data Set and its relationship to classifications for nursing practice. P. 51 in *Classification systems for describing nursing practice.* Kansas City, MO: American Nurses' Association. (Used with permission).

and touch. Intensive work is needed to both identify and adequately describe interventions so that they will be used in a consistent manner.

More precise definitions of interventions are needed in reports of nursing research studies. Although many studies provide operational definitions of independent variables, much ambiguity continues to exist about the manner in which the intervention was conceptualized by the nurse and actually used by the subject. A classification system would assist nurses in viewing an intervention in a similar fashion. A classification system provides a framework for comparing and contrasting the effectiveness of similar interventions. Are underlying mechanisms of action the same for several interventions or do these mechanisms differ?

A workable classification system would be useful to nurse educators. Being able to present categories of interventions to students would assist them in recognizing similarities between and among the various interventions. Our current practice of providing students with lists of interventions is often overwhelming for students. Being able to look at interventions within specific categories provides the students with a framework for considering possible interventions to use in a particular situation. It also allows the student to compare and contrast various interventions.

As was noted earlier, minimal attention has been given to identifying nursing interventions. What are interventions that nurses use to achieve patient outcomes. A number of strategies may be used in identifying interventions nurses use: reviewing nursing texts, journals, and care plans; observing in clinical sites; and interviewing nurses. Information obtained may reveal very circumscribed actions. These would then have to be fit into larger categories of actions. For example, applying a hot pack to a reddened intravenous site could be placed under a larger category of use of heat and cold. Observing practicing nurses and then interviewing them would provide a rich data base on interventions used in nursing practice. Interviewing the nurses being observed would be important as some of the interventions being used may not be evident to the observer. For example, use of the intervention of presence may not be readily apparent to the observer. Interviewing the nurse would verify use of this and also provide information on why a specific intervention was selected.

The process of identifying and classifying nursing interventions will take time. The progress of the nursing diagnosis movement demonstrates that from small beginnings, steady progress may be made in a relatively short period of time. Strategies that have been developed for the identification and validation of nursing diagnoses may be useful to the nursing intervention movement.

CLASSIFICATION SYSTEMS TO CONSIDER

The various theories and conceptual frameworks within nursing influence practicing nurses in the assessments made, in the interventions selected, and how these interventions are used. Kogan and Betrus (1984) note that selecting modes of care is influenced by the nurse's orientation to the nurse–patient relationship, the particular situation, and the properties of the environment, patient, and family. A nurse using Martha Rogers' unitary being framework (1970) would make very different assessments and would label the data differently than would a nurse who ascribes to Orem's self-care model (1971). Although each may elect to use the intervention "journaling" to achieve a patient outcome, the intervention would, most likely, be used for different purposes. The nurse using the Rogerian model may have the patient use journaling to discover patterns, whereas the nurse operating within the Orem model may have the patient use journaling to determine self-care deficits and strengths. Thus, it is important to consider the various nursing theories and models in formulating a classification system for nursing interventions.

In discussing domains within nursing, Meleis (1986) presented a list of nursing therapeutics emanating from the various nursing theories/models. These include:

- Regulating and controlling by providing protection, nurturance, or stimulation to subsystems.
- Providing comfort measures with the goal being adaptation.
- Repatterning of human and environment energy fields for more effective fulfillment of life's capabilities.
- Using transactions that inform and share in the setting of mutual goals.
- Helping the patient to meet his needs, such as suggesting, informing, questioning.
- Using a human dialogue that involves being and doing, nurturing, or experiencing.
- Using self in a therapeutic manner that enables the patient to cope with stress and suffering, and helping the patient to find meaning in these experiences.
- Creating an atmosphere in which healing can occur.
- Acting to assist the person with self-care.

Meleis' categories reflect the diversity found in nursing theories/conceptual models. Many independent nursing interventions could be placed into multiple areas. Her delineation stimulates thinking about how a classification system can be developed that incorporates these multiple perspectives on nursing.

Leininger (1977) and Watson (1988) have delineated factors related to caring. Leininger's major constructs related to care, caring behaviors, and caring processes provide categories that may be useful in the formulation of a classification system for independent nursing interventions. Constructs include comfort, support, compassion, empathy, direct helping behaviors, coping with specific stress alleviation, touching, nurturance, succorance, surveillance, protection, restoration, stimulation, health maintenance, health instruction, and health consultation.

Taylor (1989) cites the work of Benoliel and colleagues on the domain of clinical therapeutics. They identified five therapeutic modes of influence: prescriptive, structuring, mutual participation, indirect, and discretionary nonaction. The mode is the vehicle by which nursing interventions are administered. For each mode of influence, interventions are specified for the physiological and the cognitive/behavioral domains. Examples of physiological strategies are rest and exercise; strategies in the cognitive/behavioral domain include teaching/learning and cognitive restructuring. The work of Benoliel and colleagues offers much promise for future deliberations on a classification system for nursing interventions.

A system for classifying nursing technology has been proposed by Jacox and colleagues (1990). The purpose for developing the system was to more clearly depict actions in which nurses engage to policy-makers, third party payers, and administrators. Both independent and collaborative interventions are included in their schema. Seven categories of activities have been delineated: drugs, devices, biomedical procedures, behavioral/interpersonal relationships, administrative/organizational arrangements, role, and health services delivery model. Interventions/therapeutics are separated from social and functional reintegration. The authors note that the focus of their classification system is technology and does not encompass all nursing activities.

Bulechek and McCloskey (1985) organized the 26 interventions in their book into four categories: stress management, life-style alterations, acute care management, and communication. The central focus of the intervention served as the basis for classifying specific interventions into a particular category.

A study of European nursing interventions that was sponsored by the World Health Organization (1987) formulated six categories for the nursing actions observed: doing/acting for, doing/acting with, education/information giving, psychological support, information collection/observation, and coordination. An "other" category was used for classifying actions that did not seem to fit into the six specified. In another schema used in this study, objectives for which nursing care was given were classified into five categories: physiological, psychomotor, affective, cognitive, and social/interactive. Although no distinction was made between dependent and independent nursing interventions, the classification systems may provide direction for the development of a taxonomy for nursing interventions. It is imperative that the taxonomy developed be one that is useful to nurses throughout the world.

This author has used broad major classification labels for categorizing the interventions included in this book. These are movement, cognitive, sensory, and social. The mode of action of the specific intervention was considered in classifying interventions. However, in many instances this was suppositional as research is lacking on the mode of action for many interventions. Since much remains unknown about the underlying mode of action of specific interventions, only broad categorizations could be made at this time. One major set of interventions not included in this book are those related to teaching/information giving.

CONCLUSION

Identifying independent nursing interventions and developing a classification system for them will be a difficult task given the diversity that exists in perspectives on nursing. It is critical, however, that attention be given to these tasks. Taylor (1989) states:

> The identification of a body of knowledge which is unique to nursing practice and clinical therapeutics can move nursing toward the development of a true professional discipline. The classification of nursing interventions as part of prescriptive nursing practice models will provide nursing with a means to determine therapeutic efficacy and cost-effectiveness. [p. 35]

A review of the schema presented in this chapter reveals some commonalities upon which work can progress. A question can be asked, "Is it possible to have categories that are mutually exclusive?" This is one of the many questions that nursing will need to address in working on a classification system for nursing interventions. Although the task may be difficult, it will be exciting as nursing interventions capture the essence of nursing.

REFERENCES

American Nurses' Association. (1989). *Classification systems for describing nursing practice.* Kansas City, MO: American Nurses' Association.

Bulechek, G., & McCloskey, J. (1985). *Nursing interventions: Treatment for nursing diagnoses.* Philadelphia: W. B. Saunders.

Jacox, A., Pillar, B., & Redman, B.K. (1990). A classification of nursing technology. *Nursing Outlook* 38:81-85.

Kogan, H., & Betrus, P. (1984). Self-management: A nursing mode of therapeutic influence. *Advances in Nursing Science* 7:55-72.

Leininger, M. (1977). The phenomenon of caring, Part V. Caring: The essence and central focus of nursing. *Nursing Research Report* 2(1): 2, 14.

Meleis, A.I. (1986). Theory development and domain concepts. Pp. 3-21 in P. Moccia ed., *New approaches to theory development.* New York: National League for Nursing.

Orem, D.E. (1971). *Nursing: Concepts of practice,* New York: McGraw-Hill.

Peplau, H.E. (1988). The art and science of nursing: Similarities, differences, and relations. *Nursing Science Quarterly* 1:8-14.

Rogers, M.E. (1970). *An introduction to the theoretical basis of nursing.* Philadelphia: F.A. Davis.

Taylor, D. (1989). Interventions. Pp. 31-36 in *Classification systems for describing nursing practice.* Kansas City, MO: American Nurses' Association.

Watson, J. (1988). *Nursing: Human science and human care.* New York: National League for Nursing.

Werley, H.H., & Zorn, C.R. (1989). The nursing minimum data set and its relationship to classifications for nursing practice. Pp. 51-54 in *Classification systems for describing nursing practice.* Kansas City, MO: American Nurses' Association.

World Health Organization. (1987). *Summary of a European study.* Copenhagen: World Health Organization.

CHAPTER 3

NURSING DIAGNOSES

The development and use of diagnoses have had a major impact on the practice of nursing. Many articles in practice journals address the use of nursing diagnoses with specific patient populations; these articles provide evidence that nursing diagnoses are used in practice settings. Diagnoses have furnished a means for nurses to consider patient concerns that fall within the scope of nursing practice and to move toward a more autonomous practice of nursing. Having a common nomenclature allows nurses to more effectively communicate with each other and with other health professionals. Although much work remains, nursing diagnoses have made a significant contribution to nursing and to health care.

Tanner and Hughes (1984) contend that nursing diagnoses have made a significant contribution to nursing by defining and organizing knowledge that serves as a basis for nursing practice. What, then, is the relationship of nursing diagnoses to independent nursing interventions? Are specific interventions related to particular nursing diagnoses? How can the development of classification systems for nursing diagnoses and nursing interventions complement each other? These are two of the issues that will be discussed in this chapter.

CURRENT STATUS OF NURSING DIAGNOSES

The North American Nursing Diagnosis Association (NANDA) has accomplished much since the first Nursing Diagnosis Conference was held in 1973. The number of approved diagnoses has grown from 22 to nearly 100. A taxonomy has been developed. This taxonomy has facilitated the use of nursing diagnoses within computer programs. Nursing diagnoses have been proposed to be a part of the World Health Organization's 10th Revision of the International Classification of Diseases (ICD-10) (Fitzpatrick et al., 1989). Several strategies for identifying and substantiating nursing diagnoses have been developed (Fehring, 1986; Grant et al., 1990; Woodtli, 1988). These have contributed to a more substantive base for specific diagnoses.

Table 3.1 lists the diagnoses that are currently accepted by NANDA. The clarity and specificity of the individual diagnoses varies greatly with some, such as those on incontinence, having very clear and precise definitions and defining characteristics. Others, such as body image, are more ambiguous. The defining characteristics for the latter do not provide nurses with clear guidance in making the diagnosis of alterations in body image.

The structure NANDA has established for accepting new diagnoses now is rigorous. This process will result in more well-founded diagnoses that will assist nurses in making accurate diagnoses. However, much work remains on verifying additional diagnoses and the defining characteristics of many diagnoses currently being used. Multiple studies relating to each diagnosis are needed; to date, the literature provides little evidence of teams of investigators conducting multiple studies on one diagnosis (Hinshaw, 1989). Such efforts are critically needed to supply an empirical base for nursing diagnoses.

Acceptance of the unitary being framework for organizing nursing diagnoses furnishes a holistic framework for using nursing diagnoses. This framework originated from the work of a group of nurse theorists who were appointed by NANDA to formulate an organizing framework for the diagnosis. The nine

Table 3.1
Approved Nursing Diagnostic Categories*

Exchanging

Altered nutrition: more than requirements

Altered nutrition: less than requirements

Altered nutrition: potential for more than body
requirements

Potential for infection

Potential altered body temperature

Hypothermia

Hyperthermia

Ineffective thermoregulation

Dysreflexia

Constipation

Perceived constipation

Colonic constipation

Diarrhea

Bowel incontinence

Altered patterns of urinary elimination

Stress incontinence

Reflex incontinence

Urge incontinence

Functional incontinence

Total incontinence

Urinary retention

Altered (specify) tissue perfusion (renal,
cerebral, cardio-pulmonary,
gastro-intestinal, peripheral)

Fluid volume excess

Fluid volume deficit

Potential fluid volume deficit

✳ Decreased cardiac output

Impaired gas exchange

Ineffective airway clearance

Ineffective breathing pattern

Potential for injury

Potential for suffocation

Potential for trauma

Potential for aspiration

Potential for disuse syndrome

Impaired tissue integrity

Altered oral mucous membrane

Impaired skin integrity

Potential impaired skin integrity

Communicating

Impaired verbal communication

Relating

Impaired social interaction

Social isolation

Altered role performance

Altered parenting

Potential altered parenting

Sexual dysfunction

Altered family processes

Parental role conflict

Altered sexuality patterns

Valuing

Spiritual distress (distress of the human spirit)

Choosing

Ineffective individual coping

Impaired adjustment

Defensive coping

Ineffective denial

Ineffective family coping: disabling

Ineffective family coping: compromised

Family coping: potential for growth

Noncompliance (specify)

Decisional conflict (specify)

Health-seeking behaviors (specify)

Moving

Impaired physical mobility

Activity intolerance

Fatigue

Potential activity intolerance

Sleep-pattern disturbance

Diversional activity deficit

Impaired home maintenance management

Altered health maintenance

Table 3.1 (Continued)
Approved Nursing Diagnostic Categories*

Moving (continued)

Feeding self-care deficit	Dressing/grooming self-care deficit
Impaired swallowing	Toileting self-care deficit
Ineffective breastfeeding	Altered growth and development
Bathing/hygiene self-care deficit	

Perceiving

Body image disturbance	Sensory/perceptual alterations (specify:
Self-esteem disturbance	visual, auditory, kinesthetic, gustatory,
Chronic low self-esteem	tactile, olfactory)
Situational low self-esteem	Unilateral neglect
Personal identity disturbance	Hopelessness
	Powerlessness

Knowing

Knowledge deficit (specify)	Altered thought processes

Feeling

Pain	Rape-trauma response
Chronic pain	Rape-trauma syndrome
Dysfunctional grieving	Rape-trauma syndrome: compound reaction
Anticipatory grieving	Rape-trauma syndrome: silent reaction
Potential for violence: self-directed or directed at others	Anxiety
	Fear
Post-trauma response	

*Diagnoses approved by North American Nursing Diagnosis Association, 1988.

patterns—exchanging, communicating, relating, valuing, choosing, moving, perceiving, knowing, and feeling—provide a structure for the individual diagnoses and give guidance for the assessments that a nurse needs to make. The unitary-being framework is not aligned with a particular theorist; this allows nurses from varying perspectives to use the framework.

Concern has been voiced about the problem-oriented nature of nursing diagnoses that makes it difficult to include diagnoses related to health promotion (Allen, 1989; Pender, 1989). Pender suggests that a taxonomy which includes the strength of the person, the potential problem, and the actual problem may be helpful. Such a method would guide nurses in establishing goals and selecting strategies to maintain the identified strength of the person. Disadvantages of the "strength" system exist. Listing a strength as a diagnosis may be very confusing for some persons. Strategies for nursing diagnoses that will include the important component of nursing, health promotion, require continued attention.

Debate continues on whether all nursing diagnoses should be independent or whether collaborative or interdependent nursing diagnoses are needed. Critical care nurses (Kim, 1985; Roberts, 1988) have noted that their realm of practice includes providing care to patients whose problems are predominantly complex physiological disturbances. Many of the interventions relating to these diagnoses require both medical and nursing interventions to achieve the established patient outcomes. Purists in nursing diagnoses believe that diagnoses requiring interventions ordered by other professionals should not be part of the nursing diagnosis nomenclature. Currently many of the diagnoses listed under Pattern #1, Exchanging, fall into the collaborative category. Discussions continue between the two groups; no immediate solution to the debate is imminent.

Despite the identified problems, significant progress has been made on identifying nursing diagnoses and verifying defining characteristics. The use of nursing diagnoses in hospitals, long-term care facilities, and community health settings is evidence of the acceptance of nursing diagnoses by nurses. The impetus to continue to develop this area of nursing is being fostered by support from the American Nurses' Association and specialty organizations.

RELATIONSHIP OF INTERVENTIONS AND DIAGNOSES

Nursing diagnoses are made after assessment data have been gathered. These data are reviewed and diagnoses made. The diagnoses may be tentative or have a great deal of certainty attached to them. Various interventions are considered that could help achieve the patient outcome(s) for a specific diagnosis. Chapter 5 details the decision-making process used in the selection of a specific intervention. There is need for continual evaluation of the effectiveness of the intervention selected. First, little empirical data exist on the effectiveness of particular interventions used within the context of nursing. Secondly, the patient's status may change, necessitating use of another intervention.

Multiple interventions are possible to achieve outcomes related to one nursing diagnosis. For example, many stress management interventions and techniques exist; each of these may be appropriate to use with the nursing diagnosis of anxiety. Fewer interventions and techniques would need to be considered for the diagnosis of hyperthermia, but there are still several that may be appropriate. Physicians consider a variety of medications for treating a particular medical diagnosis. Numerous hypertensive medications are marketed; specific guidelines exist for selecting one for a specific patient. What is lacking in nursing at this time is both clarity about many of the diagnoses and lack of data regarding the effectiveness of nursing interventions with specific populations/conditions.

An intervention may be appropriate for multiple diagnoses. For example, imagery could be used for the diagnoses of powerlessness, anxiety, ineffective breathing pattern, self-esteem disturbance, and sleep disturbance. This list is not inclusive. The "Uses" sections of the chapters in Part II indicate the many conditions for which the specific interventions have been used. The effectiveness of only a small percentage of these has been verified through research. In instances in which research studies have been conducted, the sample size is often very small.

An integral relationship exists between nursing diagnoses and independent nursing interventions. However, it is not possible to specify one intervention for a specific diagnosis. This requires that nurses use their knowledge, garnered from practice, intuition, ethics, and empirical data, to determine which intervention is best for a specific patient situation.

It is important that work on both nursing diagnoses and nursing interventions proceed as both are critical to the continuing evolvement of nursing practice. Collaborative efforts among nurses involved in diagnoses and interventions are needed because of the intertwining of the two areas. Developments in one area will have an impact on the evolvement of the other area.

REFERENCES

Allen, C.J. (1989). Incorporating a wellness perspective for nursing diagnosis in practice. Pp. 37–42 in R. Carroll-Johnson Ed., *Classification of nursing diagnoses: Proceedings of the Eighth Conference.* Philadelphia: J.P. Lippincott.

Fehring, R.J. (1986). Validating diagnostic labels: Standardized methodology. Pp. 183–190 in M. Hurley ed., *Classification of nursing diagnoses: Proceedings of the Sixth Conference.* St. Louis: C.V. Mosby.

Fitzpatrick, J.J., Kerr, M.E., Saba, V.K., Hoskins, L.M., Hurley, M.E., Mills, W.C., & Rottkamp, B.C. (1989). *American Journal of Nursing* 89:493–495.

Grant, J.S., Kinney, M., & Guzzetta, C.E. (1990). Using magnitude estimation scaling to examine the validity of nursing diagnoses. *Nursing Diagnosis* 1:64–69.

Hinshaw, A.S. (1989). Keynote address: Nursing diagnosis: Forging the link between theory and practice. Pp. 3–10 in R. Carroll-Johnson Ed., *Classification of nursing diagnoses: Proceedings of the Eighth Conference.* Philadelphia: J.P. Lippincott.

Kim, M.J. (1985). Without collaboration, what's left? *American Journal of Nursing* 85:281–282.

Pender, N.J. (1989). Languaging a health perspective for NANDA taxonomy on research and theory. Pp. 31–36 in R. Carroll-Johnson ed., *Classification of nursing diagnoses: Proceedings of the Eighth Conference.* Philadelphia: J.P. Lippincott.

Roberts, S.L. (1988). Physiologic nursing diagnoses are necessary and appropriate for critical care. *Focus on Critical Care Nursing* 15(5):42–49.

Tanner, C.A., & Hughes, A.M. (1984). Nursing diagnosis; issues in clinical practice research. *Topics in Clinical Nursing* 5(4):30–38.

Woodtli, A. (1988). Identification of nursing diagnoses and defining characteristics. *Research in Nursing and Health* 11:399–406.

CHAPTER 4

RESOLVING ETHICAL AND MORAL DILEMMAS OF NURSING INTERVENTIONS

Patricia Crisham, Ph.D., R.N.

INTRODUCTION

The premise of this chapter is that moral and ethical dilemmas contribute to the quality of nursing care. Usually, moral and ethical dilemmas present as upsetting experiences for individuals. They are described as problems and associated with confusion and struggle. The invitation here is to consider the possibility that moral and ethical dilemmas associated with nursing interventions are opportunities for individual nurses, and the profession as a whole, to rediscover and recreate their commitments in nursing.

Radical changes in health care have produced a set of problems in biomedical ethics that confront health care professionals and families every day. These biological and technological developments significantly affect nursing (Veatch & Fry, 1987). Anticipating this, the American Nurses' Association (1980) passed a resolution to clarify the ethical issues in clinical practice and to establish a process for nurses to actively participate in ethical decision making. Since that time, a surge of articles and beginning studies reflect an increased interest and concern about nurses' moral reasoning and ethical behavior. The purpose of this chapter is to identify ethical dilemmas inherent in nursing interventions, to propose a process for nurses to analyze and resolve these dilemmas, and to summarize the state of the art of research on ethical issues in nursing.

Identification of Dilemmas

Clarification of nursing dilemmas has begun. The International Council of Nurses (1977) published the descriptive statements of nurses from 25 countries identifying ethical problems in nursing practice. Examples of ethical problems are grouped according to the five main facets of the International Council of Nurses Code for Nurses: Nurses and People; Nurses and Practice; Nurses and Society; Nurses and Co-workers; and Nurses and the Profession.

Yarling and McElmurry (1986) described the focus of recurring ethical problems for nurses as care of patients in pain, cardiopulmonary resuscitation, withholding or withdrawing of life-sustaining treatment, informed consent procedures, refusal of consent to treatment, harmful care by another practitioner, and professional control of information. For nurses, ethical problems often involve varied, sometimes conflicting, obligations. In an acute care setting, the nurse is the health care professional in closest contact with the patient. It is usually the nurse who perceives ethical differences among families, physicians, and other health care professionals (Veatch & Fry, 1987).

To systematically document the ethical dilemmas nurses encounter in their practice and to characterize the ways in which nursing practitioners perceive and respond to these dilemmas, Crisham (1979) interviewed 130 staff nurses. Volunteer staff nurses were interviewed individually by the investigator during which they were asked to describe a nursing dilemma they had experienced. Without exception, they stated they had wanted an opportunity to discuss a particular dilemma. Although most of the dilemmas had occurred during the past month, some had occurred more than three years earlier. All had been troubling in terms of uncertainty of action. Most had remained unresolved.

A dilemma was classified as a recurrent nursing moral dilemma if a minimum of five nurses described the same problem. The situational form of the dilemma varied among nurses, but essentially the same elements of the dilemma were identified. Interviewing of staff nurses continued as long as new dilemmas were introduced. From 130 staff nurse interviews, 21 recurrent nursing moral dilemmas were identified and grouped according to four underlying ethical issues: (1) deciding the right to know and determining the right to decide, (2) defining and promoting quality of life, (3) maintaining professional and institutional standards, and (4) distributing nursing resources.

Examples of the first issue, deciding the right to know and determining the right to decide, are dilemmas about whether or not a patient has truly given informed consent, whether to correct biased information given to a patient by a colleague or to say nothing, whether to be an advocate for a patient against the wishes of the family or to respect the family's wishes, whether to safeguard the patient's confidence or to report a public health concern to authorities, and whether or not to give information about risks of the prescribed treatment.

The second issue, defining and promoting quality of life, includes dilemmas about: whether or not to resuscitate an individual; whether or not to support aggressive intravenous therapy, ventilator, and vaso-pressors; whether or not to take a stand about interventions for a newborn with severe anomalies; and whether or not to give a p.r.n. dosage of morphine sulfate that is capable of causing death to a terminally ill patient.

Examples of the third issue, maintaining professional and institutional standards, are dilemmas about: whether or not to accept responsibility or delegate authority to other staff members; whether or not to refuse admission of an additional patient when the census is at the maximum; whether or not to replace an experienced, competent nurse with an inexperienced nurse not oriented to the setting; whether or not to cover for a colleague's negligence; and whether or not to implement a procedure which would benefit the patient but violate agency policy.

The fourth issue, distributing nursing resources, includes dilemmas about: whether or not to implement legislative allocation and rationing guidelines for the care of the elderly; how to allocate the time of staff on duty and determine who would give direct care to the most seriously ill patients; whether or not to safeguard time for patient teaching about health promotion and prevention in a busy, acute care setting; whether or not to support legislation to increase expenditures for extraordinarily expensive, new medical technology; whether or not to intervene when decisions are made for a cesarean section rather than vaginal delivery, because vaginal deliveries are costing the hospital money and the hospital makes a profit from cesarean sections.

All of these dilemmas are situations in which the nurse believed there was a moral obligation to follow two incompatible courses of action. These situations raise numerous questions about how nurses are to use their professional expertise and their knowledge about the patient's and family's wishes on behalf of the patient. To whom are nurses accountable for their intervention: the patient, the family, the physician, themselves, the health care delivery system, the profession, or society? How can nurses best protect the patient's right to refuse or accept the intervention? Who should decide? By what criteria should decisions be made? How should the nurse decide and act?

How can the nurse create a context to experience dilemmas as an opportunity for recreating commitments? Socrates always raised questions when Athenians came to him for advice. When a nurse is grappling with ethical issues inherent in choosing and implementing nursing interventions, it will be, perhaps, the nurse's willingness to raise questions that will most significantly facilitate the resolution of ethical conflict. Ethical dilemmas are an opportunity to "live in the question," to raise basic questions such as: What are nursing's reasons for being? What is the context in which the nursing intervention is used? Who am I? What are my commitments?

MODEL FOR RESOLVING ETHICAL DILEMMAS

The specific process proposed in this section was designed to facilitate the resolution of ethical dilemmas associated with nursing interventions. The model had an unusual beginning. General hospital staff nurses who had volunteered to describe ethical dilemmas that they had experienced in nursing requested a workable ethical decision-making model in fair exchange for their participation in research on ethical dilemmas in nursing practice. Most of the dilemmas the nurses described in the research had remained unresolved. The nurses anticipated that they would continue to experience being "stuck" in conflicts of fairness, continue to be evasive about what to do, continue to wake up at night wondering about the consequences of their response. The familiar nursing process was useful with many of the decisions they were making, but it was not helpful in facilitating the resolution of ethical conflict. In the future these nurses wanted to be able to formulate a position congruent with an ethical theoretical framework and to act on their position with some degree of consistency and confidence. They requested an ethical decision-making model that would facilitate this process and work in their clinical nursing situations.

Collaborating with William Stockton, a philosopher-anthropologist, Crisham developed the following model. It has been tested and refined and used in the analysis and resolution of nursing ethical dilemmas with undergraduate and graduate students in nursing, and with numerous groups of nurses, nurse educators, and nursing administrators. The model encompasses the steps of the nursing process; the usefulness of this model is found, however, in the practical techniques associated with each step that acknowledge the nature of the nursing ethical conflict, that is, being torn between conflicting moral obligations that cannot be fulfilled at the same time.

The major purpose of the model is to facilitate a transformation in the way nurses experience moral and ethical conflict, from a dilemma to an opportunity for committed action. The model makes the decision-making process explicit, facilitates the discovery of the nurse's own implicit moral and ethical rules and principles, relates the nurse's thinking to moral and ethical theories in philosophy and developmental psychology, and links judgment, choice, and action in the nursing experience. It is not a method to determine the right answer or to eliminate the inherent conflicting loyalties in ethical dilemmas. Using the model will not yield secure and definite answers, but will raise new questions, new doubts, and new responsibilities. In the end, the nurse will have considered various alternatives in light of moral principles, and will have an opportunity to choose and to take responsibility for the choice.

A mnemonic device for remembering the steps in the process was devised, MORAL. These are shown in Figure 4.1.

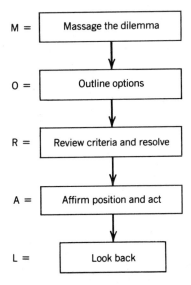

M =   Massage the dilemma

O =   Outline options

R =   Review criteria and resolve

A =   Affirm position and act

L =   Look back

Figure 4.1
Steps of the MORAL model for resolving ethical dilemmas.

M:Massage the Dilemma

The first step involves creating an image of the ethical conflict that includes all significant features about the dilemma situation. By focusing on concrete, clinical dilemmas, certain pitfalls of reasoning about general moral issues in health care are avoided.

Massaging a dilemma is like the process of temple rubbing, which results in an intricate pattern on rice paper, or like a child's technique of rubbing paper overlaying a leaf with a crayon to obtain the detailed imprint of a leaf. With the nurse's dilemma, this process includes recognizing and questioning whose interests are involved in this conflict, defining the dilemma for the individuals involved, describing the crunch of conflicting loyalties, including feelings, laws, regulations, etc. This process is often difficult in the complex health care delivery system, and some general conclusions from psychological research are relevant: (1) many people have difficulty in interpreting the issues inherent in situations, (2) striking individual differences exist among people in their sensitivity to the needs and welfare of others, and (3) the capacity to make inferences about the other's needs and wishes develops with education and age (Rest, 1982).

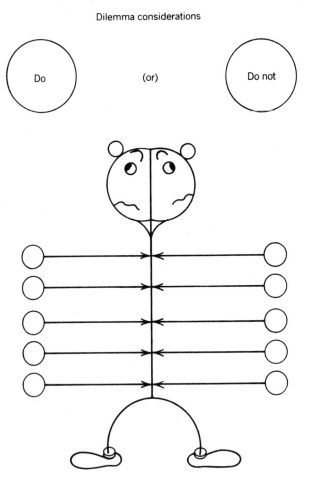

Figure 4.2
Diagram for identifying the two incompatible action choices and the forces or considerations in the ethical dilemma.

Kurt Lewin's (1969) "force field analysis" is a useful technique for graphically describing the forces or considerations in the situation. Nurses identify the two incompatible action choices that result in their being stuck in the dilemma and the forces inherent in the health care situation that influence taking either of these two actions. The force field analysis technique serves to focus attention on the horns of the dilemma and the features of the situation that are perceived to pull or push the nurse (Figure 4.2).

By completing the force field analysis, the nurse defines the dilemma and is ready to re-focus from a broader perspective on the situation by: (1) recognizing the issues that are underlying the considerations, (2) formulating a goal in relation to the major issues reflected in the considerations and the nurse's professional commitments, and (3) realigning the forces in relation to the goals.

The major issues inherent in the dilemma will be one or more of the following: (1) deciding the right to know and determining the right to decide, (2) defining and promoting quality of life, (3) maintaining professional and institutional standards, and (4) distributing nursing resources. Nurses specify the goal(s) and establish priorities if there is more than one goal, in relation to the major issues. To formulate the goal, the nurse determines the desired outcome, that is, "I would like to act in such a way that...." The focus here is on intentionality and with the question, "What is it my intention to produce in this situation?" Fundamental questions about the purpose of nursing frequently surface. The nurse has an opportunity to become clear

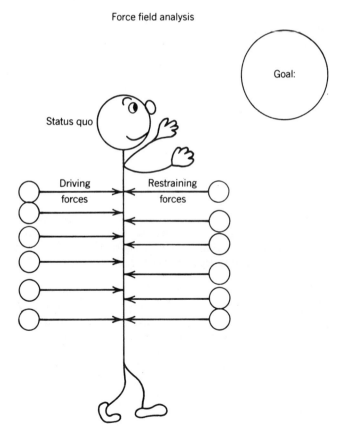

Figure 4.3
Diagram for formulating the goal in the ethical dilemma and realigning the forces in relation to the goal.

about primary commitments in nursing, and to raise questions about "who am I" as a nurse and as a human being. Once the goal is established, the forces are realigned in relation to the goal (Figure 4.3).

O:Outline Options

As a result of massaging the dilemma, the nurse has shifted from perceiving the situation as a dilemma with two incompatible responses to defining it as a problem of how to reach a goal or how to produce results, given the status quo. The focus now is on generating several effective alternatives for reaching the goal.

This second step of the model is essentially a brainstorming session to discover alternative solutions to the problem by formulating strategies that will strengthen or add to the driving forces and weaken or eliminate the restraining forces. It is most effective to approach this process in two steps. First, with each of the forces, the nurse asks what actions that could be taken to: (1) control the force, (2) influence the force, or (3) anticipate the force in the dilemma situation. This process results in numerous specific actions that could either strengthen the driving forces or weaken (or eliminate) the restraining forces. The second step of this process is simply to examine these possible actions and put together selected combinations of actions that would be likely to be effective alternatives for reaching the goal. This process usually results in the formulation of two or three general strategies that will be evaluated against selected moral criteria in the next step of the model.

R:Review Criteria and Resolve

As a result of outlining options, the nurse shifts from not knowing how to solve the problem to the question of which alternative is best. The focus is on deciding in light of ethical principles. The purpose of the "R," the third step in the model, is to identify moral principles or criteria and to select the course of action that is congruent with the criteria. This step, therefore, is crucial to resolving the dilemma and making a moral judgment. It is, likewise, pivotal in linking the moral judgment to the moral action.

The two phases, identifying the moral criteria and assessing the available options by the criteria, are often perceived by nurses as complex and difficult. The inexperienced nurse will have the greatest difficulty with this process. In studying clinical decision making of undergraduate nursing students and experienced practitioners, Grier (1983) documented a significantly lower tolerance for ambiguity among beginning students in nursing. Eberhardy (1982) studied the nursing care of terminally ill adults and found that experienced nurses identified themselves as being responsible for a decision significantly more often than undergraduate nursing students. Crisham (1981) found that nurses who were familiar with dilemmas had significantly higher principled thinking scores than nurses who were unfamiliar with the dilemmas. Using these findings, the following techniques were formulated.

Identifying Moral Principles

To identify moral criteria, two different approaches may be used. The first approach is to identify personal implicit principles and then relate these principles or rules to established ethical theory; the second approach is to critique ethical theories and then attempt to choose and order basic principles to form a personal set of principles. The end result of both approaches is the same: the identification of principles that are thought to be most basic, most important, and will be applied with some degree of conviction and confidence. When this process is repeated with successive dilemmas, a set of principles, applicable across situations, emerges.

Discovering Personal Principles

One way to facilitate the discovery of the nurse's implicit principles and rules is to follow the "O" step of the model and complete the following sentence: "I should—or should not—do (the specific action) because...." The result is a list of the nurse's implicit "shoulds," which becomes the basis of the exploration and critique of rules and principles. Nurses can examine their implicit "shoulds" in light of traditional philosophical thinking. Nurses have found it useful, for example, to contrast act and rule utilitarianism, deontological principles of Kant or Frankena, or interrelated principles from various ethical theories.

In examining their "shoulds," nurses often have difficulty distinguishing "moral shoulds" from legal, professional, and other types of "shoulds." The distinctions developed by Shweder (1980) may be useful during this process. This may also be the time to relate the distinctions among levels of moral judgment offered by Piaget (1965), Kohlberg, Levine, & Hewer (1983), Gilligan (1982), and others.

Adopting Principles from Ethical Theory

Ethical theory provides a framework to determine morally acceptable positions and actions. During recent years, two major types of ethical theory have been the focus of moral philosophy: teleological and deontological theories.

Theories that judge the worth of actions by their consequences and ends are described as teleological (from the Greek "telos" which means "end"). A feature of these theories is that one's duty and the determining of what is right are subordinated to what is good, because duty and what is right are defined in terms of good or that which will produce good. Utilitarianism is an example of a teleological theory that gauges the worth of actions by their consequences. The origins of utilitarianism are found in the writings of David Hume (1711–1776) and John Stuart Mill (1806–1873). The central principle of this theory asserts that persons ought to produce the greatest possible balance of value over disvalue for all persons involved.

Deontological theories (from the Greek "deon" which means "duty"), on the other hand, assert that the concept of duty is independent of the concept of good and that right actions are not determined by the production of good (Beauchamp & Childress, 1989). Immanuel Kant (1734–1804) is acknowledged as the first theorist to formulate an unambiguous deontological theory. Kant suggested that whatever rule of action one adopts, one must act in such a way as to preserve respect for the intrinsic value or dignity of all persons including the person performing the action. Kant (1959) stated:

> Act so that you treat humanity, whether in your own person or in that of another, always as the end and never as a means only. [p. 47]

According to Kant, this principle must serve as a separate principle against which all other ends or goals are evaluated.

Both deontological and teleological theories address the same question, "What ought I to do?" Whereas they offer different answers to this question, or similar answers with differing rationale, they share a common concept: Individuals face ethical dilemmas, and the task of ethics is to explicate moral principles so that individuals can determine duties and responsibilities in these dilemmas.

To complete the "R" step of the model, the nurse identifies and systematically examines the moral principles involved in the situation. Moral duties are determined by careful examination and reflection on selected moral principles (Beauchamp & Childress, 1989; Frankena, 1973; Muyskens, 1982). The following are four basic moral principles: autonomy, nonmaleficence, beneficence, and justice. (See Beauchamp & Childress, 1989, for a thorough explication of each principle.)

The duty inherent in the principle of autonomy is to respect all persons, including oneself, as autonomous beings with a right to their own views and the freedom to act in their judgments. In nonmaleficence, one's duty is to avoid intending, causing, permitting, or imposing harm or the risk of harm to any person. The duty of beneficence is that one should act to prevent harm, remove harmful conditions, and promote positive benefits for others. Justice, in the broadest sense, is giving to each person what is due or owed. Aristotle's concept of justice is that equals ought to be treated equally and unequals, unequally. Justice is concerned with credentialing moral persons and determining the relevant properties or criteria for distributing burdens and benefits. According to Rawls (1971), justice is determining what is fair.

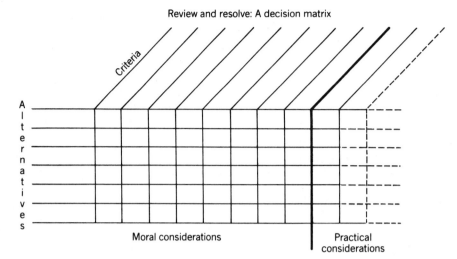

Figure 4.4
A decision-making grid to determine which alternative most adequately respects the moral principles.

A decision-making grid using criteria to determine the action to be taken is useful in determining which alternative most adequately respects the moral principles (Figure 4.4). The focus is on the moral and ethical criteria, but the grid also allows the nurse to consider professional-technical and pragmatic criteria. When two or three alternatives seem relatively equal in terms of the moral criteria, the pragmatic considerations become the deciding criteria.

Although this assessment process cannot be quantified, a number of approaches are useful in clarifying which alternative to choose. The assessment might focus on whether the moral criterion is met (+), violated (−), or not relevant (0). Another approach is to focus on ranking each alternative with each criterion, indicating the rank of "1st," "2nd," "3rd," or "4th" to show which alternative met the criterion to the greatest (or least) degree. Individuals may disagree in their assessment of alternatives chosen in relation to the moral criterion used, but each person will be in a position to present the basis of his/her differing interpretation. What is important here is that the significant questions are raised. Determining the weight and priority of various criteria will bring fundamental issues to light at this point in the process.

A: Affirm Position and Act

As a result of reviewing the criteria, the nurse has shifted from not knowing which alternative is best to making a judgment or decision about which alternative is best according to moral principles. However, a decision or judgment is not a choice. To know what is best, to make a judgment about which alternative is the best solution, is not necessarily a commitment to act on that judgment. The shift that occurs in affirming the position and acting is from deciding to choosing. To decide means "to cut off" (from the Latin, "decidere") the other alternatives; whereas, choosing means to take a stand in the full realization that reasonable people could take another stand.

The first three steps of the model result in a moral judgment, namely, a decision that a particular alternative is most congruent with one's specified moral criteria. Based on the outcome of the decision matrix, the nurse decides what should be done. The "A" step of the model, then, moves beyond cognitive clarity to acting on a commitment. Developing a moral judgment is the essential preparation for the moral action; the moral judgment is "necessary but not sufficient" in following through with the process of the model. Affirming one's position and acting calls forth the courage to act out of a choice.

The mnemonic, ACT, may be helpful in lessening the complexity of acting according to one's moral perspective in the health care delivery system.

A — Anticipate the objections and obstacles to the action.

C — Clarify own position and plan action to respond to anticipated objections and obstacles.

T — Test your choice by acting on it.

Psychologists have studied the virtues necessary to act on a resolve—competence, resoluteness, perseverance, inner strength—in terms of "ego strength." This concept, however, is not well defined. How an individual develops or chooses to use these qualities is not clear at this stage of the research.

Research in cognitive developmental psychology that examines moral judgment level, real-life decision-making, and behavior has been reviewed by Blasi (1984). He concludes that the difficulty of studying complex situations in which moral judgments are implemented is reflected in the lack of research in this area. Assessment techniques for studying the implementation of moral judgment in real-life situations have not been developed.

According to moral philosophers, the first three steps of the model concentrate on cognitive clarity about delineating the nursing ethical dilemma and identifying principles used to make a moral judgment. The "affirm and act" step concentrates on other aspects of morality that influence what nurses ought to do and be: conscience (consciousness and reflection on autonomously accepted action guides), virtue (acquired habit to do what is right), and integrity (acting consistently with one's resolve). Numerous contemporary philosophers, like the classical tradition of Plato and Aristotle, have concluded that the fundamental question is: Who should I be? Morality does not consist in adherence to principles and rules, in their view, but in the expression of conscience, virtue, and integrity internal to the person.

The "A" step of the model is about choosing, after having deliberated about alternatives and principles, and taking responsibility for the choice. It is about reversing the trends of apprenticeship and paternalism documented by Ashley (1976), and creating, through committed action, a context through which all parties to a dilemma are supported in choosing from their commitments to the health and well being of the patient.

L:Look Back

In acting from commitment, the nurse inevitably experiences confusion and doubt, and the shift called for in looking back is on completing the experience of acting from commitment. As nurses pay attention to their own data—their perception of the ethical conflict, their resourcefulness in generating options, their clarification of moral criteria and assessment of options by these criteria, their implementation of the resolve—the experience of ethical dilemmas will bring new insights and new responsibilities.

It is useful to focus the evaluation on the linkage between the moral judgment ("M-O-R") and the moral action of the "A" step. The evaluation process includes an examination of each step in the model. A focused assessment on the "M" clarifies the most recurrent ethical dilemmas in a particular clinical area of practice. The focus on the "O" includes an assessment of the nature and adequacy of the alternative strategies. Evaluating the "R" encompasses reviewing the process of defining the set of basic moral principles, the priority that is consistently given to specific principles, and the effectiveness of the process of using the moral criteria to judge various alternatives.

In summary, the purpose of the MORAL model is to facilitate a transformation in the way nurses experience moral and ethical conflict. The model starts with the nurse's experience of being stuck in a dilemma with two unacceptable options. It facilitates the discovery of the nurse's implicit moral principles and links the nurse's thinking with ethical theories. With a position, formulated by comparing alternative strategies with specified moral criteria, the nurse has an opportunity for acting from commitment and enhancing the quality of health care.

RESEARCH

Research contributing to the understanding of how nurses' resolutions of ethical dilemmas with nursing interventions contribute to quality health care could be characterized as arising from three major questions: (1) How should nurses reason about moral and ethical issues? (2) How do nurses reason about moral and ethical dilemma situations? and (3) What is the relationship between moral reasoning and judgment about dilemmas in nursing practice and actions taken in actual nursing situations? Empirical research related to these questions has focused on the second and third questions. The first question, how should nurses reason about moral and ethical issues, is a philosophical question that is not amenable to research. The continuing relevance of this philosophical research has been presented in the previous section. The review of research will include empirical research related to moral judgment and action with nursing interventions.

Judgment About Moral and Ethical Dilemmas

During the early 1980s, the number of significant studies within psychology based on cognitive theory of moral development was impressive. These studies, however, focused on moral judgment rather than moral action, and were based almost entirely on subjects' responses to hypothetical general dilemmas. Piaget (1965) and Kohlberg (1976) used hypothetical stories in their interviews; Rest (1982) based his Defining Issues Test on six hypothetical moral dilemmas. Two related questions important to the further development of existing theory are: (1) What are the patterns of correspondence between reasoning and judgment about recurrent nursing situations of moral conflict and reasoning and judgment about hypothetical, nonnursing situations? and (2) What is the relationship between moral reasoning and judgment about dilemmas in nursing practice and actions taken in actual nursing situations?

Judgment About Nursing Ethical Dilemmas

The relationship of subjects' developmental level of moral judgment to decision making in the practice of nursing has been studied by Crisham (1979). Based on interviews with staff nurses, recurrent moral dilemmas in nursing practice were identified. Six of these recurrent nursing dilemmas representing various moral issues and clinical areas of nursing were selected for her Nursing Dilemma Test. A series of studies was done to determine the important considerations of staff nurses in responding to recurrent dilemmas with nursing interventions. Moral judgment experts classified the moral issues identified in interviews with nurses using Rest's (1979) stage definitions. The frequently mentioned representational moral issues and practical considerations were selected for the Nursing Dilemma Test which included three tasks for each of the six dilemmas: (1) deciding what the nurse should do, (2) ranking the moral and practical considerations in order of importance, (3) indicating the degree of previous involvement with a similar dilemma.

Relationship of Judgment in Hypothetical and Real Situations

Based on cognitive theory of moral development, Crisham's (1981) research investigated the difference between nurses' responses to hypothetical moral dilemmas and their responses to real-life nursing dilemmas. The purposes of the research were to measure nurses' responses to nursing dilemmas and the importance given to moral issues and practical considerations; to relate staff nurses' responses to nursing dilemmas in the Nursing Dilemma Test and responses to hypothetical moral dilemmas in the Defining Issues Test to two subject variables (level of nursing education and length of clinical nursing experience); and to compare moral judgments, both hypothetical general and nursing specific, of five subject groups: staff nurses with associate degrees and baccalaureate degrees in nursing, nurses with masters' degrees in nursing, college junior prenurses, and graduate level nonnurses. Findings verified the significance of formal education and previous involvement with similar dilemmas in enhancing principled thinking and raised questions about the relative strength of practical considerations in the hospital milieu for the nurse choosing and implementing nursing interventions.

The Nursing Dilemma Test measured the relative importance of moral issues and practical considerations; it did not measure the relative strength of other values and conflicting claims in the clinical milieu. It had the limitations of a paper and pencil ranking of given considerations and choices, and it emanated from the perspective of justice which has been challenged for its lack of relevance to women. Clearly, new methodologies are needed to examine the complexity of ethical issues in nursing. A comparative study of the situation for American and Australian nurses (Lawrence & Crisham, 1984a, b) documented the need for more qualitative data to examine the nature of health care ethical choices.

Numerous examples, within and apart from clinical nursing experience, show how carefully considered judgments were altered by situational pressures. In interviews that focused on the important considerations in responding to recurrent nursing dilemmas, staff nurses readily enumerated distractions and pressures in the hospital setting: hospital policy that conflicted with their own concepts of fairness; time constraints for a broad range of services; opposing loyalties to the nursing profession, the hospital, and the patient; confusion about the most effective way to utilize the vast and expanding body of professional knowledge; lack of clarity about their own responsibilities and authority; and contrary expectations from patients, administrators, and peers.

Relationship Between Moral Judgment and Action

To advance knowledge of moral judgment, it is necessary to clarify the role of variables such as situational pressures, conflicting loyalties, and contexts of professional dilemmas in making a judgment, and to investigate the interaction of these milieu effects with the practitioner's concepts of fairness and ethical behavior.

Ketefian (1981) found that the higher the nurses' critical thinking, the higher their moral reasoning was likely to be. Ketefian's findings, as well as numerous studies using the Nursing Dilemma Test, are consistent with existing theory on moral judgment development. Scores of principled thinking are significantly higher with additional years of formal education. There is evidence, therefore, of some systematic investigations of nurses' moral judgment. The relationship between moral reasoning about recurrent dilemmas in nursing practice and actions taken in actual nursing situations currently is assumed but untested.

Ketefian (1981) developed an instrument, Judgments About Nursing Decisions (JAND), to measure two components, moral behavior and perception of realistic moral behavior. This self-administered, objective test presents seven stories of nurses in ethical dilemmas. The subjects are asked to check whether they thought the nurse experiencing the dilemma in the story should or should not engage in first action; and, secondly, whether they thought the nurse experiencing the dilemma is likely to engage in the nursing action. The correlation between moral judgment (scores on the Defining Issues Test) and knowledge and valuation of ideal moral behavior in nursing yielded a coefficient of .28, significant at the .01 level. The correlation between scores on the Defining Issues Test and nurses' perceptions of realistic moral behavior in nursing dilemmas yielded a coefficient of .19, significant at the .05 level. Ketefian's Judgments About Nursing Decisions and Crisham's Nursing Dilemma Test direct subjects to make judgments about ethical conflict in nursing. Both tests yield a low positive correlation when scores are related to a standard measure of general moral judgment, Rest's Defining Issues Test. Nurse researchers, therefore, have begun to document the generally assumed, but previously untested tenet that moral reasoning in hypothetical situations (Defining Issues Test) is positively correlated with moral reasoning in situations in which subjects actually make actual decisions.

Ketefian (1981) and Crisham (1981) raise a series of related questions: Ketefian questions whether subjects in her study responding to their "perception of realistic moral behavior" may have been in the position of predicting someone else's behavior or giving their assessment of what they thought would actually happen, as opposed to what they themselves would do in the dilemmas. She recommended alternative modalities and instrumentation be explored to measure this construct.

Blasi (1980, 1984) presented a broad discussion of the conceptual and empirical issues that concern the relationship between moral reasoning and moral action. He reviewed research relating moral reasoning to delinquency, honesty, altruism, conformity, and other real-life moral behaviors and summarized problems of design, measurement, and interpretation. Although Blasi concluded that overall these studies seem to support the cognitive–developmental perspective, this support needs to be qualified and interpreted. The importance of studying the consistency between moral cognition and moral action and the need for a process approach to research in this area were emphasized. Blasi (1984) recommended a different focus and different questions to begin to more accurately elucidate the relationship between a concrete moral judgment and its corresponding action. What appears to be needed, according to Blasi, is an explicit and direct focus on the nature of integrity, that is, on the psychological processes and skills related to the capacity to act in ways that are consistent with personally validated moral insights. This relationship between moral judgment and moral action seems important from a common sense viewpoint, and one would expect any theory that emphasizes cognitive structures to account for the interaction between judgment and action. Yet, as the series of reported studies testify, cognitive–developmental history has neglected the issue of consistency between resolution and implementation.

Nurses and philosophers have advocated a systematic process to analyze and resolve ethical conflict in nursing situations (Gadow, 1980; Davis & Aroskar, 1983; Silva, 1984; Jameton, 1984; Crisham, 1986; Murphy & Thompson, 1986; Veatch & Fry, 1987). The relationship of these approaches and models to ethical theory has been explicated. Gortner (1985), in a review of research on ethical inquiry in nursing, recommended empirical testing of the effectiveness of ethical decision-making models. To date, there has been little or no opportunity to test whether a particular process increases the nurse's: (1) recognition of the moral dimension of dilemma situations, (2) knowledge of principled thinking, and (3) ability to act consistently with moral principles.

The summary statements in the proceedings of the workshop, Bioethics and Clinical Practice: Examining Research Outcomes and Methods (Moritz, 1990), encouraged and supported philosophically based empirical research efforts. After reviewing and summarizing research conducted from a nursing perspective, Davis (1990) concluded that there is a lack of interdisciplinary research in the area of nursing and bioethics and a need for larger studies as well as studies that examine professional socialization influences on nurses; population groups such as patients, nurses, physicians, and other health care professionals should be included in this research.

A large body of literature on professional practice within organizations suggests there are inherent features in institutional practices, structures, and relationships that influence ethical decision making. After reviewing research literature related to nurses' moral reasoning and ethical practice, Ketefian (1989) recommended that future studies include an examination of institutional relationships, practices, and rules that relate to ethical decision making. She also recommended studying the nature of ethical conflict in the context of the clinical situation.

CONCLUSION

In summary, nurses experience ethical dilemmas about the right to know and decide, defining and promoting quality of life, maintaining professional and institutional standards, and distributing nursing resources in choosing and implementing nursing interventions. The MORAL model begins with the nurse's experience of the dilemma, facilitates the formulation of a position based on moral principles, and creates a challenge to act from commitment. Research has focused on hypothetical, general dilemmas rather than on real-life professional dilemmas, on reasoning about dilemmas in paper-and-pencil testing situations rather than reasoning about dilemmas in clinical nursing settings, and, consistently, on moral judgment rather than moral action. What is missing is a cultural ecology of nursing moral judgment and action grounded in observations of nurses' interventions in clinical settings. Such an approach would call for openness to a wider variety of methodologic strategies. What is clearly missing is any research examining the relationship between the resolution of ethical dilemmas with nursing interventions and quality health care. That the quality of health care is enhanced when nurses transform dilemmas into committed action is apparent from widespread experience with nurses. What is needed are studies of the processes and skills related to acting from commitment as well as research that focuses on the interaction among moral judgment, moral action, and quality nursing care.

REFERENCES

American Nurses' Association. (1980). Resolution Adopted by the House of Delegates, National Conference, San Francisco.

Ashley, J. (1976). *Hospitals, paternalism and the role of the nurse.* New York: Teachers College Press.

Beauchamp, T., & Childress, J. (1989). *Principles of biomedical ethics.* New York: Oxford University Press.

Blasi, A. (1980). Bridging moral cognition and moral action: A critical review. *Psychological Bulletin* 88:1–45.

_____. (1984). Moral identity: Its role in moral functioning. Pp. 128–140 in W. Kurtines & J. Gewirtz eds., *Morality, moral behavior, and moral development.* New York: John Wiley and Sons.

Crisham, P. (1979). *Moral judgment of nurses in hypothetical and nursing dilemmas.* Unpublished doctoral dissertation, University of Minnesota.

_____. (1981). Measuring moral judgment in nursing dilemmas. *Nursing Research* 30:104–110.

_____. (1986). Ethics, economics, and quality. *Journal of Nursing Quality Assurance* 1(1):26–35.

Davis, A. (1990). Bioethics and clinical practice research from the nursing research perspective. Pp. 9–11 in P. Moritz ed., *Bioethics and clinical practice: Examining research outcomes and methods. Proceedings of the workshop sponsored by the National Center for Nursing Research.* Bethesda, MD: NIH.

Davis, A. J., & Aroskar, M.A. (1983). *Ethical dilemmas and nursing practice* (2nd ed.). Norwalk, CT: Appleton-Century-Crofts.

Eberhardy, J. (1982). *An analysis of moral decision making with nursing students facing professional problems.* Unpublished doctoral dissertation, University of Minnesota.

Frankena, W. (1973). *Ethics.* Englewood Cliffs, NJ: Prentice-Hall.

Gadow, S. (1980). Existential advocacy: Philosophical functioning of nursing. Pp. 79–101 in S. Spicker & S. Gadow eds., *Nursing: Images & Ideals.* New York: Springer Publishing Co.

Gilligan, C. (1982). *In a different voice.* Cambridge, MA: Harvard University Press.

Gortner, S. R. (1985). Ethical inquiry. Pp. 193–214 in H. H. Werley & J. J. Fitzpatrick eds., *Review of nursing research,* vol. 3. New York: Springer Publishing Co.

Grier, M. (1983). Decision-making process with undergraduate nursing students. Presented at Research Conference, University of Minnesota, January 1983.

International Council of Nurses. (1977). *The nurse's dilemma ethical considerations in nursing practice.* Geneva: International Council of Nurses.

Jameton, A. (1984). *Nursing practice: The ethical issues.* New Jersey: Englewood Cliffs.

Kant, I. (1959). *Foundations of the metaphysics of morals* (trans. Lewis White Beck). New York: Bobbs-Merrill.

Ketefian, S. (1981). Critical thinking, educational preparation, and development of moral judgment. *Nursing Research* 30:98–103.

_____. (1989). Moral reasoning and ethical practice. Pp. 173–195 in J. Kitzpatrick, R. L. Taunton, & J. Benoliel eds., *Annual review of nursing research,* vol. 7. New York: Springer Publishing Co.

Kohlberg, L. (1976). Moral stages and moralization: The cognitive-developmental approach. Pp. 31–53 in T. Lickona ed., *Moral development and behavior.* New York: Holt, Rinehart, & Winston.

Kohlberg, L., Levine, C., & Hewer, A. (1983). Moral stages: A current formulation and a response to critics. Pp. 1–10, 65–66 in J. Meacham Ed., *Contributions to human development,* vol. 10. New York: Karger Publishers.

Lawrence, J., & Crisham, P. (1984a). A study in resolutions. *Nursing Times* 80(30):53–56.

_____. (1984b). Making a choice. *Nursing Times* 80(29): 57–59.

Lewin, K. (1969). Quasi-stationary social equilibria and the problem of permanent change. Pp. 235–238 in W. Bennis, K. Benne, & R. Chin eds., *The planning of change.* New York: Holt, Rinehart, & Winston.

Moritz, P. (ed.). (1990). Bioethics and clinical practice: Examining research outcomes and methods [Summary]. *Proceedings of the workshop sponsored by the National Center for Nursing Research.* Bethesda, MD: NIH.

Murphy, C. P., & Thompson, J. E. (1986). Ethical reasoning. Pp. 51–53 in *Proceedings application of ethical principles to nursing practice.* Washington, DC: George Washington University Medical Center.

Muyskens, J. (1982). *Moral problems in nursing.* Totowa, NJ: Rowman & Littlefield.

Piaget, J. (1965). *The moral judgment of the child.* (trans. M. Gabain). New York: Free Press. (First published in English, London: Kegan Paul, 1932).

Rawls, J. (1971). *A theory of justice.* Cambridge, MA: Harvard University Press.

Rest, J. (1979). *Development in judging moral issues.* Minneapolis: University of Minnesota Press.

Rest, J. R. (1982). Morality. In P. Mussen (Ed.), *Handbook of child psychology* (4th ed.): Pp. 556–629 in vol. 3, *Cognitive development* (J. Flawell & E. Markham vol. eds.). New York: John Wiley and Sons.

Shweder, R. A. (1980). Rethinking culture and personality theory. *Ethos* 8(2):60–94.

Silva, M. (1984). Ethics, scarce resources and the nurse executive. *Nursing Economics* 2(1):11–18.

Veatch, R. M., & Fry, S. T. (1987). *Case studies in nursing ethics.* Philadelphia: Lippincott.

Yarling, R., & McElmurry, B. (1986). The moral foundation of nursing. *Advances in Nursing Science* 8(2):63–73.

CHAPTER 5

ANALYTICAL DECISION-MAKING STRATEGIES FOR CHOOSING NURSING INTERVENTIONS

Sheila Corcoran Perry, Ph.D., R.N.

It is well documented that nurses make many clinical decisions under conditions of uncertainty and complexity (Tanner, 1987). Two major types of clinical decisions made by nurses are: (1) identification (diagnosis of clients' responses, interpretations, strengths, and problems related to their health; and (2) selection of nursing interventions to help clients achieve their short- and long-term goals. Such decisions are often made in collaboration with clients.

Many factors contribute to uncertainty in clinical decision making. Clients' responses and preferences in relation to health care are often unique and dynamic, yet they need to be taken into account. In addition, the relationships between client cues and nursing diagnoses and between nursing interventions and client outcomes are probabilistic; that is, the relationships are probable or likely rather than certain (Hammond, 1966; Tanner, 1984). Other variables that contribute to this uncertainty and the resulting complexity of decision making include the nature of the context, the expertise of the nurse, and the amount, accuracy, and relevance of the data and knowledge available (Benner, 1984; Corcoran, 1986a, b; Grier, 1981, 1984; Hammond, 1966).

This chapter addresses analytical decision-making strategies for selecting nursing interventions, particularly independent nursing interventions. Several conditions make the complex process of clinical decision making even more difficult when choosing among independent nursing interventions. One condition is the lack of objective data concerning the probable consequences of these interventions. Without such objective data, one must rely on subjective estimates of probable consequences.

Another condition which makes selection of independent nursing interventions difficult is that often the interventions being considered are not mutually exclusive; selection of one does not exclude others. For example, when working with a person experiencing pain, a nurse might consider and eventually select a combination of interventions such as progressive relaxation, imagery, and therapeutic touch. Less is known about cognitive strategies used for selecting multiple interventions than about those used for selecting an intervention from among mutually exclusive ones. In addition, little is known about the comparative efficacy of each intervention alone or in combination.

In the remainder of this chapter, a frame of reference is established for addressing analytical decision making in choosing nursing interventions, related research is described, selected strategies are applied to a client situation, and research questions are posed.

FRAME OF REFERENCE

Nurses have come to recognize the limitations of the nursing process as the formalization of clinical judgment (Tanner, 1988). In the 1960s, the delineation of the nursing process as a cognitive, systematic process was significant in emphasizing that nurses were thinkers and decision makers, not simply doers. This step-by-step procedure provided a framework for collecting and interpreting data, developing intervention plans, and evaluating patient outcomes. However, the nursing process did not describe how the steps were to be carried out. This cognitive, linear process did not represent the dynamic, interactive nature of clinical decision making.

In the late 1970s and the 1980s numerous nursing researchers investigated aspects of nurses' clinical decision making and found: (1) there is no single process for making clinical decisions; (2) task characteristics and contexts are major determinants of processes used; (3) successful clinicians use both analytical and intuitive processes; (4) when being analytical, clinicians often use an iterative (repetitive) process rather than a linear, step-by-step method; and (5) students and nurses new to a decision task rely on established rules and analytical processes, but as they gain experience with similar tasks they rely more on their past experience and intuitive processes (Benner, 1984; Benner & Tanner, 1987; Corcoran, 1986a, b; Grier, 1976, 1977; Tanner et al., 1987).

As a result of these findings, Tanner (1989) developed an integrated conceptual model of clinical judgment (see Figure 5.1). Although the model includes both analytical and intuitive processes, the focus of this chapter is on *analytical* strategies for choosing nursing interventions. This limited focus is selected because formal strategies for using analytical processes can be described and generalized to some extent, but intuitive processes are of little use if they are described free of the context in which they are implemented.

The theoretical framework selected for addressing the analytical processes is a combination of an information-processing model and a behavioral-decision model of decision making. An information-

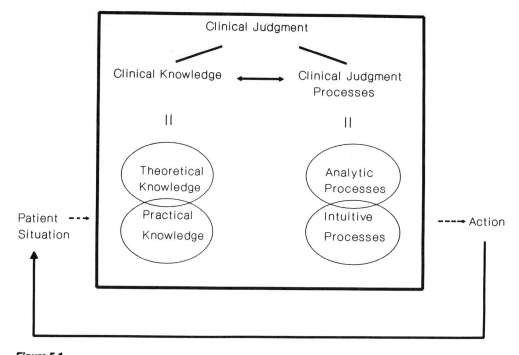

Figure 5.1
Tanner's model of clinical judgment. (From C. Tanner and C. Lindeman. (1989). Use of research in clinical judgment. In C. Tanner and C. Lindeman (Eds.), *Using nursing research* (p. 28). New York: National League for Nursing. Used with permission.)

processing model of decision making is a descriptive model based on the work of Newell and Simon (Newell & Simon, 1972; Simon, 1979). The goal of this model is to characterize the sequence of cognitive processes used by persons faced with particular problem-solving tasks and to explain those processes in terms of psychological concepts and principles.

In this problem-solving model, problem solving is described as an interaction between a problem solver and a problem task. Humans are viewed as information-processing systems operating in a complex environment. It is assumed that humans have two memory structures—a short-term memory that is the working memory, and a long-term memory where knowledge is stored in organized networks. A major concept within this model is bounded rationality. This concept emphasizes the limitations of human capacity for rational thought because of the relatively small capacity of short-term memory as compared to the essentially infinite capacity of long-term memory (Elstein & Bordage, 1979; Newell & Simon, 1972).

One contribution of the research based on the information-processing model is identification of cognitive strategies used by humans to adapt their limited information-processing capacities to the complex tasks they confront. These strategies include processing data serially, selecting data carefully, and representing problems in simplified ways (Elstein & Bordage, 1979; Newell & Simon, 1972). Such strategies reduce the cognitive strain imposed by complex tasks.

In contrast to an information-processing model, a behavioral-decision model of decision making is prescriptive in that it deals with the fundamental question of what decisions should be made, rather than on how they are made. In this model, humans are viewed as intuitive statisticians faced with the problem of combining imperfect information concerning the likelihood and value of certain consequences after given actions. A basic assumption is that a rational person chooses the alternative with the highest expected value, the best consequences (Edwards & Tversky, 1967; Elstein & Bordage, 1979; Raiffa, 1968).

A behavioral-decision model represents a decision situation as having four major components: (1) a set of possible actions, (2) consequences associated with those actions, (3) judgments concerning the likelihood that the consequences will occur if a given action is taken, and (4) judgments concerning the value of the consequences to the person(s) involved in the decision. The model provides: (1) a structure for representing the relationships among alternative actions, chance events, and their consequences; and (2) a method for combining judgments concerning likelihoods and values to prescribe the best alternative from among those being considered.

Another aspect of a frame of reference for addressing decision making in choosing nursing interventions is the client's involvement in the process (Corcoran, 1988). Conceptual frameworks for nursing practice view clients as competent, responsible persons who have a right to be involved in making decisions about their own care. Therefore, nurses often involve clients in decision making about interventions.

RELATED RESEARCH

A major finding in a classic psychology study by Miller (1956) was that the capacity of humans' short-term memory (working memory) is seven plus or minus two (7 ± 2) symbols or "chunks" of information. This limited capacity seems to be invariant across a wide range of tasks.

Many studies have investigated how humans adapt their limited processing capacity to the demands of decision-making tasks. Findings have indicated that information processing in decision making is highly contingent on the demands of the task (Corcoran, 1986a, b; Gordon, 1980; Payne, 1976, 1982). Task complexity is one factor that determines the cognitive strategies used. Characteristics which make a task complex include: (1) the number of alternatives considered, (2) the number of dimensions used to define alternatives, and (3) the amount of time available to make a decision (Payne, 1982).

In studies of complex decision tasks involving mutually exclusive alternatives, subjects were found to use cognitive strategies, which quickly reduces the complexity of the task. For example, Payne (1976) used an information-processing model for a study in which he varied the number of alternatives available to subjects in the task of choosing an apartment. When faced with many apartments, subjects used strategies to eliminate some alternatives as quickly as possible based on limited information search and evaluation. When the task was simplified to consideration of a few (often two) apartments, then subjects evaluated alternatives more thoroughly, examining the same amount of information on each alternative.

Payne (1976) described four types of cognitive strategies that might be used when choosing among alternative actions: (1) an elimination-by-aspect strategy, (2) a conjunctive strategy, (3) an additive strategy, and (4) an additive difference strategy. Payne found that subjects used an elimination-by-aspect or a conjunctive strategy early in the decision-making process when multiple alternatives were being considered.

In the elimination-by-aspect strategy, a decision maker selects a desirable dimension and eliminates all alternatives which do not possess that dimension. The process is continued until all but one alternative has been eliminated. In the conjunctive strategy, a decision maker establishes a minimum value on all relevant dimensions. Alternatives that do not have the minimum value on all dimensions are eliminated. These two strategies can be used to quickly reduce the number of alternatives being considered.

Payne (1976) also found that subjects used an additive or additive difference strategy to choose between two alternatives. In an additive strategy, each alternative is evaluated separately. A value is assigned for each dimension of an alternative, and the values for all dimensions summed for each alternative. The alternative with the highest overall value is chosen. In the additive difference strategy, both alternatives are compared directly on each dimension. A difference is determined and the results are summed to reach a decision.

Gordon (1980) had findings similar to those of Payne (1976). In a study in which nurses were given a diagnostic task, Gordon found that nurses who make more accurate diagnoses used multiple-hypothesis testing strategies in the first half of the decision-making process to quickly reduce the number of alternative hypotheses. Then, in the second half of the process, they switched to single-hypothesis testing in which they more thoroughly tested remaining hypotheses about the state of the client.

Most of the research on clinical decision making has focused on diagnostic reasoning (for example, Aspinall, 1979; Elstein et al., 1978; Gordon, 1980; Tanner et al., 1987). Little research has been done on the planning process in which interventions are chosen. In three studies, Grier and colleagues (Grier, 1976, 1977; Grier et al., 1979) used a behavioral-decision model to investigate nurses' decision making when choosing among mutually exclusive alternatives.

In a 1976 study, Grier used four client situations. In each situation, subjects were given a written case description and several mutually exclusive actions. Subjects were asked to choose the best action for the client. Subjects next were asked to assign probabilities and values to a list of possible consequences for each possible action. Then Grier calculated the expected value of each alternative, based on the probabilities and values assigned to each consequence by each subject. There was significant agreement between the calculated expected values and the rankings of the actions. Grier concluded that a behavioral decision model is applicable to nursing practice and that nurses can order consequences of their actions according to their desirability and likelihood of occurrence.

In a study concerning decision making about placement of elderly persons, Grier (1977) found that hospital nurses, visiting nurses, and elderly people differed significantly in their initial intuitive choice of living arrangement; however, there was no significant difference in their quantitative choices. That is, when the nurses and the elderly persons assigned probabilities and values to possible consequences for each alternative placement, there was significant agreement on which placement had the highest expected value.

Grier et al., (1979) studied nurses' decision making in administering narcotic analgesics to terminally ill patients. The method used was similar to that used in the earlier studies by Grier (1976, 1977). However, in this study, subjects were asked to select their goal when caring for patients in pain. A major finding was that the quantitative choices (choices made after assigning probabilities and values to possible consequences of mutually exclusive analgesics) were more goal related than were initial choices. The work of Grier and colleagues provides support for use of a behavioral-decision model of decision making in which possible consequences of mutually exclusive alternative actions are identified and probabilities and values are assigned to those consequences.

Corcoran (1986a, b) used an information-processing model of decision making to study the planning process used by hospice nurses. Subjects were given written case descriptions of clients experiencing severe pain and were asked to think aloud as they developed drug administration plans to control the clients' pain. The subjects had to generate alternatives to consider; none were given to them, except those mentioned in the case description. Alternatives were not necessarily mutually exclusive; that is, subjects could choose more that one alternative to control the clients' pain. A major finding was that all subjects evaluated alternatives as they were generated, and no subject generated all alternative actions before evaluating any of them. In this way, subjects reduced the number of alternatives under consideration by quickly rejecting some of them. In addition, subjects overtly evaluated all alternatives when few were generated and only a portion of them when many were generated. This was another strategy used to reduce cognitive strain.

In summary, findings of research studies support the conclusion that information processing in decision making is contingent on the demands of the tasks. A variety of strategies are used by subjects to reduce cognitive strain. When multiple alternatives are being considered, cognitive strategies are used to quickly reduce the number of alternatives; different types of cognitive strategies are used to evaluate a few alternatives. There is evidence to support the use of a behavioral-decision model of decision making. Several studies by Grier and colleagues indicated that decisions are more goal related and more consistent among subjects when a quantitative approach is taken. There is little research on the decision-making processes used when alternatives are not mutually exclusive.

APPLICATION OF SELECTED STRATEGIES

In this section, some of the cognitive strategies described earlier in this chapter will be applied to a situation in which a nurse is choosing independent nursing interventions for a client experiencing tension headaches. The client, Laura Olson, is 39 years old. During an initial interview with the nurse, Laura describes her headaches as steady, bilateral pain that originates in the frontal region. She says she has had headaches at least three times per week for 11 years. When asked about the intensity of the headaches on a scale of 1 to 100, with one being barely noticeable and 100 being extremely painful, Laura indicates they are usually at 60 or 70. When asked about her goal for treatment, Laura says she wants relief from her headaches and, if possible, a sense of control over them.

Elimination-By-Aspect Strategy

The nurse indicates that there are a number of interventions that might help Laura achieve her goal. The nurse immediately thinks of the following ones: progressive relaxation, biofeedback, therapeutic touch, acupressure, imagery, heat or cold, meditation, or massage. Before describing the alternatives to Laura, the nurse quickly reduces the number using an elimination-by-aspect cognitive strategy. The nurse does not have the expertise needed for using therapeutic touch, acupressure, imagery, or meditation, so those alternatives are eliminated.

Decision Analysis

At a later time, the nurse and Laura wonder if the best alternative was selected. The nurse realizes that in assigning numbers to the dimensions for each alternative, information about the likelihood that a dimension would be associated with the alternative was combined with information about the value of that dimension to Laura. The nurse realizes that in quantitative decision making, estimates of likelihood and value should be independent. So the nurse offers to do a decision analysis and to involve Laura in the process.

The nurse describes decision analysis to Laura as one method used within a behavioral-decision model of decision making that provides: (1) a structure for representing the relationship between alternative actions, chance events, and consequences and (2) a simple procedure for mathematically combining estimates of likelihood of chance events and value of consequences. The four steps in decision analysis are:

1. Structure a decision flow diagram in which there is a chronological arrangement of choices controlled by the decision maker and choices controlled by chance.
2. Assign values to each set of possible outcomes at the distal tip of each branch of the diagram.
3. Assign probabilities to chance events.
4. Calculate the expected value of each alternative. Start with the distal forks and calculate the sums of the probabilities times the values, $\Sigma(p \times v)$. Then move backward in the flow diagram to each preceding fork and calculate $\Sigma(p \times v)$.

(See Corcoran, 1986c; Kassirer, 1976; Raiffa, 1968; Schwartz et al., 1973 for more detailed descriptions of decision analysis.)

Step One

The nurse and Laura begin by structuring a decision flow diagram including: (1) alternatives which are under their control and (2) events that are under the control of chance. The nurse remembers reading a number of research articles in which the alternatives of progressive relaxation and biofeedback are compared (Chesney & Shelton, 1976; Cox et al., 1975). The research findings indicate differing effects of these interventions on the frequency, duration, and intensity of tension headaches. Consequently, frequency, duration, and intensity are separated as possible chance events in the decision flow diagram. In addition, the nurse recalls that electrical shock is a possible consequence of the use of biofeedback; so the chance of injury is introduced to the decision flow diagram (See Figure 5.2.)

After completing the portion of the decision flow diagram represented in Figure 5.2, the nurse and Laura realize that the diagram is too unwieldy to use. Laura indicates that she is most concerned about the frequency and intensity of the headaches, so the diagram is simplified to that represented by Figure 5.3.

Step Two

The second step is to assign values to each set of possible outcomes at the distal tip of each branch of the diagram. The values should be Laura's values because she will be the person experiencing the outcomes. The nurse uses a two-step procedure to help Laura assign values. First, ranks are assigned to each set of outcomes, giving a rank of one to the set of outcomes most preferred, a rank of two to the set next preferred, and so on. To do this, the nurse has each set of possible outcomes on a separate index card. Laura is asked to place the cards in the order in which she prefers the outcomes, putting the set of outcomes that she most prefers first. It takes Laura about 10 minutes to assign ranks. The rankings she assigns are those in the rank column of Figure 5.4.

In the second phase of the two-step procedure for assigning values, the nurse asks Laura to think about the strength of her preferences for the outcomes by assigning values to them ranging from +100 to −100. This allows Laura to indicate varying intervals among her preferences. The values she assigns are those in the value column of Figure 5.4.

Step Three

The nurse assigns subjective probabilities to the chance events of the decision flow diagram. To assign the probabilities, the nurse reflects on the findings of research studies (Bowles et al., 1979; Chesney & Shelton, 1976; Cox et al., 1975) and on experience in using these interventions. The probabilities assigned are represented by the numbers on each branch in Figure 5.4; the probabilities for each fork total 1.0.

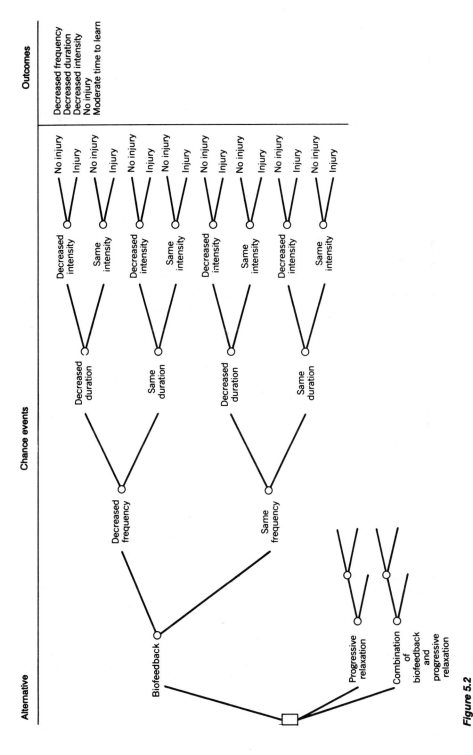

Figure 5.2
Portion of a decision flow diagram. Choices controlled by the decision maker (squares); choices controlled by chance (circles).

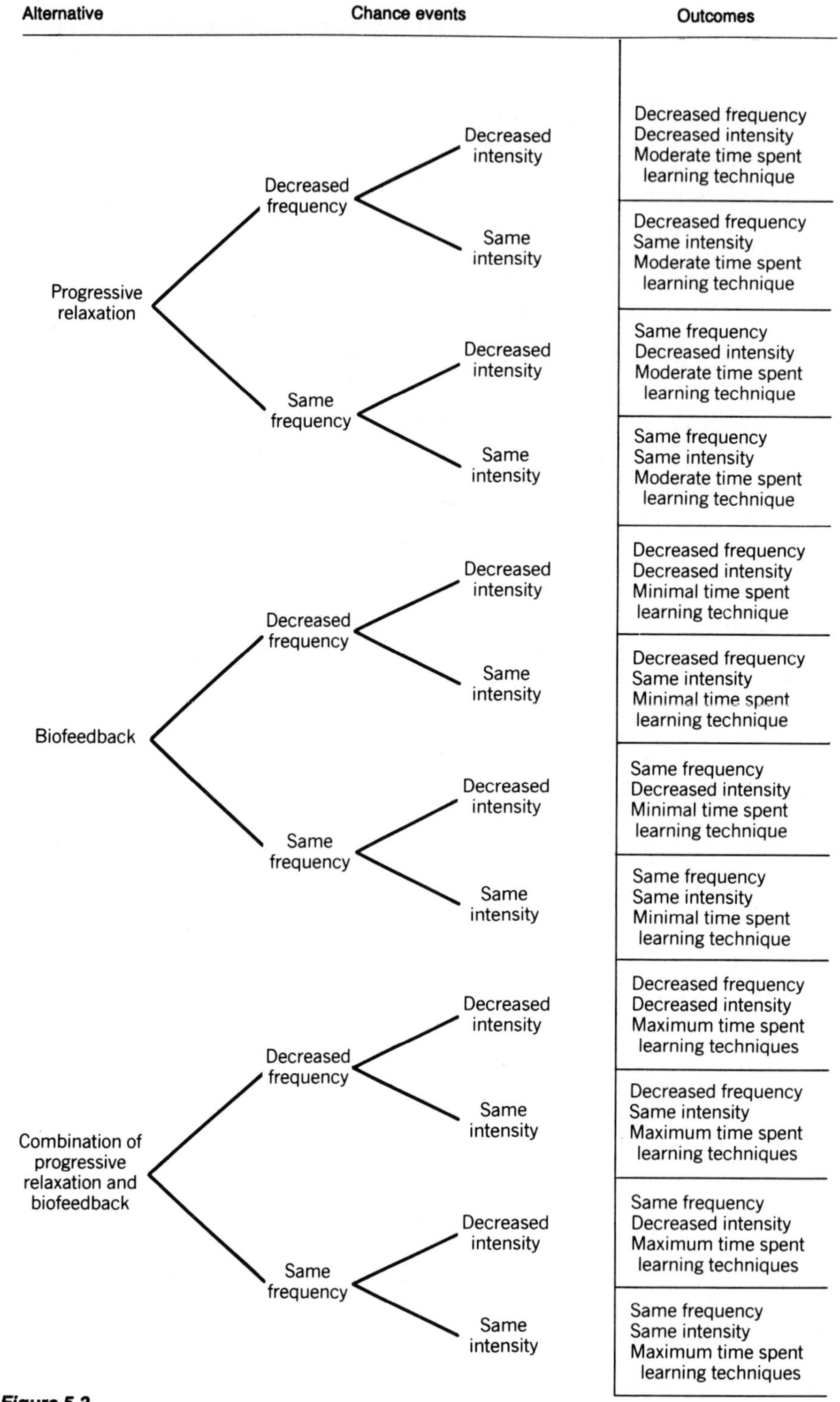

Alternative	Chance events	Outcomes

Figure 5.3
Revised decision flow diagram for treating a tension headache.

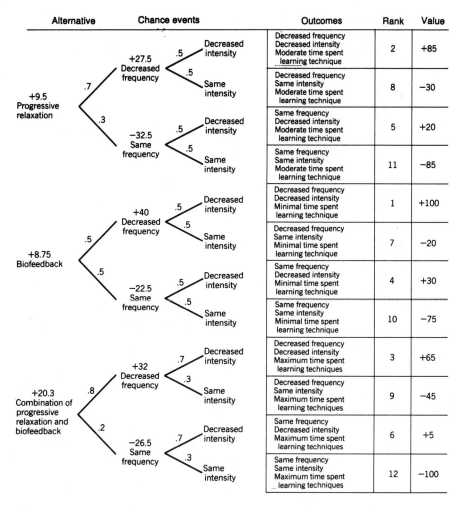

Figure 5.4
Decision flow diagram with probabilities, values, and expected values added. (The numbers on each branch represent subjective probabilities that the chance events will occur. The numbers within the circles represent the expected value of each fork.)

Step Four

The function of this last step in decision analysis is to identify the best alternative, the intervention with the highest expected value. For this step, the nurse works backward through the decision flow diagram to calculate the expected values, $\Sigma(p \times v)$, for each fork. For example, in the top distal fork of Figure 5.4, the nurse calculates the expected value of having decreased or the same intensity with decreased frequency of headaches, $.5(+85) + .5(-30) = +27.5$. A similar calculation is done for the next distal fork, $.5(+20) + .5(-85)$ $= -32.5$. After the expected value is calculated for all distal forks, then the nurse moves backward in the diagram to the preceding forks to calculate their expected values. For example, in the top middle fork, the calculation is $.7(+27.5) + .3(-32.5)$ to arrive at an expected value of $+9.5$ for the alternative of progressive relaxation.

When all calculations are completed, the alternative with the highest expected value is chosen. In this case, the prescribed alternative is a combination of progressive relaxation and biofeedback. This prescription of decision analysis confirms the earlier choice made using the additive strategy.

In actual situations where the author has worked with nurses using decision analysis, she has observed numerous benefits (Corcoran, 1986c, 1988). In addition to providing a structure for decision making and a procedure for prescribing the best alternative among those considered, nurses state that use of decision analysis helps them become more aware of the alternatives available to them. They recognize the importance of identifying chance events over which they have no control and distinguishing those chance events from consequences. This recognition helps them appreciate that they can make good decisions and still have bad outcomes. In addition, the nurses indicate that assignment of values to outcomes makes them more conscious of patients' preferences and the significance of patient input into decision making. In several instances, nurses and clients have chosen to not perform the final step of calculating the expected value. Structuring the decision task in the form of decision flow diagram was adequate.

Thinking Aloud Strategy

By now the reader is probably concluding that the knowledge of analytical processes involved in clinical judgment is far from complete and there will never be prescribed approaches for clinical decision making. Such conclusions are warranted and highlight the need to reflect on the nature, efficiency, and effectiveness of one's own decision-making processes. One strategy for promoting such reflection is "thinking aloud."

"Thinking aloud" has been used successfully in research as a method for revealing nurses' cognitive processes. Clinicians are usually unable to describe how they perform decision-making tasks. Their knowledge and cognitive skills are tacit; that is, unavailable to consciousness (Johnson, 1983). However, such cognitive processes can be inferred from behavior when actually performing the task.

In using this strategy for the situation described earlier, the nurse who is working with Laura Olson "thinks aloud" while making a decision about interventions to control Laura's headaches. The "thinking aloud" verbalizations are audiotape recorded.

Analysis of such recordings or transcriptions reveals the information to which the nurse attends, the sequence in which information is processed, the heuristics or rules-of-thumb used to combine information and make decisions, and the degree to which Laura's preferences and values are taken into account. From such data, the nurse can gain insights into the types of decisions made, the knowledge required, and the effectiveness and efficiency of the cognitive processes used in her own clinical practice.

This strategy can be used independently or with colleagues. Corcoran, Narayan, and Moreland (1988) proposed that "thinking aloud" be used among experienced nurses to gain a better understanding of the knowledge they have and how they use it. These authors also suggested that "thinking aloud" might be used when experienced nurses are serving as mentors for inexperienced nurses in an area of practice. Either the mentor or the inexperienced nurse can "think aloud" about a particular case while selecting independent nursing interventions. Then the mentor and nurse can listen to the tape recording together, stopping whenever desired to reflect on: (1) goals; (2) relevant issues; (3) methods of selecting, eliciting, and interpreting data; (4) rules for combining data; and (5) arguments used to arrive at a decision.

RESEARCH QUESTIONS

Numerous investigators have studied individuals' use of analytical decision-making processes for planning. However, few nursing studies have been done in this area. The following questions identify some areas for further research to provide a more scientific basis for choosing independent nursing interventions:

1. Under what conditions do nurses use various analytical decision-making strategies to choose among independent nursing interventions?
2. Do the strategies vary according to area of practice, level of expertise, nature of interventions being considered, level of uncertainty, or degree of complexity?

3. Can nurses effectively implement strategies such as decision analysis to choose independent nursing interventions? More specifically, can they appropriately structure a problem, assign probabilities, and assess preferences?
4. Is the use of analytical strategies to choose independent nursing interventions associated with better decisions, better client outcomes, and greater self-confidence in decision-making abilities than use of other methods?
5. What factors promote and/or inhibit nurses' use of analytical decision-making strategies for choosing independent nursing interventions?
6. To what extent, when in the decision-making process, and in what ways do nurses involve clients in choosing independent nursing interventions?
7. What factors promote and/or inhibit nurses' involving clients in choosing independent nursing interventions?
8. How do the cognitive processes used by nurses to choose among mutually exclusive nursing interventions compare with those used to choose among nonmutually exclusive ones?
9. Are nurses' and patients' choices of independent interventions consistent with their stated goals and their judgments about probabilities and preferences? If not, how might the inconsistency be explained?

REFERENCES

Aspinall, M. (1979). Use of a decision tree to improve accuracy of diagnosis. *Nursing Research* 28(3):182–185.

Benner, P. (1984). *From novice to expert: Excellence and power in clinical nursing practice.* Menlo Park, CA: Addison-Wesley Publishing.

Benner, P., & Tanner, C. (1987). Clinical judgment: How expert nurses use intuition. *American Journal of Nursing* 87(1):23–31.

Bowles, C., Smith, J., & Parker, K. (1979). EMG feedback and progressive relaxation training: A comparative study of two groups of normal subjects. *Western Journal of Nursing Research* 1(3):179–189.

Chesney, M., & Shelton, J. (1976). A comparison of muscle relaxation and electromyogram biofeedback treatments for muscle contraction headache. *Journal of Behavior Therapy and Experimental Psychiatry* 7:221–225.

Corcoran, S. (1986a). Task complexity and nursing expertise as factors in decision making. *Nursing Research* 35(2):107–112.

_____. (1986b). Planning by expert and novice nurses in cases of varying complexity. *Research in Nursing & Health* 9:155–162.

_____. (1986c). Decision analysis: A step-by-step guide for making clinical decisions. *Nursing and Health Care* 7(3):148–154.

_____. (1988). Toward operationalizing an advocacy role. *Journal of Professional Nursing* 4(4):242–248.

Corcoran, S., Narayan, S., & Moreland, H. (1988). Thinking aloud as a strategy to improve clinical decision making. *Heart & Lung* 17(5):463–468.

Cox, D., Freundlich, A., & Meyer, R. (1975). Differential effectiveness of electromyograph feedback, verbal relaxation instructions, and medication placebo with tension headaches. *Journal of Consulting and Clinical Psychology* 43(6):892–898.

Edwards, W., & Tversky, A. (1967). *Decision making.* England: Penguin Books.

Elstein, A., & Bordage, G. (1979). Psychology of clinical reasoning. Pp. 333–367 in G. Stone, F. Cohen, and N. Adler Eds., *Health psychology.* San Francisco: Jossey-Bass.

Elstein, A., Shulman, L., & Sprafka, S. (1978). *Medical problem solving.* Cambridge, MA: Harvard University Press.

Gordon, M. (1980). Predictive strategies in diagnostic tasks. *Nursing Research* 29(1):39–45.

Grier, M. (1976). Decision making about patient care. *Nursing Research* 25(1):105–110.

_____. (1977). Choosing living arrangements for the elderly. *International Journal of Nursing Studies* 14:69–76.

_____. (1981). The need for data in making nursing decisions. Pp. 15–31 in H. Werley and M. Grier eds., *Nursing information systems.* New York: Springer.

_____. (1984). Information processing in nursing practice. Pp. 265–287 in H. Werley and J. Fitzpatrick eds., *Annual review of nursing research*, vol. 2. New York: Springer.

Grier, M., Howard, M., & Cohen, F. (1979). Beliefs and values associated with administering narcotics and analgesics to terminally ill patients. In *Clinical and scientific sessions*. Kansas City: American Nurses' Association.

Hammond, K. (1966). Clinical inference in nursing: Psychologist's viewpoint. *Nursing Research* 15(1):27–38.

Johnson, P.E. (1983). What kind of expert should a system be? *Journal of Medicine and Philosophy* 8:77–97.

Kassirer, J. (1976). The principles of clinical decision making: An introduction to decision analysis. *The Yale Journal of Biology and Medicine* 49:149–164.

Miller, G. (1956). The magical number seven, plus or minus two. *Psychological Review* 63:81–97.

Newell, A., & Simon, H. (1972). *Human problem solving*. Englewood Cliffs, NJ: Prentice-Hall.

Payne, J. (1976). Task complexity and contingent processing in decision making: An information search and protocol analysis. *Organizational Behavior and Human Performance* 16:366–387.

_____. (1982). Contingent decision behavior. *Psychological Bulletin* 92(2):382–402.

Raiffa, H. (1968). *Decision analysis: Introductory lectures on choice under uncertainty*. Reading, MA: Addison-Wesley.

Schwartz, W., Gorry, G., Kassirer, J., & Essig, A. (1973). Decision analysis and clinical judgment. *American Journal of Medicine* 55:459–472.

Simon, H. (1979). Information processing model of cognition. *Annual Review of Psychology* 30:363–396.

Tanner, C. (1984). Factors influencing the diagnostic process. Pp. 61–82 in D. Carnevali, P. Mitchell, N. Woods, & C. Tanner eds., *Diagnostic reasoning in nursing*. Philadelphia: J. B. Lippincott.

_____. (1987). Teaching clinical judgment. Pp. 153–173 in J. Fitzpatrick, & R. Taunton eds., *Annual review of nursing research*, vol. 5. New York: Springer Publishing.

_____. (1988). Curriculum revolution: The practice mandate. *Nursing and Health Care* 9:427–430.

_____. (1989). Use of research in clinical judgment. Pp. 19-34 in C. Tanner, & C. Lindeman eds., *Using research*. New York: National League for Nursing Publication (#15–2232).

Tanner, C., Padrick, K., Westfall, U., & Putzier, D. (1987). Diagnostic reasoning strategies of nurses and nursing students. *Nursing Research* 36:358–363.

SECTION 2

MOVEMENT INTERVENTIONS

CHAPTER 6

PROGRESSIVE RELAXATION

BACKGROUND

Progressive relaxation, a technique developed by Edmund Jacobson (1938), is an intervention that has been used extensively to reduce high levels of stress and to promote health. Progressive relaxation provides the patient with a means for exerting control over the body's responses to tension and anxiety. Thus, the intervention is congruent with conceptual frameworks used in nursing in which independence and self-care are key beliefs. This chapter provides the basis for the use of progressive relaxation as a nursing intervention.

Definition

Progressive relaxation requires that a person tense and then relax successive muscle groups. Attention is focused on discriminating between the feelings experienced when the muscle is relaxed as compared to when it was tensed. As the person continues to use the technique over time, discrimination between tenseness and relaxation can be noted without actually tensing individual muscle groups. When experiencing a very stressful situation, a person can reduce the stress response by relaxing the muscles of the body and unconsciously maintaining muscles in a relaxed state, unless tension is needed for the performance of a specific activity.

Many variations of progressive relaxation have evolved. Table 6.1 presents relaxation procedures that are often referred to as relaxation techniques. Numerous articles and research studies fail to specify the specific technique that is used, placing all under the rubric of relaxation techniques. Major differences exist between these various techniques. Progressive muscle relaxation techniques are frequently incorporated into other relaxation interventions.

Comparison with Other Relaxation Interventions

Progressive relaxation and autogenic training contain some similar features. Schultz & Luthe (1969) developed the autogenic technique; this technique includes the element of autosuggestion in addition to the relaxation of muscles. The technique entails being in an undisturbed environment, relaxing in a comfortable

Table 6.1
Variations of the Progressive Relaxation Technique

Progressive muscle relaxation (Jacobson, 1938)
Progressive muscle relaxation (Bernstein & Borkovec, 1973)
Progressive relaxation plus cue-controlled relaxation (Paul, 1980)
Passive relaxation (Haynes, Moseley, & McGowan, 1975)
Autogenic training (Schultz & Luthe, 1969)
Rapid relaxation (Deffenbacher & Snyder, 1976)
Self-control relaxation (Lichstein, 1988)

position, and passively concentrating on verbal suggestions of warmth and heaviness of one's limbs (Davis et al., 1980). Shapiro and Lehrer (1980) compared the psychophysiological effects of autogenic therapy and progressive relaxation with two groups of college students. They found that both groups had significant decreases on the SCL-90 scales of anxiety, depression, number of symptoms, and intensity of symptoms. Some people may be hesitant to engage in autogenic training because of its close association with hypnosis.

In cue-controlled relaxation, the person uses a word or phrase that prompts the remembrance of feelings of complete muscle relaxation. The person must have first acquired the skills necessary to relax the muscles of the entire body.

Benson's (1975) relaxation response and progressive relaxation are often confused. Progressive relaxation incorporates specific attention to the contraction and relaxation of muscles, whereas the relaxation response contains the four elements of a quiet environment, an object to dwell upon, a passive attitude, and a comfortable position. Muscle relaxation may occur subsequent to the person assuming a quiet and passive state. The technique is more akin to meditation than progressive relaxation and will be discussed in Chapter 18.

Biofeedback, the use of sensory information to assist the person to gain control over body functions, may be used alone or as an adjunct in teaching progressive muscle relaxation (Chapter 24). Somatosensory biofeedback gives the person sensory feedback on the tenseness of specific muscle groups. The frontalis and the forearm extensor muscles are the groups most frequently used for teaching muscle relaxation with biofeedback. Numerous studies have compared the relative effectiveness of using only EMG biofeedback or only progressive relaxation training (Beiman et al., 1978; Bowles et al., 1979; Chesney & Shelton, 1976). Bowles et al. (1979) found biofeedback to be superior to progressive relaxation. Others, (Beiman et al., 1978; Chesney & Shelton, 1976) found progressive relaxation to be superior to biofeedback. Lehrer (1982) reported that live training in progressive relaxation appeared to be more powerful in reducing various measures of physical arousal and in treating stress-related problems than EMG biofeedback; EMG biofeedback added little to improve the effects when it was added to live progressive relaxation training.

Scientific Basis

When a person perceives a situation or event to be a stressor, the body reacts; this is the fight-flight or sympathetic response. This response provides humans with the immediate extra strength necessary to handle short-term stressful situations. The stress response is needed for survival, but if the perceived stressor is of a long duration, this response has deleterious effects on body systems. Selye's (1956) research identified the harmful effects that long-term high stress levels could have on the body. A variety of body responses occur in the fight-flight response: Pupils dilate, respirations become more shallow, heart rate increases, and muscles tense. Brown (1977) emphasized the psychophysiological relationship that occurs when stressors are perceived. She stated:

> In essence this circular mental activity is part of a closed feedback loop between muscles and the mind, i.e., the mental activity is also a feedback loop, operating between sensory mechanisms subserving perceptions and brain mechanisms concerned with the integration and synthesis of information. Since these cerebral mechanisms also process the information about muscle activity and the cerebral-muscle system can operate automatically as a feedback control system, the integrative brain mechanisms can be viewed as providing two interfaces, interacting on the one side with muscle control activity and on the other side with perceptual recognition processes. Within the integrative brain, information is exchanged between the two feedback loops. Thus, as the cerebral processes are engaged in rumination, there is a stream of emotional stimuli impinging upon the muscle control systems, activating and tensing the muscles. The tense muscles in turn send streams of information about the tension to the cortical appreciation areas which simply continue the stimulation to ruminate. [p.45]*

*From *Stress and the Art of Biofeedback* by B. Brown, Copyright © 1977 by Barbara Brown. Reprinted with permission of Bantam Books, Inc. All rights reserved.

Relieving muscle tension reduces the stimuli being sent to the brain, thus reducing the person's anxiety. Brown further stated:

> Inducing relaxation by focusing awareness on muscle effect—such as Jacobson's tense-relax exercises—results in fewer muscle tension impulses being sent to the central nervous system and so there are fewer stimuli to affect the cortex, keeping it alerted and this in turn decreases the cortical action on the lower-brain areas which have been maintaining the muscle tension. [p.48]

Lichstein (1988) questions how pervasive muscle relaxation is in reducing anxiety and other emotional states. He views it as one of the factors that interacts with the various biochemical and cognitive factors to reduce the negative effects of stressors.

Jacobson (1964) found that progressive relaxation decreased the body's oxygen consumption, metabolism, respiratory rate, heart rate, muscle tension, premature ventricular contractions, systolic and diastolic blood pressure, and increased alpha brain waves. Such responses promote health.

Edmund Jacobson is called the father of progressive relaxation. Jacobson taught patients to tense and relax 218 muscle groups. He later reduced this number to 15 muscle groups. The person learned to relax each muscle group during 56 hour-long sessions. Jacobson viewed the technique as a purely muscular skill and did not incorporate suggestion in his training. He believed that suggestion encouraged the trainee to feel relaxed during the training session even when muscle tension remained high (Lehrer, 1982).

Wolpe (1958) incorporated aspects of Jacobson's technique into his systematic desensitization technique for counterconditioning in persons with fear responses. He shortened the technique; his training consisted of six 20-minute sessions. The patient was instructed to practice twice daily for 15 minutes. The therapist in Wolpe's technique directs the sessions and gives suggestions on feelings that may be experienced by the patient. Wolpe also focused on the factors that may be precipitating the stress. His work has served as the basis for the development of a myriad of progressive relaxation procedures.

INTERVENTION

A considerable number of procedures for teaching progressive relaxation have evolved since Jacobson first publicized the intervention. The method for relaxing the muscle groups, the groups to be relaxed, the number of sessions to be used, and the role of the instructor (live versus taped instructions) are variables that differ in the various reported uses (Snyder, 1984, 1988). Studies present conflicting evidence on the relative effectiveness of the various techniques. Little research has been done to identify the characteristics of persons for whom a particular technique would be most advantageous. More attention to the characteristics of persons who do and do not benefit from a technique is needed before definitive prescriptions on the technique to use can be made.

Technique

A quiet environment is needed for teaching (and practicing) progressive relaxation. A soundproof room is ideal, but this is rarely available. In addition, a comfortable setting is needed including a restful, attractive room and a moderate temperature. Lighting should be subdued, but too little lighting may prevent the teacher from viewing the patient to determine if relaxation has occurred. Too dark a room may also cause uneasiness on the part of both the patient and the instructor. The patient may get the message that the purpose of the sessions is to promote sleep instead of creating a relaxed body and a refreshed mind. Precautions to prevent interruptions are necessary: no ringing of the telephone, no knocks, no conversations, and no other loud noises.

A reclining chair gives adequate support of the body while also providing comfort. A bed or couch may be used, but the tendency to sleep increases in the supine position. Patients who are bedfast can be taught the technique; adjustments for tensing certain muscle groups will need to be made. Pender (1985) used lawn recliners when teaching the technique to groups. These are relatively inexpensive and yet provide comfort during the training session. The instructor is seated in a manner so as to be able to view the patient and be able to determine reactions and degree of relaxation achieved.

Comfortable, unrestrictive clothing should be worn. Slacks or shorts allow the person to tense muscle groups and move extremities without exposure. Glasses and contact lenses are removed. Shoes are removed as they restrict movement; they also may produce external stimulation and draw the patient's attention away from the task at hand. Since the sessions, especially the initial ones, last 45–60 minutes, the patient may wish to use the bathroom before beginning a session.

The procedure developed by Bernstein and Borkovec (1973) will be presented. Other techniques for progressive relaxation will be compared and contrasted with this widely used procedure.

Procedure

Bernstein and Borkovec (1973) begin their ten training sessions by providing the client with the rationale for progressive relaxation. (Table 6.2 presents the content included in each session.) The scientific basis

Table 6.2
Content Included in Each of the Ten Training Sessions

Session	Content
1	Rationale for technique Demonstration for tensing 16 muscle groups Practice of tensing and relaxing muscles Determination of time for home practice
2	Practice tensing and relaxing muscles Discussion of problems encountered
3	Practice tensing and relaxing muscles Discussion of problems encountered
4	Introduction of seven muscle group technique Demonstration of technique Discussion of concerns and adaptations
5	Practice tensing and relaxing seven muscle groups
6	Introduction of four muscle group technique Demonstration of technique Discussion of concerns and adaptations
7	Practice tensing and relaxing four muscle groups
8	Practice of four muscle group technique Discussion of problems encountered Introduction to recall technique Discussion to life situations
9	Practice of four muscle group technique Use of recall technique Discussion to life situations
10	Introduction to counting technique Practice of counting technique Discussion of problems Arrangement for follow-up session Practice of tensing and relaxing muscles

Table 6.3
Instructions for Tensing the Sixteen Muscle Groups

The trainer asks the person to tense the muscle group when he states, "Tense," and to release the tension when he says, "Relax." Tension is held for seven seconds.

Dominant hand and forearm: Make a tight fist and hold it.

Dominant upper arm (biceps): Push elbow down against the arm of the chair.

Instructions repeated for arm of nondominant side.

Forehead muscles: Lift eyebrows as high as possible.

Muscles of central face (cheek, nose, and eyes): Squint eyes and wrinkle nose.
Lower face and jaw: Bite teeth together and extend corners of mouth wide.

Neck: Pull chin down toward chest, but prevent it from touching chest.

Chest, shoulders, and upper back: Take deep breath, hold it, pull shoulder blades back.

Abdomen: Pull stomach in and try to protect it.

Thigh of dominant side: Lift leg and hold it out straight.

Calf muscles of dominant side: Point toes toward ceiling.

Foot of dominant side: Curl toes down. Tension is only held for five seconds or less because cramps can easily occur. If this is a problem, this muscle group can be excluded.

Instructions repeated for leg of nondominant side.

for progressive relaxation is presented in terms patients can understand. This varies depending on their background. Information on stress in everyday life, the effects it has on our body, and signs and symptoms of stress are incorporated into the sessions. The patient is asked to identify situations that cause stress and how he or she has felt and reacted to them. Demonstration of the method for tensing each of the 16 muscle groups is done at a slow pace. If a person has difficulty tensing a muscle group, alternate ways can be presented. If the teaching is done in a group, the instructor needs to be aware of patients being self-conscious in tensing muscle groups, particularly those of the face.

Table 6.3 presents the instructions for tensing each of the 16 muscle groups. *Progressive Relaxation* (Jacobson, 1938), and *Relaxation Skills* (Robert J. Brady Company, 1976) provide illustrations for other ways to tense specific muscle groups. Bernstein and Borkovec (1973) present alternative methods for muscle groups that are difficult to relax. The patient may devise other methods for relaxing muscles by experimenting with several of the suggested ways and making adaptations.

The following instructions are used to teach the tensing and relaxing of each muscle group (Bernstein & Borkovec, 1973):

1. The patient's attention is focused on the muscle group.
2. At a predetermined signal from the instructor, the muscle group is tensed.
3. Tension is maintained for a period of 5–7 seconds with the duration shorter for the feet; instructor patter draws attention to accompanying feelings.
4. At a predetermined cue from the instructor, the muscle group is relaxed.
5. Suggestions from the instructor focus the patient's attention on the relaxed muscle group.

In the initial sessions, each muscle group is tensed and relaxed twice. Assessment is made by the instructor to determine if the muscles are relaxed. The patient is asked to raise the little finger of the right hand if the right hand and forearm are relaxed. As each subsequent group is tensed and relaxed, it is compared with the previous group. After 45–60 seconds, the instructor ascertains if the muscle group is relaxed. If deep relaxation is not experienced, the muscle group can be tensed again. The instructor also makes objective assessments to determine if the patient is truly achieving relaxation. Movement, uneasy breathing, and talking or coughing are indicators that the person has not achieved relaxation of the muscles even though he or she reports relaxation. The instructor informs the person that it takes time to become adept at relaxing muscles and that practice will increase the speed with which this is achieved. Alternate ways of tensing the muscle could be tried if relaxation is not obtained.

During the session, the instructor uses phrases that assist the patient to achieve relaxation and to keep attention focused on a specific muscle group. These phrases (patter) differ for each instructor and are ones with which he or she feels comfortable. Phrases used may include:

Relax, let all the tension go.

Notice what it feels like as the muscles become relaxed.

Compare these feelings to what the muscles felt like when they were tensed.

Enjoy the feelings as the muscles become more and more relaxed. Just enjoy it.

Enjoy the feelings as your muscles relax, unwind, become loose.

Give attention to the sensations of relaxation.

Patter is interspersed with periods of quiet. Constant chatter may create pressure and increase anxiety.

After all the muscle groups have been progressed through, the instructor asks the patient to identify if any tension remains in each muscle group as it is named. This is interspersed with focusing on relaxing all muscle groups. The instructor also observes if the patient is relaxed; slowed breathing is a good indicator of overall body relaxation. The patient is asked to signal if he or she feels completely relaxed. If the person signals that total relaxation has not been achieved, then the names of each muscle group are repeated and extra time is given for relaxing those causing a problem. An example of a checklist used for evaluating the degree of relaxation is presented in Table 6.4.

Two or three minutes are provided at the conclusion for the patient to enjoy the feelings associated with overall body relaxation. Suggestions are made to concentrate on the feelings in the body, to focus on breathing deeply and slowly letting the breath and tension out. Instructions to recall these feelings when situations producing stress occur during the day are provided.

Termination of relaxation is done gradually. The instructor begins counting backwards from four to one. With four, the patient moves hands and feet; with three, arms and legs; with two, head and neck; and with one, opens eyes. The patient is given an opportunity to express feelings concerning the technique or problems experienced. Because the patient may be unfamiliar with sensations of deep relaxation, the person may question if certain feelings experienced are normal. Reassurance is often necessary. Allowing adequate time for the patient to discuss feelings and concerns contributes to the continuing use of the intervention.

Practice Sessions

Practice between sessions is essential to the success of progressive relaxation. Hillenberg and Collins (1982) found a greater reduction in anxiety and tension scores in the group who practiced at home than in the group assigned not to practice at home. Establishing a time and place for practice is done during the first session. However, Luiselli (1981) notes that the setting and time should be varied so that the relaxation experience is not solely associated with one time or place. At least one 15-minute practice session a day is necessary for mastering the technique. Two practice sessions a day would be ideal, but a person may find this demand to be overwhelming. Some persons prefer to practice in the morning as it helps them maintain reduced tension throughout the day; others practice during lunch or coffee breaks. Persons who practice in the evening need to overcome tiredness, but they may find it beneficial in ridding themselves of the stress and tension of the day. Taped instructions may be helpful for home practice sessions. Written instructions with illustrations for relaxing muscle groups also provide guidance for home practice.

Lichstein (1988), based on a review of the literature on relaxation, found the following to be factors for persons not continuing to use a relaxation technique:

Table 6.4
Relaxation Checklist

Tense		Relaxed
Forehead	5 4 3 2 1	
Deeply furrowed or wrinkled		Smooth
Eyes	5 4 3 2 1	
Deeply wrinkled, squeezed tightly		Loosely closed, almost fluttering
Neck	5 4 3 2 1	
Veins or muscles visible, extended		Smooth
Head	5 4 3 2 1	
Held straight, centered		Tilted to side or forward
Arms	5 4 3 2 1	
Closed to body or shoulders raised		On chair arms or lap or away from body, shoulders forward
Hands	5 4 3 2 1	
Closed fist, clenching chair, tapping		Open, palms up, resting on lap or chair arms
Legs	5 4 3 2 1	
Close together, swaying, wiggling		Apart, knees out, no movement
Feet	5 4 3 2 1	
Together, flat on floor, tapping		Apart, resting on heels, toes pointing out
Breathing	5 4 3 2 1	
Rapid, uneven		Slow, even

From J. Luiselli, D. Steinman, D. Marholin, & W. Steinman. (1981). Evaluation of progressive muscle relaxation with conduct-problem learning-disabled children. *Child Behavior Therapy* 3:47. Used with permission.

Not enough time
Forget to use it
Unsure of relaxation procedure
Unsuccessful in achieving relaxation
Lack of a quiet place for practice
Changing interest in relaxation

Technique Variations

Bernstein and Borkovec's (1973) technique proceeds from the tensing and relaxing of 16 muscle groups to combining these into seven and then four groups. This reduces the length of time required to attain overall body relaxation. Table 6.5 indicates these combinations. Teaching the seven muscle groups procedure is begun in session four. Initially, the patient may not experience the level of relaxation achieved during the 16 muscle groups technique, but with practice this level is again reached.

Teaching the four muscle group technique is begun in session six. Again, the person needs to practice the method before the previous level of relaxation is achieved. After this procedure has been mastered, approximately ten minutes are needed for achieving overall body relaxation. Information about the time saving factor may serve as a motivator to persons when they are faced with "learning something new again." Pender (1987) cautioned against using the four muscle grouping with persons who have hypertension.

Table 6.5
Combination of Sixteen Muscle Groups to Seven and Four Groupings

7	Dominant hand and forearm Dominant biceps	
7	Nondominant hand and forearm Nondominant biceps	4
7	Forehead Upper cheeks and nose Lower cheeks and jaw	4
7	Neck and throat	
7	Chest, shoulders, and upper back Abdomen and lower back	4
7	Dominant thigh Dominant calf Dominant foot	
7	Nondominant thigh Nondominant calf Nondominant foot	4

Tensing large muscle groups may increase the blood pressure; this does not occur when smaller muscle groups are tensed and relaxed.

Achieving relaxation by recall and counting are also part of Bernstein and Borkovec's training. In recall, the person focuses attention on each of the seven muscle groups and recalls the feelings experienced when the muscle group was relaxed. The person strives to release any remaining tension in that particular muscle group. After overall relaxation is obtained, the person concentrates on these feelings. Many people find that this method is useful in everyday stressful situations.

The counting technique and cue-controlled relaxation are similar. In the counting technique, the instructor or the patient counts from ten to one. When each number is said, attention is focused on a particular muscle group and the sensations associated with the relaxation of that muscle group. Eventually, by counting from ten to one, the patient is able to achieve overall body relaxation. In cue-controlled relaxation, using a word or phrase prompts the remembrance of feelings of complete muscle relaxation.

Many variations of progressive relaxation procedures are reported in the literature. The number of sessions for teaching the technique vary from one to over 50. Borkovec and Sides (1979) reviewed 25 studies that had used progressive relaxation as the independent variable. The average number of training sessions was 4.57 for studies in which progressive relaxation was effective in achieving the desired outcome. Several sessions are needed just to determine if the person has mastered the technique. Lehrer (1982) commented that the superficiality of training may have been the contributing factor in studies in which progressive relaxation has been ineffective.

Garrison (1978) recommended a follow-up session to be held approximately two months after the last training session. A major problem encountered in health teaching is maintaining the gains after teaching sessions have ended. The objectives of the follow-up session are to evaluate progress, support maintenance of skills, and to help the person with problems encountered with the technique. Smith (1985) suggests use of a daily calendar for recording relaxation and results achieved.

One variation that has been tested in several nursing studies (Flaherty & Fitzpatrick, 1978; Horowitz, Fitzpatrick, & Flaherty, 1984) is the jaw drop technique. This technique incorporates a small portion of Jacobson's relaxation technique. After general instructions on relaxation are provided, the person's attention is directed to the muscles around his/her mouth. First, the person is told to smile as widely as possible and to hold the tension for several seconds. The tension is then released. Next, instructions are given to press one's lips together into an "O" formation and to concentrate on the tension created in the muscles; this tension is held for several seconds. Lastly, tension in the throat muscles is achieved by clenching the jaw, biting down hard, and pressing the tongue against the roof of the mouth; again, tension in these muscles is held for several seconds. After the tension in each muscle group is "let go," the person is asked to concentrate on the difference between the feelings when the muscles are tensed and when they are relaxed. This short technique can be easily used by persons to prevent high levels of stress.

Presentation of Content

Live (by an instructor) and taped instructions have been used in teaching progressive relaxation. Whereas taped instructions save both time and money, studies have shown that they are not as effective as live instructions. Paul and Trimble (1970) reported that persons receiving instructions via tapes showed significantly less response than persons who had been taught with live instructions. In a review of studies that had used progressive relaxation as an intervention, Borkovec and Sides (1979) noted that significant differences between the experimental and control groups occurred in 73% of the studies in which live instruction had been used, whereas no differences were found between the control and experimental groups in studies of taped instruction use. Live instructions allow the instructor to individualize the technique for the patient and to provide immediate feedback on problems encountered (Lehrer & Woolfolk, 1982). Interaction between the instructor and the patient may help to motivate the patient to continue to use the technique.

The voice of the instructor is important to the success of the intervention (Corah et al., 1981). How the instructions are given is as crucial as what is said. A conversational tone is used at the beginning of the session, but as time progresses, volume and speed are reduced. The voice should not be so soft that the patient has to strain to hear the instructions. The tone used is smooth and quiet but not monotonous or hypnotic. Directions to tense muscle groups is given at a louder pitch than instructions to relax the muscles. This assists the patients in noticing differences between tension and relaxation. After the second session the instructor requests feedback about the tone, pace, and other aspects of the instructions. Patients differ in the style that is most helpful for achieving relaxation.

Before beginning to teach progressive relaxation, an instructor benefits from personal practice of the technique. Unless the instructors know the sensations associated with tenseness and relaxation, they will find it difficult to help patients and to evaluate progress. The instructor also should be knowledgeable concerning the effects of stress on the body and the rationale for the use of progressive relaxation. Most importantly, the instructor needs to be aware of precautions for the use of progressive relaxation. These will be addressed later in the chapter. Lastly, the instructor needs to be able to determine the effectiveness of the intervention, and thus needs knowledge about parameters to assess.

Measurement of Effectiveness

A variety of measurements has been used to judge the effectiveness of progressive relaxation. Because the technique has been used as an intervention for very diverse conditions, the measurement appropriate for each varies. If the purpose for teaching the technique is to decrease overall anxiety, then a test to measure the level of anxiety is appropriate. On the other hand, if insomnia is the problem, the instructor will want to determine if the person's ability to sleep has improved. In addition, determination of the overall stress level may also be desired. Baseline determinations need to be ascertained before instruction is begun. Measurement indices will be discussed according to somatic, cognitive/emotional, and overall indices.

Somatic Measurement

Some general indices of reduced stress include a slowed and regular breathing pattern, a restful demeanor such as in peaceful sleeping, a slackened jaw, and feet at 45-degree angles to each other. These measurements can be used by the instructor to determine if a patient is mastering the technique.

Other physiological measurements include reduced muscle tension, decreased heart rate, lowered blood pressure, decreased respiratory rate, and an altered galvanic skin response (GSR). Electromyogram readings of the frontalis or forearm muscles are taken to determine the degree of tension present. It is postulated that relaxation of these muscles is an indication that muscles throughout the body are relaxed. Jones and Evans (1981), however, contended that decreased tension in the frontalis muscle is not indicative of generalized reduction of tension throughout the body. Use of the skin resistance measurement (GSR) is based on the premise that increased perspiration during high levels of stress alters the resistance of the skin to electrical transmission.

Changes in vital signs is a widely used physiological measurement. Because the autonomic nervous system is intimately involved in the stress response, reduction of the level of stress should be manifested in reduced blood pressure, heart rate, and respirations. Shapiro and Lehrer (1980) stated, however, that significant changes in vital signs would not occur in persons who did not have high levels of stress. Underlying pathology may also affect the changes in vital signs. Broussard (1979) noted that a reduction in blood pressure did not occur in patients with congestive heart failure who were taught progressive relaxation; she attributed this to the presence of right ventricular hypertrophy. Reduction of heart rate and lowering of blood pressure are easily obtained indices in the clinical setting. In many studies, electrocardiogram leads were used to monitor changes in heart rate, which eliminated the effect that touch can have on a person's response.

Cognitive

Numerous tests have been used to measure changes in anxiety level: Adjective Affective Check List (AACL) (Zuckerman, 1960); SCL-90 (Gough & Heilburn, 1965); State-Trait Anxiety Self-Questionnaire (Spielberger et al., 1984); and Taylor Manifest Anxiety Scale (Taylor, 1953). Validity and reliability of these tests have been established. The Profile of Moods States (POMS) (McNair et al., 1971) has been used to measure changes in other emotions. Various depression inventories have been used in detecting alterations in this emotion.

Yesavage (1984) used cognitive and memory tests to determine the effectiveness of relaxation strategies in improving memory in the elderly. Problem-solving ability has also been used as an indicator of relaxation.

Overall

Patient reports on the degree of relaxation experienced have been used to measure the effectiveness of the intervention. This is important because, if the patient does not perceive a state of relaxation, test results or measurements are going to do little to prove to the person that he or she is relaxed. The degree of subjective relaxation experienced also serves as a strong determinant on whether or not the person will continue to practice progressive relaxation. Comments from the patient and use of a subjective scale are methods that have been used to obtain data on perceived levels of relaxation.

Other Considerations

The majority of measurements reported have been done immediately after training sessions. Determination of the long-term effectiveness of progressive relaxation is needed. Snyder (1983) queried persons with epilepsy six months after they had been taught the technique; seven of the 16 persons had continued to use the technique on a regular basis and reported that it was helpful in reducing anxiety in a variety of ways.

Another aspect of measurement is choosing evaluation methods that are feasible for use in the clinical setting. Kallio (1983) noted that paper and pencil tests take time to administer and questioned if busy nurses would find the time to administer them correctly. Also, the patient's condition may not permit him or her to accurately complete the test because of fatigue or pain. Use of additional equipment, such as an EMG machine, add expense and time plus being another intrusive modality with which the patient is faced. Nurses need to consider the purpose for which progressive relaxation is being taught, the nature of the population, and the time required for the measurement when choosing the method(s) for evaluating the effectiveness of progressive relaxation. Not only consistency in teaching the technique, but also careful evaluation of the effectiveness of the technique, will help to develop prescriptive uses for progressive relaxation.

USES

Progressive relaxation has been used for many conditions. Table 6.6 lists patient populations in which the technique has been used. In the majority of populations, the focus has been the reduction of anxiety, but other outcomes include pain relief, improved mental state, and health promotion. Davis et al. (1980) indicated that progressive relaxation was an appropriate intervention to use for anxiety, hostility, anger, fears, muscular tension, hypertension, headaches, muscle spasms, tics, ulcers, fatigue, and insomnia. Attention in this chapter will focus on its use for health promotion, relief of pain, and reduction of stress in specific conditions.

Health Promotion

In the past decade much attention has been given to health promotion. Educating persons on practices that will assist them in staying healthy has included instruction on ways to manage tension or high stress levels. Progressive relaxation is one of the techniques used to accomplish this purpose. The technique is easily taught and requires no additional equipment. A review of studies done on healthy persons has shown the technique to have little or no effect on reduction of heart rate, blood pressure, or other measurements of fear and anxiety (Glaister, 1982). Shapiro and Lehrer (1980) concluded that significant changes in vital signs do not occur in "normal" persons who are taught relaxation. These findings do not negate the use of the

Table 6.6
Conditions In Which Progressive Relaxation Has Been Used As an Intervention

Stress Reduction
    Insomnia (Borkovec et al., 1975)
    Asthma (Alexander, 1972; Freedberg et al., 1987)
    Phobias (Green et al., 1981)
    Psychiatric conditions (Sheer, 1980)
    Reduction of seizures (Snyder, 1983; Whitman et al., 1990)
    Hypertension (Beiman et al., 1978; Pender, 1985)
    General anxiety (Borkovec et al., 1978; Woolfolk et al., 1982)
    Chronic obstructive pulmonary disease (Renfroe, 1988)

Pain Reduction
    Postoperative (Flaherty & Fitzpatrick, 1978; Wells, 1982)
    Headache (Cox et al., 1978)
    Chronic pain (Greziak, 1977)

Health Promotion
    Anger control (Davis et al., 1980)
    Relief of nausea and vomiting (Cotanch, 1983)
    Diagnostic procedures (Rice et al., 1986)

technique for health promotion. Rather, use of the technique will assist persons in handling stressful situations without becoming unduly disturbed. Measurement of the technique's success would be ascertained over a period of time rather than determined by immediate changes.

Pain

Progressive relaxation has been used in the treatment of several types of pain: headache, postoperative pain, labor pain, and chronic pain such as with low-back pain. Muscle tension increases pain; reduction of this tension contributes to the lessening of pain. Anxiety heightens the perception of pain; a decrease in a person's anxiety level through the practice of progressive relaxation decreases the level of pain. Using the technique provides the person with a sense of control over the pain which in turn may decrease anxiety.

The intervention has been used in the treatment of tension headaches. Cox et al. (1978) found progressive relaxation to be as effective as EMG biofeedback in relieving tension headaches. Because tension in the large neck muscles contributes significantly to the cause of the pain, reduction of tension in these muscle groups should decrease the occurrence of headaches. Progressive relaxation is useful also in preventing headaches.

Flaherty and Fitzpatrick (1978) taught progressive relaxation preoperatively to general surgery patients for use postoperatively when getting out of bed. They found that these patients had less of an increase in heart rate, blood pressure, and respiratory rate when getting out of bed than patients in the control group. The patients also reported less distress and used fewer analgesics. Despite only limited training sessions on the day prior to surgery (four), the patients were able to master the technique sufficiently to use it effectively postoperatively. Teaching progressive relaxation to surgical patients could begin at the time the decision to have surgery is made, in the doctor's office. The person could be given a tape to guide home practice; review of the technique and application to postoperative use would then be done before surgery.

The effectiveness of progressive relaxation in the treatment of patients with chronic pain is based partially on decreasing the level of anxiety. The gate-control theory of Melzack and Wall (1965) supports the premise that anxiety increases the perception of pain. When muscles are relaxed, blood flow to the tissues is improved, which also contributes to pain reduction. Focusing on relaxing of muscles can serve as a distraction from the pain stimulus. Greziak (1977) reported that after paraplegics with chronic pain had been taught progressive relaxation, they experienced some relief from pain and had an improved outlook.

Careful assessment of the person with pain, particularly the person with chronic pain, needs to be made. McCaffery (1979) stated that focusing attention on the body may heighten the person's perception of pain instead of reducing it. The type of persons in whom this occurs has not been identified; instructor alertness to alterations in pain when teaching the technique to persons with chronic pain is vitally important.

Reduction of Stress

Respiratory conditions. Progressive relaxation has been used in the treatment of several types of respiratory conditions. Broussard (1979) used the technique with a patient who had emphysema. The heart rate and respirations decreased significantly over time after progressive relaxation had been taught. In addition, the patient experienced an overall sense of well being. Alexander (1972) taught progressive relaxation to children with asthma. Significant differences in the vital capacity existed between children in the experimental and control groups. Freedberg et al. (1987) likewise found that progressive muscle relaxation reduced anxiety in persons with asthma. Relaxation of the striated muscles is believed to generalize to the smooth muscles, thus reducing the spasms in the bronchi and bronchioles. Difficulty in breathing is very stressful; if persons know that they can alleviate some of the symptoms themselves, stress is diminished. Teaching progressive relaxation to persons with respiratory problems may require modifications in the technique. Instead of a reclining position, the persons may be more comfortable in an upright position. The addition of breathing techniques to the progressive relaxation procedure may also be helpful for persons with respiratory conditions.

Reduction of seizures. Several studies have reported that progressive relaxation is beneficial as a means for reducing seizures. Snyder (1983) reported that persons who practiced progressive relaxation had a greater reduction in the number of seizures than those who did not practice it. Rousseau et al. (1985) and Whitman et al. (1990) likewise found that persons with epilepsy who practiced progressive muscle relaxation experienced a reduction in the occurrence of seizures. A 54% reduction was found in the study by Whitman and colleagues. It is not advocated that anticonvulsants be eliminated, but that progressive relaxation be used as an adjunct.

Psychoses and neuroses. Progressive relaxation has been used in persons with high anxiety due to phobias and in persons suffering from depression. One reason for its success in phobia cases may be that the person concentrates on the process and thus blocks out stimulation from the perceived stressor. Persons also have reported an improvement in overall sense of well-being, particularly in having increased energy. Additional training sessions may be needed for persons who have extremely high levels of anxiety as they may be unable to fully concentrate on the content during the initial sessions. Careful monitoring of depressed persons is necessary; they may use the technique as a method of escape and use it for more than the 15–30 minutes prescribed each day. Caution is also needed in the use of progressive relaxation in persons with schizoid tendencies as the technique may intensify symptoms.

Hypertension. Many stress management techniques have been used for persons with hypertension. Because anxiety has an effect on increases in blood pressure, reducing anxiety should produce a reduction in blood pressure. Beiman et al. (1978) reported that the use of progressive relaxation resulted in significant decreases in blood pressure. Pender (1985) likewise reported reductions. One important measurement in the use of progressive relaxation is its long-term effect on the blood pressure. The majority of studies have used pressure readings taken immediately after the conclusion of the training sessions. Long-term measurements and patient adherence to practice of the technique are needed to evaluate its effectiveness.

Insomnia. Increased anxiety precipitates sleep problems. Because progressive relaxation is an easy technique to use, it can be learned easily and used by many persons. Borkovec et al. (1975) found progressive relaxation to be effective for persons with insomnia. Participants in Snyder's study (1983) noted that use of progressive relaxation helped them get to sleep. Sleep disturbances, as indicated by the large volume of sleeping medications sold each year in this country, are a major health problem. Informing persons being taught progressive relaxation about its application for insomnia may be beneficial to many of them.

Precautions

A number of uses for progressive relaxation have been identified and the potential for its use as a nursing intervention is evident. Although it may seem to be a relatively benign intervention, nurses need to have an awareness of populations requiring careful assessment and monitoring when progressive relaxation is used with them. Occurrence of harmful side effects is possible.

Trophotropic reactions may occur when persons practice progressive relaxation. The trophotropic state potentiates the effects of a medication resulting in toxic levels of the drug. This is particularly true for insulin, in which case a hypoglycemic state results. Because of the relaxed state, lowered dosages of medications may be required.

Total relaxation may produce a hypotensive state. Persons need to be taught to remain seated for a period of time after practicing progressive relaxation. Movement in place and gradual resumption of activity helps alleviate hypotension. Some persons may be more prone to becoming hypotensive than others. Taking blood pressure at the conclusion of early teaching sessions helps to identify these individuals.

Herman (1987, 1989) studied the effect of progressive relaxation on inducing the Valsalva response in healthy adults. Her findings indicated that the Valsalva response occurred in 43% of subjects. However, the percentage in the second study was less (18%). Subjects in the first study had tensed their muscles for a shorter time than in the second study. Findings from these studies make it imperative that the instructor be attentive to the breathing patterns of patients during the tensing phase.

Progressive relaxation is not suggested for persons who have hallucinations or delusions. The technique may increase out-of-reality reactions. The exact reason why this occurs is not known, but it may be the result of the intense concentration on the body demanded during the procedure. Care also is needed when progressive relaxation is used for persons in a depressed state as it may be used as a means of further withdrawal. Heide and Borkovec (1984) reported the possible occurrence of relaxation-induced anxiety (RIA) in persons practicing progressive relaxation, particularly in persons experiencing pervasive generalized anxiety. Symptoms include intense restlessness, profuse perspiration, shivering, trembling, and rapid breathing.

Some persons with chronic pain find that the technique heightens the experience of pain in which case use should be abandoned. As the person concentrates on the muscles of the body to achieve relaxation, he or she is drawn more to the pain sensation than to the feelings of tension and relaxation.

Persons with hypertension should not practice the seven or four muscle group relaxation techniques. Relaxing the large muscle groups after they have been tensed forces large volumes of blood to be returned to the heart which increases the blood pressure. Whereas tight tensing of muscles is to be avoided by all persons, this caution is particularly important for persons who have had a myocardial infarction. The damaged heart is unable to handle the sudden return of a large volume of blood.

RESEARCH QUESTIONS

Several reviews of the use of progressive relaxation have been done in nursing (Hyman, et al., 1989; Snyder, 1988) and in other fields (Lichstein, 1988; Woolfolk & Lehrer, 1984). These reviews indicate numerous areas in which further information about the use of progressive relaxation is needed. This is particularly true in relation to nursing studies. These areas include:

1. What are the characteristics of persons who would benefit most from progressive relaxation?
2. What are the conditions for which progressive relaxation is the intervention of choice?
3. Does progressive relaxation decrease the need for pain and/or other medications?
4. What are the long-term effects of progressive relaxation?
5. What are the characteristics of persons who continue to use progressive relaxation as compared to persons who do not continue to use it?
6. What are reliable and valid evaluation methods that are useful in the clinical area for determining the effectiveness of progressive relaxation?
7. Do persons who learn progressive relaxation for one purpose generalize it to other life situations?
8. Are comparable findings found from use of the various progressive relaxation techniques?

REFERENCES

Alexander, A. (1972). Systematic relaxation and flow rates in asthmatic children: relationship to emotional precipitants and anxiety. *Journal of Psychosomatic Research* 16:405–410.

Beiman, I., Graham, L., & Ciminero, A. (1978). Self-control progressive relaxation training as an alternative nonpharmacological treatment for essential hypertension: therapeutic effects in the natural environment. *Behavior Research and Therapy* 16:371–375.

Benson, H. (1975). *The relaxation response.* New York: Avon Press.

Bernstein, D., & Borkovec, T. (1973). *Progressive relaxation training.* Champaign, IL: Research Press.

Borkovec, T., Grayson, J., & Cooper, K. (1978). Treatment of general tension: subjective and physiological effects of progressive relaxation. *Journal of Consulting and Clinical Psychology* 46:518–528.

Borkovec, T., Kaloupek, D., & Slama, K. (1975). The facilitative effect of muscle tension-release in the relaxation treatment of sleep disturbance. *Behavior Therapy* 6:301–309.

Borkovec, T., & Sides, J. (1979). Critical procedural variables related to the physiological effects of progressive relaxation: a review. *Behavior Research and Therapy* 17:119–125.

Bowles, C., Smith, J., & Parker, K. (1979). EMG biofeedback and progressive relaxation training: a comparative study of two groups of normal subjects. *Western Journal of Nursing Research* 1:179–189.

Broussard, R. (1979). Using relaxation for COPD. *American Journal of Nursing* 79:1962–1963.

Brown, B. (1977). *Stress and the art of biofeedback.* New York: Bantam.

Chesney, M., & Shelton, J. (1976). A comparison of muscle relaxation and electromyogram biofeedback treatments for muscle contraction headache. *Journal of Behavior Therapy and Experimental Psychiatry* 7:221–225.

Corah, N., Gale, E., Pace, L., & Seyrek, S. (1981). Evaluation of content and vocal style in relaxation instructions. *Behavior Research and Therapy* 19:458–460.

Cotanch, P. (1983). Relaxation training for control of nausea and vomiting in patients receiving chemotherapy. *Cancer Nursing* 6:277–282.

Cox, D., Freundlich, A., & Meyer, R. (1978). Differential effectiveness of electromyograph feedback, verbal relaxation instructions, and medication placebo with tension headaches. *Journal of Consulting and Clinical Psychology* 43:892–898.

Davis, M., McKay, M., & Eshelman, E. (1980). *The relaxation and stress reduction workbook.* Richmond CA: New Harbinger Publications.

Deffenbacher, J., & Snyder, A. (1976). Relaxation and self-control in the treatment of test and other anxieties. *Psychological Reports* 39:379–385.

Flaherty, G., & Fitzpatrick, J. (1978). Relaxation technique to increase comfort level of postoperative patients: a preliminary study. *Nursing Research* 27:352–355.

Freedberg, P.D., Hoffman, L.A., Light, W.C., & Kreps, M.K. (1987). Effect of progressive relaxation on the objective symptoms and subjective responses associated with asthma. *Heart & Lung* 16:24–30.

Garrison, J. (1978). Stress management training for the handicapped. *Archives of Physical Medicine and Rehabilitation* 59:580–585.

Glaister, B. (1982). Muscle relaxation training for fear reduction of patients with psychological problems: a review of controlled studies. *Behavior Research Therapy* 20:493–504.

Gough, H., & Heilbrun, A. (1965). *The adjective checklist manual.* Palo Alto: Consulting Psychologists Press.

Green, K., Webster, J., Beiman, I., Rosmarin, D., & Holliday, P. (1981). Progressive and self-induced relaxation training: their relative effects on subjective and autonomic arousal to fearful stimuli. *Journal of Clinical Psychology* 37:309–315.

Greziak, R. (1977). Relaxation techniques in treatment of chronic pain. *Archives of Physical Medicine and Rehabilitation* 58:270–272.

Haynes, S., Moseley, D., & McGowan, W. (1975). Relaxation training and biofeedback in the reduction of frontalis muscle tension. *Psychophysiology* 12:547–552.

Heide, F., & Borkovec, T. (1984). Relaxation-induced anxiety: mechanisms and theoretical implications. *Behavior Research and Therapy* 22:1–12.

Herman, J. (1987). The effect of progressive relaxation on valsalva response in healthy adults. *Research in Nursing and Health* 10:171–176.

———. (1989). Valsalva response during progressive relaxation: An extension study. *Scholarly Inquiry for Nursing Practice* 3:217–232.

Hillenberg, J., & Collins, F. (1982). A procedural analysis and review of relaxation training research. *Behavior Research Therapy* 20:251–260.

Horowitz, B.F., Fitzpatrick, J.J., & Flaherty, G.G. (1984). Relaxation techniques for relief of pain after open heart surgery. *Dimensions of Critical Care Nursing* 3:364–371.

Hyman, R.B., Feldman, H.R., Harris, R.B., Levin, R.F., & Malloy, G.B. (1989). The effects of relaxation training on clinical symptoms: A meta-analysis. *Nursing Research* 38:216–220.

Jacobson, E. (1938). *Progressive relaxation.* Chicago: University of Chicago Press.

———. (1964). *Anxiety and tension control: A physiologic approach.* Philadelphia: J. B. Lippincott.

Jones, G., & Evans, P. (1981). Effectiveness of frontalis feedback training in producing general body relaxation. *Biological Psychology* 12:313–320.

Kallio, J. (1983). Anxiety. Pp. 291–306 in M. Snyder ed., *Guide to neurological and neurosurgical nursing.* New York: John Wiley & Sons.

Lehrer, P. (1982). How to relax and how not to relax: a re-evaluation of the work of Edmund Jacobson—I. *Behavior Research Therapy* 20:417–428.

Lehrer, P., & Woolfolk, R. (1982). Self-report assessment of anxiety. *Behavioral Assessment* 4:167–177.

Lichstein, K.L. (1988). *Clinical relaxation strategies.* New York: John Wiley & Sons.

Luiselli, J.K. (1981). Facilitating transfer of clinical biofeedback training: A review. *Behavioral Engineering* 7:1–6.

Luiselli, J.K., Steinman, D.L., Marholin, D., & Steinman, W.M. (1981). Evaluation of progressive muscle relaxation with conduct-problem learning disabled children. *Child Behavior Therapy.* 3:41–55.

McCaffery, M. (1979). *Nursing management of the patient with pain.* Philadelphia: J. B. Lippincott.

McNair, D.M., Lorr, M., & Droppleman, L.F. (1971). *Profile of moods.* San Diego: Educational and Industrial Testing Service.

Melzack, R., & Wall, P. (1965). Pain mechanisms: a new theory. *Science* 150:971–978.

Paul, G. (1980). Relaxation training—the misunderstood and misused therapy. Pp. 223–229 in F. McGuigan, W. Sime, & J. Wallace eds., *Stress and tension control.* New York: Plenum Press.

Paul, G., & Trimble, R. (1970). Recorded vs. live relaxation training and hypnotic suggestion: comparative effectiveness for reducing arousal and inhibiting stress response. *Behavior Therapy* 1:285–302.

Pender, N. (1985). Effects of progressive muscle relaxation training on anxiety and health locus of control among hypertensive adults. *Research in Nursing and Health* 8:67–82.

_____. (1987). *Health promotion in nursing practice.* Norwalk, CT: Appleton-Century-Crofts.

Relaxation skills. (1976). Bowie, MD: Robert J. Brady Co.

Renfroe, K. (1988). Effect of progressive relaxation on dyspnea and state anxiety in patients with chronic obstructive pulmonary disease. *Heart & Lung* 17:408–413.

Rice, V.H., Caldwell, M., Butler, S., & Robinson, J. (1986). Relaxation training and response to a cardiac catheterization. *Nursing Research* 35:39–43.

Rousseau, A., Hermann, B., Whitman, S. (1985). Effects of progressive relaxation on epilepsy: Analysis of a series of cases. *Psychological Reports* 57:1203–1212.

Schultz, J., & Luthe, W. (1969). *Autogenic training: A psychophysiologic approach in psychotherapy.* New York: Grune and Stratton.

Selye, H. (1956). *The stress of life.* New York: McGraw Hill.

Shapiro, S., & Lehrer, P. (1980). Psychophysiological effects of autogenic training and progressive relaxation. *Biofeedback and Self-Regulation* 5:249–255.

Sheer, B. (1980). The effects of relaxation training on psychiatric inpatients. *Issues in Mental Health Nursing* 2(6):1–15.

Smith, J.C. (1985). *Relaxation dynamics.* Champaign, IL: Research Press.

Snyder, M. (1983). Effect of relaxation on psychosocial functioning in persons with epilepsy. *Journal of Neurosurgical Nursing* 15:250–254.

_____. (1984). Progressive relaxation as a nursing intervention: an analysis. *Advances in Nursing Science* 6(3):47–58.

_____. (1988). Relaxation. Pp. 111–128 in J. Fitzpatrick, R. Taunton, & J. Benoliel eds. *Annual Review of Nursing Research* (vol. 6). New York: Springer.

Spielberger, C., Gorusch, R., Luschene, R., Vagg, P., & Jacobs, G. (1984). *Manual for STAI.* Palo Alto: Consulting Psychologists Press.

Taylor, J. (1953). A personality scale of manifest anxiety. *Journal of Abnormal Psychology* 48:285–295.

Wells, N. (1982). The effect of relaxation on postoperative muscle tension and pain. *Nursing Research* 31:236–238.

Whitman, S., Dell, J., Legion, V., Eibhlyn, A., & Statsinger, J. (1990). Progressive relaxation for seizure reduction. *Journal of Epilepsy* 3:17–22.

Wolpe, J. (1958). *Psychotherapy in reciprocal inhibition.* Stanford, CA: Stanford University Press.

Woolfolk, R.L., & Lehrer, P.M. (1984). *Principles and practice of stress management.* New York: Guilford Press.

Woolfolk, R., Lehrer, P., Mc Cann, B., & Rooney, A. (1982). Effects of progressive relaxation and meditation on cognitive and somatic manifestations of daily stress. *Behavior Research and Therapy* 20:461–467.

Yesavage, J.A. (1984). Relaxation and memory training in 39 elderly patients. *American Journal of Psychiatry* 141:778–781.

Zuckerman, M. (1960). The development of an adjective checklist for the measurement of anxiety. *Journal of Consulting Psychology* 24:457–462.

CHAPTER 7

BREATHING

BACKGROUND

For many years nursing has used breathing techniques to achieve various outcomes, but nursing has given little attention to breathing as a specific intervention. Fundamentals of nursing texts provide instructions on using deep breathing as part of the postoperative care regimen. Nursing also has made considerable use of breathing patterns as part of relaxation techniques, such as the incorporation of breathing techniques into the LeMaze strategy. Nursing has used techniques for breathing for various purposes, but nursing has given little attention to breathing as a specific intervention. This chapter will discuss some of the possible uses of breathing.

During her student days, this author observed expert nurses instructing postoperative patients who were experiencing nausea to take several deep breaths. Often this practice was effective in decreasing feelings of nausea. Various hypotheses for the effectiveness of the breathing intervention in reducing nausea were generated: Is the proximity of the respiratory and vomiting centers responsible for the effect? Does concentrating on breathing serve as a distractor? Is breathing effective because it produces relaxation? No studies were done to verify the scientific basis for the intervention; however, interest in the use of breathing as a nursing intervention has persisted.

Breathing techniques have been used as forms of therapy since ancient times (Jencks, 1984). Reports on the use of breathing therapy by the Chinese date to the sixth century B.C. Records from the second century B.C. in India reveal that Hatha Yoga incorporated breathing techniques to achieve hypnosis. Early Christian monks used a rhythmic form of breathing during prayers. Breathing was not an important component of Western medicine until the 1900s when psychotherapy began to incorporate breathing techniques. Bonnet (cited in Jencks, 1984) instructed his patients to repeat hypnotic formulas in rhythm with their breathing patterns. Schultz (1932), the father of the autogenic technique, observed that irregular breathing was present during stress. He incorporated, "It breathes me," into the autogenic technique; this provided for a passive focusing on breathing.

Definition

Breathe is defined as drawing air into and expelling it from the lungs. Inhalation and exhalation comprise the process.

Breathing is sometimes preceded by an adjective that identifies the muscles being used in respiration: diaphragmatic, intercostal, or accessory muscles. The diaphragm is innervated by the phrenic nerve which exits from the spinal cord at the level of cervical 2–4 vertebrae. Diaphragmatic breathing is the most efficient and relaxed type of breathing. Damage to the spinal cord in the high cervical region damages the phrenic nerve and often necessitates continuous ventilator assistance. Intercostal muscles are involved in the expansion of the chest cavity. However, reliance on the intercostal muscles is very taxing. Accessory muscles are used primarily when there is interference with diaphragmatic breathing.

Others have classified breathing according to the emotional state associated with particular patterns of breathing. Smith (1985) notes that a person breathes quickly and choppily when angry, holds one's breath when fearful, and gasps when shocked. Thus breathing reveals much about a person's emotional state. The effect that fear or anxiety has on breathing is very pronounced.

Scientific Basis

The character of one's breathing has a profound influence on a person's quality of life (Speads, 1986). Proper breathing improves circulation, normalizes muscle tone, and enhances clearer thinking. These effects often result in the person having a more positive mood. According to Speads, the effect of breathing on physiological and psychological functioning indicates the total unity of human beings.

Breathing is an automatic, self-regulatory function. However, many variables influence the breathing pattern of an individual. Attention to these variables will assist the person in being able to change his or her breathing patterns to promote more effective and healthy breathing.

INTERVENTION

Breathing techniques vary depending on the purpose for which they are used. Most fundamentals of nursing texts include descriptions of deep breathing techniques to use for postoperative and immobilized patients. Speads (1986) describes a number of "experiments" that assist persons to become more aware of their breathing. Numerous breathing techniques have been incorporated into relaxation interventions. Breathing techniques are an integral part of yoga (Hittleman, 1988). Some techniques are very simple, such as having the patient focus on inhalation and exhalation. An accompanying message is, "To let tension escape with the exhalation." Other breathing techniques, such as the integrative breathing technique of Smith (1985), are more complex. This latter technique will be described.

Technique

Table 7.1 lists the phases of the integrative breathing technique. The patient is seated comfortably in a chair with feet flat on the floor. Initial instructions are to close one's eyes and let the body become comfortable. The person is told to take a deep breath and slowly exhale. This is repeated several times. Instructions for the arm swing breathing include circling the arms behind the body as the person inhales and circling the arms to the front of the body as the person exhales. These actions are repeated several times, with attention

---

Table 7.1
Exercises of Integrative Breathing Technique

Deep breathing
Arm swing breathing
Body arch breathing
Bowing and breathing
Bowing and stretching
Stomach squeeze breathing
Active diaphragmatic breathing
Inhaling through nose breathing
Exhaling through lips breathing
Focused breathing
Thinking the word "one"
Thinking a relaxing word

Source: Smith, J.C. (1985). *Relaxation dynamics.* Champaign, IL: Research Press.

given to inhaling at an unhurried pace. At the completion of the last circling, persons are instructed to let their arms hang by their sides.

In the third step of the integrative breathing technique, persons stretch their backs and let their heads tilt back as they inhale. The arms remain hanging at the person's side. With each exhalation, persons are instructed to relax and bring their bodies back into a comfortable upright position. The head may bend slightly forward. These actions are repeated several times.

For the breathing and bowing segment, the back is arched as in the previous segment, but during the exhaling portion persons bend forward with the head and chest moving toward their knees. The arms hang limply at the person's side. Several shorter breaths may be taken while the person is leaning forward. A deep breath is taken as the person sits upright. Several deep breaths are taken in the sitting position with the exhalations being very slow and deliberate. The bowing and stretching segment follows. Persons are instructed to arch their backs and gently circle both arms toward the sky, like the wings of a bird. When ready to exhale, the person lets the arms slowly circle down so that they are hanging heavily at his/her sides. Then persons bow forward and remain in that position for a short period of time during which they breathe at whatever pace feels most comfortable. The sequence is repeated twice. This is followed by placing the arms in the lap and breathing in a natural manner.

During the stomach squeeze breathing segment, the palms of the hands are spread across the abdomen with the thumbs touching the bottom of the chest. After taking a deep breath, the hands are pressed firmly against the abdomen as if assisting in expelling the air from the lungs. The fingers are relaxed as the person inhales. This segment is repeated several times. Active diaphragmatic breathing follows. In this segment the hands remain gently on the stomach during both inhalation and exhalation. After the exhalation the person is instructed to pull his/her stomach in as if to push out any remaining air. These actions are repeated several times.

In the inhaling through the nose segment, persons are instructed to imagine that they are sniffing a delicate flower as they inhale; the inhalation should be smooth and gentle. Exhalation is done naturally. The actions are repeated several times. Attention is drawn to feeling the air moving through the nostrils and into the body. Instructions for the exhaling through the lips segment request persons to gently blow out through their lips as if blowing at a candle flame; the intensity should only be enough to make the candle flicker and not to extinguish it. Inhalation is done through the nose. Inhalations and exhalations are repeated several times.

In the last three segments of the technique, a more relaxed and inner focused state is emphasized. In the focus on breathing segment, the person's attention is drawn to the air being drawn into and leaving the body. Instructions are to let breathing be effortless; the person is instructed to relax and just think of the word "one" with each exhalation. This is done for about a minute. In the last segment, the person uses a word of his/her choosing to repeat during exhalation. Suggestions, such as letting the word repeat effortlessly as you breathe in and out, are provided. To conclude the integrative breathing exercise, it is suggested that the person let the word quietly float away like a cloud. Time for enjoying the relaxation that has been achieved is provided.

Although the integrative breathing technique of Smith (1985) comprises 12 segments, any one or combination of the segments may be used for producing relaxation. Modifications may need to be made for certain patients. For patients on bed rest or with functional deficits, the stretching exercises would not be feasible. However, the focused breathing segment and thinking a relaxing word segment could easily be used with these patients.

Imagery is often used in conjunction with breathing techniques. This combination is frequently used in hypnosis. Jencks (1984) noted that imagery with breathing produced positive effects in children.

Measurement of Effectiveness

Parameters that can be used to measure the effectiveness of breathing include emotions, overall well-being, and behavioral indices of relaxation. Subjective reports of well-being may be the most useful indicator. Table 6.4 provides a checklist to use for observing behavioral indices of anxiety.

USES

Breathing techniques have been used with a wide variety of patient populations. One of the most frequent uses has been to decrease anxiety and the symptoms associated with increased anxiety. Jencks (1984) reported that breathing and relaxation directions were helpful in reducing anxiety associated with blood drawing in adults. In a comparison of three stress management techniques, DiSorbio (cited in Jencks, 1984) found significantly lowered anxiety when breathing or breathing and electromyogram (EMG) biofeedback were used as compared to the group who only received EMG biofeedback.

Few reports of nursing studies on the use of breathing were found. Often the breathing was incorporated into another intervention, making it difficult to determine the specific effectiveness of breathing. Populations for whom it would seem to have particular relevance would be persons with asthma or other chronic obstructive pulmonary conditions. Attention to breathing may decrease anxiety and improve overall respiration.

Miller and Perry (1990) described use of a simple, slow, rhythmic, deep-breathing technique to decrease pain in subjects who had undergone coronary artery bypass graft surgery. The authors did not provide a full description of the technique used. Statistically significant but not clinically significant decreases in systolic and diastolic blood pressure occurred in the experimental group. The majority of the persons using the breathing relaxation technique reported that the technique was beneficial in lessening postoperative pain.

Precautions

Breathing patterns and techniques need to be personalized for each patient. Helping the person gain awareness of his/her breathing will assist the person in developing the technique with which he/she is most comfortable. During the initial sessions, the nurse needs to be attentive to how the patient is breathing to avoid shallow breathing and hyperventilation.

RESEARCH QUESTIONS

As was indicated earlier, few nursing researchers have specifically explored breathing as an intervention. Therefore, studies are needed to:

1. Compare the effectiveness of breathing with other relaxation techniques and determine with which populations it is the intervention of choice.
2. Determine more about problems encountered in the use of the intervention so that complications can be avoided.
3. Compare and contrast the effectiveness of the various breathing techniques.

REFERENCES

Hittleman, R. (1988). *Yoga—28 day exercise plan.* New York: Bantam.

Jencks, B. (1984). Using the patient's breathing rhythm. Pp. 29–41 in W.C. Wester & A. Smith eds., *Clinical hypnosis: A multidisciplinary approach.* Philadelphia: J.B. Lippincott.

Miller, K.M., & Perry, P.A. (1990). Relaxation technique and postoperative pain in patients undergoing cardiac surgery. *Heart & Lung* 19:136–146.

Schultz, J.H. (1932). *Das Autogene Training.* Leipzig: G. Theime Verlag.

Smith, J.C. (1985). *Relaxation dynamics.* Champaign, IL: Research Press.

Speads, C. (1986). *Ways to better breathing.* Great Neck, NY: Felix Morrow.

CHAPTER 8

EXERCISE

BACKGROUND

Exercises, such as passive and active range of motion exercises and ambulation, have been part of nursing's repertoire for many years. Not only the positive effects of exercise on body systems but also its influence on overall feelings of well-being make it an important intervention for nurses to use. This chapter will go beyond these frequently used exercise modes and present information on other forms of exercise that nurses can prescribe.

More than 2000 years ago, Temesau counseled Socrates that moderate exercise brings order to the affinities, the particles and affections which are wandering about the body (in Fox et al., 1971). Physical exercise has received increased attention as a means for reducing the risk of illness and promoting well-being. More than 20 million Americans now jog (Lamb, 1984) and over 55 million Americans are fitness walkers (Porcari et al., 1988). The number of health spas and athletic clubs has increased. Nurses often plan and coordinate cardiac rehabilitation programs in which exercise plays a prominent role. Likewise, nurses are integrally involved in implementing exercise programs for many other patient populations including the elderly, persons with rheumatoid arthritis, and persons with neuromuscular conditions. Thus the intervention, exercise, is widely used by nurses in numerous settings from critical care units to long-term care.

Definition

According to Albrecht and colleagues (1989), exercise is a complex concept, and there is no consensus regarding an overall definition for it. Definitions vary according to the group or discipline describing it. Exercise is defined by Halfman and Hojnacki (1981) as

> Regular or repeated appropriate use of physical activity for the purpose of training or developing the body and mind for the sake of health. [p. 1]

Merikas (1982), addressing the philosophy of exercise, noted that exercise promotes the optimum psychophysiological development of humans. According to Licht (1984), therapeutic exercise is the movement of the body or its parts to relieve symptoms of pathology or to improve function. These definitions allow for many activities to be included as part of exercise.

Several classification systems for exercise exist. Isotonic, isometric, or isokinetic is a classification system based on the type of muscle contraction involved. In isotonic exercise, the length of the entire muscle changes; the muscle may become longer or shorter and in so doing causes movement in the parts of the body where it is attached (Fletcher, 1982). Isotonic exercise is synonymous with dynamic exercise. Isometric exercise, on the other hand, does not result in changes in the length of the total muscle, but rather contraction of muscle fibers occurs with considerable increase in the tension of the muscle. This type of exercise is used when extremities cannot or should not be moved, such as when a leg is in a cast. Isometric exercise is a static form of exercise. An increase in diastolic pressure occurs in isometric exercise while pressure increases minimally in isotonic exercise. Isokinetic contractions occur when there is a constant rate of resistance in response to the contraction of a muscle (Halfman & Hojnacki, 1981).

Aerobic and anaerobic is another method used for classifying exercise. Exercise also is classified according to oxygen consumption; aerobic and anaerobic are the two categories. Oxygen consumption is increased in aerobic exercise; the aim is to increase or the body's ability to use oxygen maximally. This type of exercise promotes efficient functioning of the heart, lung, and circulation and aids in preventing heart disease. The body is able to more efficiently utilize energy during aerobic exercise. In contrast, anaerobic exercise consumes minimal oxygen. Its aim is the building up of specific muscle groups through, for example, weight training (Lamb, 1984). This chapter will primarily address aerobic exercise.

Scientific Basis

Cooper (1981) identified the following as outcomes of aerobic exercise:

1. Strengthens the muscles of respiration and tends to reduce the resistance to air flow, facilitating the flow of air in and out of the lungs.
2. Improves strength and pumping efficiency of the heart, enabling more blood to be pumped with each stroke to more rapidly transport oxygen from the lungs to the heart and to other parts of the body.
3. Tones muscles throughout the body, thus improving circulation, and helping to reduce blood pressure.
4. Increases the total amount of blood circulating in the body and the hemoglobin level.

Use of aerobic exercise has resulted in improved overall well-being (Compton et al., 1989). The effects aerobic exercise has on many of the systems of the body are presented in Table 8.1.

According to Fletcher (1982), four response phases to exercise occur in the cardiovascular system: anticipatory, initiation, adjustment, and drift. Each of these will be discussed.

Autonomic changes occur as the person anticipates beginning exercise resulting in an increase in heart rate. The initial increases are due to vagal withdrawal. An increase in heart rate is one of these changes.

The initiation phase begins eight to ten seconds after exercise has begun. A large sympathetic outburst occurs and the heart overshoots the rate needed, but then returns to the rate required for increased activity. Impulses from muscles being exercised are sent to the brain; an increase in the heart rate is initiated. Increased venous return activates the Bainbridge reflex resulting in an increased heart rate. The increase is greater when both the arms and legs are exercised simultaneously. Cardiac output increases during exercise due to increased venous return, increased heart rate, increased myocardial contractability (from positive inotropic sympathetic impulses to the heart), and a decreased peripheral resistance offered by the exercising muscles (Fletcher, 1982). Blood pressure increases are the result of increased cardiac output and the sympathetic vasoconstriction of vessels in the nonexercising muscles, viscera, and skin.

Oxygen consumption increases markedly from 250 ml/min to 61 per minute. The Metabolic Equivalent System (MET), although not a precise method for measuring oxygen consumption, is frequently used as a basis for prescribing exercise for an individual. Each MET is equal to 3.5 ml/kg per minute of oxygen consumption. One MET is equal to the energy expended while sitting quietly in a chair. Exercising muscles may extract 20 times more oxygen from the blood than occurs during sedentary activities.

During the adjustment phase, the body integrates central and peripheral mechanisms to maintain cardiac output, venous return, and output to working muscles. Shunting of blood from the abdominal organs to the exercising muscles continues. Plasma volume decreases during the first 10 to 15 minutes of exercise due to a functional increase in the systemic capillary pressure of the working muscles.

Table 8.1
Positive Influences of Chronic Endurance Physical Exercise

Blood Vessels and Chemistry
    Increase blood oxygen content
    Increase blood cell mass and blood volume
    Increase fibrinolytic capability
    Increase efficiency of peripheral blood distribution and return
    Increase blood supply to muscles and more efficient exchange of oxygen and carbon dioxide
    Reduce serum triglycerides and cholesterol levels
    Reduce platelet cohesion or stickiness
    Reduce systolic and diastolic blood pressure, especially when elevated
    Reduce glucose intolerance

Heart
    Increase strength of cardiac contraction (myocardial efficiency)
    Increase blood supply (collateral) to heart
    Increase size of heart muscle
    Increase blood volume (stroke volume) per heart beat
    Increase heart rate recovery after exercise
    Reduce heart rate at rest
    Reduce heart rate with exertion
    Reduce vulnerability to cardiac arrythmias

Lungs
    Increase blood supply
    Increase diffusion of oxygen and carbon dioxide
    Increase functional capacity during exercise
    Reduce nonfunctional volume of lung

Endocrine and Metabolic Function
    Increase tolerance of stress
    Increase glucose tolerance
    Increase thyroid function
    Increase growth hormone production
    Increase lean muscle mass
    Increase enzymatic function in muscle cells
    Increase functional capacity during exercise (muscle oxygen uptake capacity)
    Reduce body fat content
    Reduce chronic catecholamine production
    Reduce neurohumeral overreaction

Neural and Psychic
    Reduce strain and nervous tension resulting from psychologic stress
    Reduce tendency for depression
    Euphoria or "joie de vivre" experienced by many

Source: From R. Cantu (1980). *Toward fitness: Guided exercise for those with health problems.* New York: Human Sciences Press. Used with permission.

During the cardiovascular drift phase there is a gradual increase in sympathetic activation. Vasodilation of skin vessels occurs helping to eliminate heat from the body. A gradual decrease in venous pressure, stroke volume, and arterial pressure is found; cardiac output remains relatively constant.

A desired outcome of aerobic exercise is an increase in the body's maximal consumption of oxygen (VO_2). The usual criteria for determining the maximum VO_2 are that no further increases in oxygen uptake occur despite a further increase in workload, and the blood lactate is above 70–80 mg per 100 ml. The maximal cardiac output after exercise training is largely the result of an increase in stroke volume produced by an increase in venous return, a reduction in total peripheral resistance due to vasodilatation in the exercising muscles, cardiac hypertrophy, tachycardia, an increase in blood volume, and a possible increase in myocardial contractility. Discussion of the effects exercise has on other body systems will be presented in the section on Uses.

INTERVENTION

There are countless activities and exercises that persons can use. Finding the one or ones that a specific patient likes and that fits with the capabilities of the person and the purposes for which exercise is being prescribed is key to the success of the intervention (Gavin, 1988). Table 8.2 lists some aerobic exercise activities that can be prescribed. Exercise should involve prolonged rhythmic contractions of the large muscle groups (Smith, 1989).

An exercise program needs to be individually tailored for each person. Whereas a treadmill stress test is ideal for everyone beginning an exercise program, it is essential for persons 35 years of age or older. The test provides an accurate picture of the individual's cardiovascular system and the presence of pathology. The stress test consists of walking on a treadmill with the belt speed increased every three minutes. The person exercises to maximum endurance in the absence of any abnormality or to the maximum tolerance without abnormal symptoms (Fletcher, 1982). The patient is closely monitored (EKG recording) during the exercise and examined thoroughly at the conclusion. Emergency equipment is always present during stress testing. An arm exercise test may be used with persons who have physical disabilities that preclude their using the treadmill.

Pender (1987) noted that the activities selected for an individual's program should:

Be enjoyable.
Be vigorous enough to use 400 calories.
Sustain the heart rate at 70–85% potential for 20–30 minutes.
Produce rhythmical motions.
Be repeated four–five times a week for 30–60 minutes.
Be integrated into life style.

Table 8.2
Aerobic Exercise Activities

Jogging	Brisk walking
Cycling	Stationary running-treadmill
Swimming	Crosscountry skiing
Aerobic dance	Rowing
Jazzercise	Rope skipping
Handball/racquetball	

Technique

To be effective and not be harmful, aerobic exercise should include a warming-up period, stretching exercises, endurance exercises, and a cooling down period. Many variations for performing these steps can be used; some basic exercises for these phases will be given.

Warming Up

Warming-up exercises should be done for 5–7 minutes. Activities frequently used for warming up include walking briskly for a minute, jogging in place for a minute, doing jumping jacks, making arm circles, bending, rotating the head, and doing leg raises. The specific activities can be varied, but inclusion of ones that involve all parts of the musculoskeletal system is important. Warm-up activities serve to decrease tension, increase blood flow to the heart and muscles, and strengthen muscles.

Stretching Exercises

Stretching exercises help maintain a full range of motion in all body joints and strengthen tendons, ligaments, and muscles. Because stretching exercises put more strain on muscles than do the warm-up exercises, it is important that they follow the warm-up exercises. Stretching exercises are done at a slow, steady pace. The back, hamstring, calf, feet, and ankles require special attention. Greenberg (1990) provides excellent diagrams and directions for stretching exercises for muscle groups.

Endurance Exercises

The aim of endurance exercises is to promote the optimal functioning of the cardiovascular, pulmonary, and musculoskeletal systems. Target heart rate is used in prescribing the amount and intensity of exercise. This is the beats per minute at which a subject should exercise on a regular basis to achieve a training effect. The rate is just below the level at which the myocardial oxygen consumption exceeds the oxygen supply; when oxygen consumption exceeds the supply, myocardial ischemia occurs. The target heart rate is approximately 70–85% of one's maximum heart rate; this varies for each age group. To indirectly determine a person's maximal heart rate, subtract the person's age from 220, then take 70–85% of that number. If a person has deficits, adjustments may be necessary.

Walking. Walking is one activity that persons of all age groups and with varying disabilities can use for improving endurance. A major advantage is that it requires no special equipment or facilities. Brisk walking at 50–85% of one's functional capacity is done for 20–60 minutes, three to five times a week (Porcari et al., 1989). This intensity corresponds to 60–90% of the maximum heart rate. The speed of walking and the distance walked are gradually increased. Degree of fatigue and breathlessness are indicators used for determining the endurance level of an individual. If a person is tired for more than an hour after completing the walk, the distance and rate should be decreased for a period until endurance has improved.

Pender (1987) suggested the following guidelines for walking:

Walk naturally.
Wear good shoes that give good support.
Let arms hang loosely at one's sides.
Hands, knees, and ankles should be relaxed.
Heels should strike the surface first.
Push off with the toes.
Use heel-to-toe rolling motion.
Breathe naturally.

Using relaxation techniques prior to walking may assist the person in gaining maximum benefit from the exercise. Walking has a positive effect on aerobic power, changes in body mass and fat, and the cardiovascular system (Porcari et al., 1989).

Cool Down

Immediately following the endurance exercises, the person engages in a cooling down period. This allows the body to adjust to normal conditions and to eliminate the lactic acid that accumulated in the muscle tissue during exercise. Five to ten minutes are needed for the body to adjust to a slower pace. Cooling down exercises may include walking slowly and deep breathing, straight arm and leg stretches, Achilles stretching, half knee bends, bent-knee half-curls, or any stretching exercises.

Maintenance

Maintaining the exercise program is the key to the effectiveness of the intervention. Setting both short- and long-term goals helps improve adherence. The person can see accomplishments when short-term goals are met while still striving for overall goals. Keeping a record or graphing progress helps the person see progress or determine reasons why success is or is not being attained.

Having a specific time and place for exercising helps assure adherence. Selecting new paths for walking or jogging and varying the exercises used for warming up and cooling down help in minimizing monotony. Alternating intensive and light exercise days also helps the person maintain an exercise program.

Measurement of Effectiveness

Effectiveness of aerobic exercise can be measured by a reduction in the symptoms of the condition for which the exercise was prescribed, such as depression, cardiac pathology, or decreased joint flexibility. Improvement in flexibility, endurance, strength, and motor skill coordinations also may be used as parameters for the measurement of the effectiveness of aerobic exercise.

Effect on the cardiovascular system is often used to determine the effectiveness of an aerobic exercise program. The results of sustained aerobic exercise include an improved oxygen uptake at both maximum and submaximal levels due to more efficient delivery of oxygen to muscles, strengthened cardiac muscles manifested by lowered heart rates both at rest and during exercise, a more efficient peripheral vascular system resulting in improved oxygen extraction, and an increased collateral circulation (Halfman & Hojnacki, 1981). Ability to exercise for longer periods of time without tiring, or simply to be able to work without tiring, would be gross ways to measure the effect of exercise on the cardiovascular system. The rapidity with which the heart rate returns to normal after exercise is another parameter that can be used. The effect of exercise on the musculoskeletal system is another indicator of the effectiveness of exercise. Improved joint mobility, prevention or reduction of osteoporosis, and improved strength are several parameters that may be measured (Compton et al., 1989). Studies on the effectiveness of exercise in the elderly have frequently used these parameters as desired outcomes.

USES

Exercise is a frequently prescribed nursing intervention. Numerous ways in which it has been used can be found in the literature. Table 8.3 lists some of the conditions for which exercise has been used. Four areas in which exercise has been used—to promote health, to decrease the symptoms of a chronic condition, to increase mobility/movement, and to promote psychological well-being—will be discussed.

Health Promotion

Optimal health for each person is an aim of nursing. Initiating exercise programs with children and young people will have a major impact on the health of the nation. Engaging in regular exercise will decrease cardiovascular disease, which is the leading cause of death in the United States (Cantwell, 1984).

Table 8.3
Uses of Exercise

Health Promotion
Weight reduction (Kostrubala, 1984; Porcari et al., 1989)
Osteoporosis reduction (Halfman & Hojnacki, 1981)
Reduction in overall cholesterol (Cook et al., 1986)
Pregnancy (Wolfe et al., 1989)

Decrease Symptoms of Chronic Illness
Hypertension (Fletcher, 1982)
Diabetes (Soman et al., 1979)
Pulmonary conditions (Fletcher, 1982)
Cardiac rehabilitation (Alling-Berne, 1987)
Decrease nausea and vomiting in chemotherapy (Winningham & MacVicar, 1988)
Prevent thrombophlebitis

Increase Mobility/Movement
Elderly (Benison & Hogstel, 1986; Holm & Kirchoff, 1984)
Parkinson's disease (Hurwitz, 1989; Van Oteghen, 1987)
Rheumatoid arthritis (Byers, 1985)

Promote Psychological Well-Being
Physical disabilities (Compton et al., 1989)
Decrease depression (Kostrubala, 1984)
Overall well-being (Sime, 1984)

Paffenbarger et al. (1978) found that persons who exercised infrequently had a greater risk of heart attack than a comparable group who exercised regularly. Increased physical activity beginning in youth and continuing throughout one's life will decrease the occurrence of osteoporosis (Dalsky et al., 1988).

Exercise is advocated as one method for preventing and/or reducing stress. Bahrke (1979) found that exercise reduced tension; walking is a particularly good exercise to use for achieving this goal. DeVries and colleagues (1981) found that exercise had a tranquilizing effect on persons who performed 20 minutes of exercise on a bicycle ergometer three times a week. Long and Haney (1988) found that exercise and progressive relaxation were equally effective in reducing anxiety and improving self-efficacy in a group of sedentary women. If anxiety can be reduced by exercise, continuous high levels of stress can be prevented by exercise and thus the deleterious effects caused by high levels of stress avoided.

Decrease Symptoms of Chronic Illness

The positive effect of exercise on the pathology underlying diabetes has been documented by numerous researchers. Exercise serves to potentiate the metabolic effects of insulin and reduces blood sugar levels; thus, dosages of insulin can be reduced. Wahren and colleagues (1982) noted that exercise mobilizes carbohydrates and fat substrates. This results in an increased utilization of both blood glucose and glycogen in the muscle and liver during exercise. An improved tolerance to carbohydrate ingestion occurs during the post-exercise period. Exercise increases insulin sensitivity and insulin binding to monocytes. Insulin sensitivity is correlated with an increase in oxygen consumption that occurs during exercise (Soman et al., 1979).

Vigorous aerobic exercise is contraindicated for diabetics who lack metabolic control of their diabetic condition, who have not been taught to prevent hypoglycemia, or who have complications from neuropathy (Hollmann et al., 1982). The exercise program is terminated if the person shows signs of hypoglycemia, has subjective complaints of cardiovascular problems, has large increases or decreases in blood pressure, or has electrocardiogram changes (Hollmann et al., 1982). When prescribing an exercise program for a person with diabetes, the person is instructed concerning the effects that exercise may have on the insulin requirements. Close monitoring of the person is necessary (Wasserman & Abumrad, 1989).

Exercise has been widely prescribed for patients with cardiovascular disorders. It is an integral component of all cardiac rehabilitation programs. Alling-Berne (1987) details an exercise program to be used with persons who have had coronary artery bypass surgery. Beginning exercise soon after the surgery has produced positive results. Fletcher (1984) presented considerable substantiating data regarding the effects of exercise on both primary prevention and rehabilitation of the post-myocardial infarct patient. Persons who exercised regularly had lower serum triglycerides, had an increase in their exercise oxygen consumption rate, and had no recurrent infarctions as compared with persons who had discontinued their exercise program. Persons with cardiac pathology require close supervision during the initiation and carrying out of their exercise program. Exercise often results in weight reduction which promotes more effective cardiovascular functioning.

Promote Mobility/Movement

The elderly are especially prone to the "hazards of immobility" which affect many of the body's systems. Exercise results in increased bone strength. Smith and Reddan (1976) found that elderly who exercised regularly had a 4.2% increase in bone mass as opposed to a 2.5% increase in those who did not exercise. An increase in total body calcium was found in postmenopausal women who participated in regular exercise (Dalsky et al., 1988).

It is also hypothesized that exercise promotes coordination which may result in a reduction in falls. Bassett et al. (1982) conducted a 10-week exercise program with senior citizens; improvement in hip, shoulder, and knee flexibility was found. Such improvements would facilitate movement and activities and promote self-care by the elderly. Blumenthal et al. (1982) reported significant changes in tolerance in elderly who participated in regular aerobic exercise for an 11-week period.

While it is important to tailor exercise programs for all persons, this is particularly significant for the elderly who may have specific limitations. Exercise needs to be initiated more gradually and attention given to fatigue. Group exercise may be especially appealing to the older person. Benison and Hogstel (1986) and Bassett et al. (1982) describe exercise programs they have adapted for elderly populations.

Exercise programs have been used with other populations in whom mobility deficits are often found. Byers (1985) found that subjects with rheumatoid arthritis who participated in evening exercise reported less morning stiffness and had more mobility than when evening exercises were not carried out. To determine if an exercise program improved agility and the ability to carry out self-care functions, Hurwitz (1989) taught exercise to a group of persons with Parkinson's disease. Subjects in the exercise program demonstrated significant improvements in sucking ability and decreased incontinence. Compton and colleagues (1989) present an excellent review of research that has been done on exercise and persons with disabilities.

Promote Overall Well-Being

Numerous investigators have reported the positive effects of exercise on depressive states (Greist et al., 1979; Kaplan et al., 1983; Kostrubala, 1984). Kostrubala, a psychiatrist, used jogging as an adjunct to psychotherapy with his patients. Jogging was used by Griest and colleagues to lessen symptoms of moderate depression.

The "runner's high" is a known phenomenon; it is thought to result from the release of endorphins in intense exercise. Exercise improves body functioning and as such improves one's body image; this, in turn, affects morale. Merikas (1982) noted that the fundamental nature of human life is movement; exercise enhances movement and improves overall well-being. Blumenthal et al. (1982) reported that 40% of the elderly in their study who exercised felt healthier, were more satisfied with life, had more self confidence, and were in a better mood than before the program began.

Precautions

Although exercise has many positive effects, caution is needed before prescribing an exercise regimen. Exercise testing (stress test) is mandatory for those over 35 years of age to rule out persons with potential coronary disease. Persons under 35 who have a family history of coronary heart disease should also have a stress test before an exercise program is initiated. Information on warning signs of cardiac problems is an essential component to include in teaching persons about exercise.

Consistency in exercising is essential. Persons who are sedentary all week and then participate in strenuous exercise on weekends frequently experience problems. Exercise needs to be initiated gradually and then be regularly carried out. There is always the temptation to be over-enthusiastic at the beginning of an exercise program. Moderation needs to be emphasized. The body, particularly the cardiovascular system, is overly taxed by spurts of activity. Exercise tailored to the individual is more likely to be followed than merely handing the person an exercise book.

Some of the noncardiac dangers of exercise include heat-induced illness, sprains, stress fractures, soft tissue bleeding, exacerbations of arthritis, runners' trots, exercise asthma, myoglobinuria, and petechiae (Fletcher, 1982). While proper instructions and practice of exercise can do much to alleviate these, they may occur. Persons need to be alerted to the possibility of their occurrence; medical attention should be sought if problems arise.

Environmental factors affect responses to exercise (Johnston, 1982). Caution is necessary when persons exercise at either very high or very low temperatures or in high humidity. High humidity levels interfere with evaporation of sweat, preventing dissipation of body heat. Outside exercise should be cancelled if the temperature is below 5° or above 95° F (Fletcher, 1982). Persons moving to high altitudes need to acclimatize to the decreased oxygen concentrations. Air pollutants adversely affect the pulmonary system; outside activity is contraindicated when the air pollution index is high.

RESEARCH QUESTIONS

Considerable research has been done on the effects of exercise in cardiac rehabilitation programs. Sports medicine has also conducted studies on aspects of exercise. Mason-Hawkes (1989) and Smith (1989) have reviewed a significant amount of the research related to exercise, particularly adherence to exercise regimens. Their reviews provide an excellent starting point for nurses wishing to conduct research related to exercise. Albrecht and colleagues (1989) detail areas in which nursing research is needed. Some of their suggestions are incorporated into the questions that follow.

1. What are the long-term effects of regular exercise on body systems? Longitudinal studies are needed. School nurses and community nurses have excellent opportunities to initiate such research.
2. Does the use of groups promote adherence to exercise regimens? Kostrubala (1984) believed that this is true. Additional studies are needed.
3. What effects does exercise have on women? Until recently, exercise and its effects have been largely studied in males. It is not known if these findings are transferable to women.
4. What are the characteristics of persons who find exercise to be the best method for reducing stress?
5. Since more persons are participating in exercise programs earlier in life, do the same cautions for exercise by the elderly continue to apply? Also, research related to use of exercise in the elderly needs to group elderly into various age groups rather than designating them as the category of persons over 65 years of age.

REFERENCES

Albrecht, M., Aaronson, L., Lasky, P., & Loveland-Cherry, C.J. (1989). Panel response to paper presentations regarding interventions to improve exercise behaviors. Pp. 70–73 in M. Lobo & C. Loveland-Cherry eds., *Individual, family and community interventions to improve exercise and nutrition behaviors.* Indianapolis, IN: Sigma Theta Tau International.

Alling-Berne, L. (1987). The nurse's role: Early supervised exercise following coronary artery bypass surgery. *Focus on Critical Care* 14(6):11–16.

Bahrke, M. (1979). Exercise, meditation, and anxiety reduction: A review. *American Corrective Therapy Journal* 33:41–44.

Bassett, C., McClamrock, E., & Schmelzer, M. (1982). A 10-week exercise program for senior citizens. *Geriatric Nursing* 3:103–105.

Benison, B., & Hogstel, M.O. (1986). Aging and movement therapy: Essential interventions for the immobile elderly. *Journal of Gerontological Nursing* 12(12):8–16.

Blumenthal, J., Schocken, D., Needles, T., & Hindle, P. (1982). Psychological and physiological effects of physical conditioning on the elderly. *Journal of Psychosomatic Medicine* 26:505–510.

Byers, P.H. (1985). Effect of exercise on morning stiffness and mobility in patients with rheumatoid arthritis. *Research in Nursing and Health* 8:275–281.

Cantu, R. (1980). *Toward fitness: Guided exercise for those with health problems.* New York: Human Sciences Press.

Cantwell, J. (1984). Exercise and coronary heart disease: Role in primary prevention. *Heart and Lung* 13:6–13.

Compton, D.M., Eisenman, P.A., & Henderson, H.L. (1989). Exercise and fitness for persons with disabilities. *Sports Medicine* 7:150–162.

Cook, T.C., LaPorte, R.E., Washburn, R.N., & Trevern, N.D. (1986). Chronic low level physical activity as a determinant of high density lipoprotein cholesterol and subfractions. *Medicine, and Science in Sports and Exercise* 19:S171.

Cooper, K. (1981). *The new aerobics.* New York: Bantam.

Dalsky, O.P., Stocke, K.S., Ehsani, A.A., Slatopolsky, E., et al. (1988). Weight-bearing exercise training and lumbar bone mineral content in postmenopausal women. *Annals of Internal Medicine* 108:824–829.

DeVries, H., Wiswell, R., Bulbulian, R., & Moritani, T. (1981). Tranquilizer effect of exercise. *American Journal of Physical Medicine* 60:57–66.

Fletcher, G. (ed.) (1982). *Exercise in the practice of medicine.* Mount Kisco, NY: Futura Publishing Co.

Fletcher, G. (1984). Long-term exercise in coronary artery disease and other chronic disease states. *Heart and Lung* 13:28–46.

Fox, S., Naughton, J., & Haskell, W. (1971). Physical activity and the prevention of coronary heart disease. *Annals of Clinical Research* 3:404–432.

Gavin, J. (1988). Psychological issues in exercise prescription. *Sports Medicine* 6:1–10.

Greenberg, J.S. (1990). *Comprehensive stress management.* Dubuque, IA: Wm. C. Brown.

Greist, J., Klein, M., Eischens, R., & Faris, J. (1979). Running as a treatment for non-psychotic depression. *Comparative Psychiatry* 1:41–54.

Halfman, M., & Hojnacki, L. (1981). Exercise and the maintenance of health. *Topics in Clinical Nursing* 3(2):1–10.

Hollmann, W. Dufaux, B., & Rost, R. (1982). Some practical aspects of physical training and exercise in diabetes. Pp. 142–146 in M. Berger, P. Christocopoulos, & J. Wahren eds., *Diabetes and exercise.* Bern: Hans Huber Publishers.

Holm, K., & Kirchoff, K.T. (1984). Perspectives on exercise and aging. *Heart & Lung* 13:519–524.

Hurwitz, A. (1989). The benefit of a home exercise regimen for ambulatory Parkinson's disease patients. *Journal of Neuroscience Nursing* 21:180–184.

Johnston, B. (1982). Environmental factors on exercise and activity of cardiac patients. *Cardio-Vascular Nursing* 18:7–12.

Kaplan, K., Mendelson, L., & Dubroff, M. (1983). The effect of a jogging program on psychiatric inpatients with symptoms of depression. *Occupational Therapy Journal of Research* 3:173–175.

Kostrubala, T. (1984). Running and therapy. Pp. 112–124 in M. Sachs & G. Buffone eds., *Running as therapy—an integrated approach.* Lincoln, NE: University of Nebraska Press.

Lamb, D. (1984). *Physiology of exercise.* New York: Macmillan Publishing Co.

Licht, S. (1984). History. Pp. 1–44 in J. Basmajian ed., *Therapeutic exercise.* Baltimore: Williams and Wilkins.

Long, B.C., & Haney, C.J. (1988). Coping strategies for working women: Aerobic exercise and relaxation interventions. *Behavior Therapy* 19:75–83.

Mason-Hawkes, J. (1989). Exercise adherence: Prevalence, determinants, and interventions. Pp. 43–59 in M. Lobo & C. Loveland-Cherry eds., *Individual, family and community interventions to improve exercise and nutrition behaviors.* Indianapolis, IN: Sigma Theta Tau International.

Merikas, G. (1982). The philosophy of exercise. Pp. 13–21 in M. Berger, P. Christocopoulos, & J. Wahren eds., *Diabetes and exercise.* Bern: Hans Huber Publishers.

Paffenbarger, R., Wing, A., & Hyde, R. (1978). Physical activity as an index of heart attack risk in college alumni. *Journal of Epidemiology* 108:161–175.

Pender, N.J. (1987). *Health promotion in nursing practice,* 2nd ed. Norwalk, CT: Appleton & Lange.

Porcari, J.P., Ebbeling, C.B., Ward, A., Freedson, P.S., & Rippe, J.M. (1989). Walking for exercise testing and training. *Sports Medicine* 8:189–200.

Sime, W. (1984). Psychological benefits of exercise. *Advances* 1(4):15–29.

Smith, B.A. (1989). Exercise behavior: Physiological parameters and prescription. Pp. 60–69 in M. Lobo & C. Loveland-Cherry eds., *Individual, family and community interventions to improve exercise and nutrition behaviors.* Indianapolis, IN: Sigma Theta Tau International.

Smith, E., & Reddan, W. (1976). Physical activity—a modality for bone accretion in the aged. *American Journal of Roentgenology* 126:1297.

Soman, V., Koivisto, V., Diebert, D., Felig, P., & DeFronzo, R. (1979). Increased insulin sensitivity and insulin binding to monocytes after physical activity. *New England Journal of Medicine* 301:1200–1202.

Van Oteghen, S.L. (1987). An exercise program for those with Parkinson's disease. *Geriatric Nursing* 7:183–184.

Wahren, J., Christacopoulos, P., & Berger, M. (1982). Introduction. Pp. 11–12 in M. Berger, P. Christacopoulos, & J. Wahren eds., *Diabetes and exercise.* Bern: Hans Huber Publishers.

Wasserman, D.H., & Abumrad, N.N. (1989). Physiological bases for the treatment of the physically active individual with diabetes. *Sports and Medicine* 7:376–392.

Winningham, M.L., & MacVicar, M.G. (1988). The effect of exercise on patient reports of nausea. *Oncology Nursing Forum* 15:447–450.

Wolfe, L.A., Hall, P., Webb, K.A., Goodman, L., Monga, M., & McGrath, M.J. (1989). Prescription of aerobic exercise during pregnancy. *Sports Medicine* 8:273–301.

CHAPTER 9

MOVEMENT THERAPY

BACKGROUND

Movement is central to all human activities (Laban, 1975). Movement and stance reveal much about a person's emotional state; likewise, movement has an effect on one's emotional state (Feder & Feder, 1982). Creative movement is a health promoting activity appropriate for diverse population groups extending from those with complete independence to those with mobility problems. This chapter will present two movement therapy techniques: dance and afspaending. These are only two of a myriad of techniques that comprise movement therapy. Social dance, Bartenieff, relaxation exercises, T'ai Chi Ch'uan, creative drama, and rhythmic games are some other movement therapy techniques.

Dance places emphasis on the holism of human beings. In dance, the person through his body externalizes concepts created in his mind (Lange, 1975). Holism is a key concept in many nursing theories and models. Goldberg and Fitzpatrick (1980) contended that nursing, more than any other profession, is oriented to the wholeness of persons. Thus, interventions that promote the integration of the total person should be emphasized in nursing.

Definition

Creative movements are a gentle, enjoyable, and expressive form of exercise; these can be fitted to meet the needs of persons with varying levels of physical abilities. The creative movements provide opportunities for persons to express themselves; this may contribute to enhancement of a person's ego (Van Zandt & Lorenzen, 1985). Many dance forms exist and the definitions for each vary slightly. Laban (1975) described dance as:

> ....Movement, by which in this context I mean the interaction of effort and space through the medium of the body. Our bodily movements make shapes in space and they are charged with effort, that is energy coming from within, springing from a whole range of impulses, intentions, and desires. [p. 108]

His definition notes the unique interaction between the internal and external environments that characterizes all dance forms. Laban viewed each dance movement as consisting of a combination of effort elements: The person's attitudes toward the motion factors of weight, space, time, and flow.

According to Schoop (1974), dancing is a personally created style of physical movement that projects a person's being to be closely connected between motions and emotions. Her definition is for free or creative dance in which persons establish their own movements. The basic dance elements proposed by Schoop include alignment, centrality, tension, rhythm, and use of space. These differ from the four elements proposed by Laban; tension is akin to Laban's weight, and rhythm encompasses his time and flow. Both include space, but Schoop has added alignment and centrality, thus placing more emphasis on inner awareness. Application of these basic elements will be presented in the technique section of this chapter.

In dance therapy, movements serve as a form of nonverbal communication assisting in releasing emotions, promoting physical relaxation, and increasing awareness of self (Toombs, 1968). Emphasis is placed on the therapeutic outcomes and not on the esthetics of the movement or the perfecting of specific dance steps. This is why free dance form rather than specific dance steps are most frequently used in dance therapy; the person is not constrained by established patterns to which he/she must adapt.

Scientific Basis

Throughout history dance has played an important role in human life. Almost all cultures have special dances that are an integral part of their history. The Greek Dionysian dance was used for obtaining ecstatic experiences. Pueblo Indians believed that their dance swung the forces of nature to their purposes (Toombs, 1968). Folk dances, a key part of festive or religious celebrations, are part of our Western heritage. New dance forms that embody the prevailing spirit of the time have evolved. Some of these are the Charleston, the bunny hop, rock'n roll, disco, and the lambada.

Dance emphasizes definite rhythms and shapes of movement. According to Laban (1975), an aim of dance is to assist persons to find bodily relationships to the whole of existence. A person learns through dance to relate the inner self to the outer world. A reciprocal stimulation of the inward and outward flow of movement occurs that pervades and animates the entire person.

Five tenets underly the therapeutic effectiveness of dance. They are:

1. Persons manifest themselves in their body.
2. Mind and body are in constant reciprocal interaction.
3. Whether thoughts are rational or irrational, positive or negative, split or unified, they are manifested in the alignment of one's body, the way the body is centered, in the rhythmical patterns of the body, the tempo of the movement, the use of tension and energy in movement, and the relationship of the parts of the body to the space surrounding it.
4. Through the body a person's mind experiences reality.
5. Mind and body are fused by their reciprocal interaction. (Schoop, 1974)

Movement, particularly dance, depends on rhythmic unity. An intrinsic quality of rhythm is periodic repetition (Laban, 1975). Creating a movement sequence consists of searching for a satisfying spatial composition in which one's inner impulses or efforts find a pleasing visible form and of responding from within to the shapes that the movements of the limbs and body make in space (Laban, 1975). Many parts of the body are involved in the rhythmic patterns, and the unification of these produces a sense of cohesion in the person.

INTERVENTION

Many dance forms exist and can be used to achieve therapeutic outcomes. The form that is used most frequently in dance therapy is free or creative dance. Schoop (1974) believed that this form allows persons to investigate themselves and their relationships to the surrounding space. Creative dance is not bound by a specifically fashioned style, but it also is not chaotic. Altering and combining speed, intensity, size, and fluency of movement result in different forms of dance. An example would be increasing the size of the step and the speed of movement while lessening the intensity (muscle tension) and fluency (continuity of movement). In contrast, smaller steps and arm movements could be used with greater intensity. These two movements would produce different effects on the person.

Laban (1975) described 16 basic movement themes. These are presented in Table 9.1. There is a progression in the movements from one to 16. The first eight movements are elementary movement themes and need to be mastered before the later movement themes can be initiated.

Table 9.1
Movement Themes in Dance as Designated by Laban

Elementary Movement Themes
1. Awareness of body
2. Awareness of weight and time (sustained or sudden movements)
3. Awareness of space (narrow and wide movements)
4. Awareness of the flow of the weight of the body in space and time (twisted pathways and different speeds and rhythms)
5. Adaptation to a partner(s) (one moves and the other responds; follow movements of leader)
6. Instrumental use of limbs (hands, feet, and body used in different ways)
7. Awareness of isolated actions (press, flick, thrust parts of body; use light and strong movements and alternate these)
8. Themes associated with occupational rhythms (sawing, chopping, etc.; awareness of the rhythms of exertion and recovery)

Advanced Movement Themes
9. Shapes of movement (drawing or writing in air; difference between angular and curved patterns)
10. Combination of the eight basic effort actions—wring, press, glide, float, flick, slash, punch, and dab. Each contains three of the six movement elements: firm, light, sustained, sudden, direct and flexible. Each sequence has its own rhythm
11. Space orientation (direct movements to a certain point in space around the body; change from points so harmonious and flowing)
12. Shapes and effort using different parts of the body
13. Elevation from the ground (skips, leaps, jumps; flying movements in air)
14. Awakening of group feeling
15. Group formations (rows and circles)
16. Expressive qualities or moods of movements

Source: Laban, R. (1975). *Modern educational dance.* London: Macdonald and Evans, Ltd.

Technique

Dance

Alignment, centrality, tension, rhythm, and space were the basic elements of dance elucidated by Schoop (1974). The place each of these has in dance will be addressed along with ways to assist the person to become more aware of the existence of each element, its effects, and the feelings associated with altering it.

Alignment is the proper positioning of the body. Opposite aspects or exaggerations can be used to assist the person to become aware of the parts of the body and their normal positions. Walking pigeon-toed or using a waddling gait are exaggerations that make the person more conscious of the normal positioning of the body. A sense of correct alignment is needed for the person to create effective dance movements.

Centrality denotes the middle area of the body. An awareness of one's center is necessary for equilibrium. Engaging in a tug of war is one method that helps the person concentrate on his body's center. Swinging the extremities is another means that assists persons to gain knowledge about the location of the center of their bodies. In addition to becoming more aware of one's physical body, centering, in which the person focuses inward, also promotes internal harmony (Boots & Hogan, 1981).

Schoop (1974) defined tension as, "a person's talent to energize and de-energize his physical being" (p. 103). Creating split tensions makes persons more aware of what they do unconsciously. Examples of exercises that help to develop an awareness of tension include having the person walk with stiff, woodlike legs while making the arms limp like those of a rag doll, or relaxing the muscles of the trunk while tightly tensing the muscles of the face and neck. Making persons more conscious of the varying degrees of tension possible in the body increases feelings of a coordinated and unified self.

Rhythm is an integral part of dance. Because rhythms pervade all of life, increasing the person's awareness of these helps achieve unity. Exercises in rhythm can begin with persons taking their pulses, then chanting out loud in time with them, and eventually moving the arms and legs in tune with their heart rates. Repetition of a rhythm conveys a sense of security to the person. This may be the basis for the rocking movements that are frequently used by persons with extremely high levels of anxiety; they may be attempting to find security through these movements.

Movements occur in space. Space, according to Wigman (1966), is the dancer's domain. After becoming aware of one's center, the person is encouraged to explore the surrounding space. Kicking, poking, and moving the trunk of the body back and forth is an exercise that helps the person explore the adjacent space. Laban (1975) suggested having the person stand upright and spread the arms out sideways. This is followed by moving the legs forward and backward while simultaneously gathering and scattering the arms. The limbs are traversing space while also spreading and filling it. Other approaches that can be used for exploring space are using the body to design shapes in space (spatial architecture), to pantomime situations, or to demonstrate emotionally descriptive actions such as opening the arms to the sky and then closing them in on the body (Boots & Hogan, 1981).

Creative dance movement sessions can take many forms. Music may or may not be a part of the sessions. When music is not used, participants can more freely express their feelings and be creative in the tempo and forms that the dance movements will take. However, some persons may be hesitant to express themselves through movements without music. The climate of the group dictates the type of music to use. Dance therapy may be used on a one-to-one basis or in a group. Assessment of the individual and the time available will guide the type of setting to use. Dance movements may be done as a single form of intervention or combined with other interventions such as imagery, poetry, or drama (Adler & Fisher, 1984; Benjamin, 1983; Lange, 1975).

Bartenieff and Lewis (1980) suggested allocating 45–60 minutes for each dance therapy session. A group context was used. Participants formed a circle, but they were not bound to remain in the circle but could move in and out. Although music was played during the session, the leaders provided no particular directions on the type of dance movements in which participants should engage. Sessions flowed with the mood of the group.

Afspaending

This technique originated in Denmark; the name is a Danish word for "unbuckling" or "relaxing." The underlying principle of this therapy is that the body and psyche form an indivisible whole and the functioning of one influences the other (Haxthausen & Leman, 1987). The goal of afspaending therapy is for persons to achieve a better understanding of their bodies through changing the balance and tension that occur in the various movements.

Slowness of movements characterizes the afspaending technique. Attention is focused on the feelings experienced during the various movements. According to Haxthausen and Leman (1987),

> If you work slowly and attentively with the movements, you will be able to sense how to relax your muscles and let the movements stretch them. You will also see how you resist movement, thus preventing the muscles from stretching. You will be able to sense which groups of muscles are elastic enough that you can use them actively without tightening them unnecessarily, and which muscles and joints are stretched to the point where they slow down or block your execution of movement. [p. 11]

A person's emotional state affects the type of muscle reactions that occur. Listening to one's body is helpful in discerning one's overall true feelings. This allows for the detection of stress and the implementation of strategies to reduce tension.

Specific positions of the body and types of movements are part of afspaending. Included are lying-down, sitting, and standing. An example of one of the movements, termed the accordion, is to have the person bend at the ankles, knees, and hips while the feet are firmly planted on the ground. The knees are pointed forward and the buttocks are pulled in. The person bobs up and down, increasing and decreasing the bending of the joints so that he/she feels like an accordion being played. *Body Sense: Exercise for Relaxation* (Haxthausen & Lorenzen, 1987) provides specific instructions for the various movements and positions. The suggested movements are creative and fun to do. After the fundamental movements are mastered, the individual may use them in creative dance forms. Afspaending movements can be performed alone or in a group.

Measurement of Effectiveness

The desired outcomes, determined by assessment of the patient, dictate the criteria to use in evaluating the effectiveness of movement therapy techniques. Some of the measurements used for specific populations will be described in the next section.

Gestures/postures		Directions in space			Effort qualities		
Symbol	Definition	Symbol	Term	Definition	Symbol	Term	Definition
P	Motions involving a visible adjustment in every part of the body and usually involving a weight shift (sitting down; lifting a box; walking)	⇈	Up	Moving in a vertical direction (standing up; stretching)	⌣	Free flow	Absence of tension (floating on water ; jumping on leaves; breathing easily)
		⇊	Down	Moving downward in a vertical direction (sitting down; squatting)	o	Bound flow	Observable tension (walking cautiously; careful threading of a needle; tense breathing)
G	Motions confined to one or a few body parts (waving; kicking; nodding head)	⇥	Forward	Moving in a horizontal path directly forward (advancing toward a person)	~	Space Indirect	Movement in a spiraling, twisting path through space (tossing head; inattentive gazing around room)
		↔	Backward	Moving in a horizontal path directly backward (retreating from a person)	|	Direct	Movement in a straight, purposeful path through space (lifting a fork to mouth; pushing a doorbell)
		\/	Outward	Moving outward from center (moving arms out to side; skipping sideways)	⌄	Force Light	Gentle, weightless (holding a delicate object)
		||	Inward	Moving inward toward center (clutching self when cold; crossing arms and legs while sitting)	⌃	Strong Time	Vigorous, forceful with impact (stamping; throwing an object)
					⌣	Slow	Slow, sustained movement (dawdling walk)
					⌍	Quick	Rapid movement (startle response; nervous twitching)

Figure 9.1
Notations that can be used in recording a person's movements. (Copyrighted by the National Association for Music Therapy, Inc., Washington, D.C.) Used with permission.

Table 9.2
Uses of Movement Therapy

Communication and Interaction
　　Deaf (Wisher, 1972)
　　Sensory deprivation (Gerhart, 1979)
　　Mentally retarded (Toombs, 1968)
　　Psychiatric patients (Feder & Feder, 1982; Grodner et al., 1982; Schoop, 1974)

Unity of Being
　　Elderly (Goldberg & Fitzpatrick, 1980)
　　Health promotion (Boots & Hogan, 1981)
　　Alcoholic outpatients (Feder & Feder, 1982)
　　Reality orientation in elderly (Bumanis & Yoder, 1987)

Improved Functioning of Musculoskeletal System
　　Improved physical mobility (Hecox et al., 1976)
　　Quadriplegics (Gerhart, 1979)
　　Post-mastectomy (Molinaro et al., 1986)
　　Rheumatoid arthritis (Van Deusen & Harlowe, 1987)

Staum (1981) developed symbol notations to use in assessing and recording movements. These are shown in Figure 9.1. Because movements are dynamic, it is difficult to observe and remember all aspects of them for future reference. The notations included in Figure 9.1 assist the nurse in assessing the patient's movements and dance forms. Analysis of movements guides the nurse in making suggestions for changing specific movements (Staum, 1981).

USES

Schoop (1974) delineated four goals of dance therapy that are applicable to many of the movement therapy techniques. These are:

1. Develop functional patterns for specific parts of the body that have not been used or have been misused.
2. Establish unifying interactive relationships between mind and body, fantasy and reality.
3. Bring conflicting emotions into an objective physical form that allows the person to deal with them in a constructive manner.
4. Assist the person to adapt to the environment and to experience self as a whole.

Other purposes for which movement therapy techniques may be used are improving communication and social interaction and as a catharsis.

Minimal references to the use of movement therapy techniques in nursing were found. Dance therapy has been used extensively in the treatment of patients with psychiatric problems. Table 9.2 lists other conditions in which movement therapy techniques have been used as an intervention. Uses for three purposes, improving communication and social interactions, promoting unity of being, and improving physical functioning, will be discussed.

Communication

Many persons experience difficulty in expressing their thoughts and feelings. Dance offers a safe outlet for expressing feelings (Feder & Feder, 1982). Batzas (1982) suggested taking a feeling and working with a partner to express it. The technique assists persons in becoming more conscious of their feelings and expressing them. The partners can begin by expressing the feeling with their hands and arms and then with their entire bodies. Discussion on the feeling culminates the session. Brumanis and Yoder (1987) reported that elderly persons who used music and dance displayed improvement in social interactions and emotional states; no significant improvement in the person's orientation was found.

Communication involves interacting with others. Reaching out into the space surrounding one's body assists the person in breaking down the barriers that have prevented interactions with others. Group sessions for dance facilitate interaction between persons. Release of anxiety that may result from the physical activity makes the person less hesitant to interact with others. This would be particularly helpful for persons who are depressed and withdrawn. Grodner and colleagues (1982) used movement and art therapies with patients who had various types of psychiatric conditions. Their findings revealed that the use of these therapies resulted in improved mood. Dance has also been shown to improve communication in autistic children (Feder & Feder, 1982).

Unity of Being

Movement therapy is an appropriate intervention for use in the maintenance and promotion of health (Boots & Hogan, 1981). Espenak (cited in Toombs, 1968) believed that the value of dance resided in the conscious buildup of kinesthetic awareness and the subsequent work-back to the emotions that correspond with this awareness. A more positive mental state often accompanies improved physical harmony (Batzas, 1982). This may be due to the fact that tension is released through physical movement (Eskow, 1976). According to Feder and Feder (1982), persons under hypnosis cannot feel emotions that are contrary to their physical postures or body stances.

Schoop (1974) used dance with psychiatric patients. She found that patients with different psychiatric diagnoses had varying responses to dance. Aggressive patients, often unconscious of their pent-up hostility, found a release in expressive interpretation. Patients who were exhibitionistic tended to dance only when watched and needed much individual attention. She found that dance helped initiate emotional expression. *Won't You Join the Dance?* (Schoop, 1974) contains many anecdotal accounts of the author's work with psychiatric patients and delineates the specific approaches she used with each group.

Goldberg and Fitzpatrick (1980) found that elderly persons who participated in group movement therapy sessions showed a significant increase in morale and attitude toward aging scores than did elderly persons who did not participate in the therapy. They stated that a nursing intervention, such as movement therapy, could be used to improve attitudes about aging. Although significant differences were not found between the control and the experimental group on a self-esteem scale, improvement in scores were found in the movement therapy group. Scores were very high on the pretest, thus leaving little room for change. A number of articles have documented the use of movement therapy with elderly populations (Berryman-Miller, 1986; Sandel, 1978; Van Zandt & Lorenzen, 1985).

Physical Mobility

Hecox et al. (1976) used dance therapy with a group of patients who had mild to moderately severe physical disabilities due to orthopedic or neurologic causes. The goals of the sessions were:

1. To help the person shift from the frustration about what the body cannot do to pride in what it can do.
2. To provide an enjoyable experience for the person who seldom has an opportunity to participate in physical activities.
3. To improve functioning in daily life activities.
4. To improve physical abilities.

Weekly sessions comprising five to eight patients were held. Having persons with the same degree of mobility deficits in therapy groups was found to be helpful in structuring the exercises to use; for example, patients with Parkinson's disease and multiple sclerosis both benefited from arm swinging exercises. Centering, awareness of the center of gravity of the body, was deemed an essential component of the therapy. This exercise increased the awareness of inner space in addition to providing the person with knowledge about his body. Consciousness of space helped patients extend self into the space surrounding their bodies and to draw on unused abilities for exploring and invading it. The needs of the group dictated what areas received the most emphasis. Sessions ended with encouraging the enjoyable sensations that came from expanding into the adjacent space. Although no statistical data were provided, Hecox et al. (1976) concluded that dance therapy was an effective intervention for persons with physical disabilities.

Molinaro and colleagues (1986) found dance therapy to be an effective intervention for patients who had had a mastectomy. The authors stated that dancing provided these women with a stimulus that emphasized the women's femininity and sexuality while adjusting to changes in body image. The authors combined jazz and ballet movements in the dance therapy sessions.

A range of motion dance program was devised by Van Deusen and Harlowe (1987) for persons with rheumatoid arthritis. The eight sessions incorporated T'ai-Chi Ch'uan exercises. At four months post-teaching, members of the experimental group were more regular in performing their daily exercises than were persons who had been taught the routine exercises. Thus, the creativity aspect may be a motivation to carrying out an exercise program.

Precautions

Schoop (1974) related problems encountered when beginning to do volunteer work with patients in a psychiatric facility. Her experiences point to the critical need for initial assessment of the patient before using the intervention. If structured dance forms are being used, frenzied dances are not suitable initially for persons who have pent-up hostility as they may become violent. Withdrawn patients may be reluctant to participate if the dance is too boisterous. Assessment also provides data on whether the person would benefit most from being part of a group session or whether one-to-one sessions are best.

Discussion of the feelings that the dance elicits helps the person to integrate physical and emotional elements. Again, assessment of the patients would dictate whether this is done as a group or on an individual basis.

The qualities of the therapist were addressed by Toombs (1968). A dynamic therapist influences the outcomes achieved. Other essential therapist qualities include the ability to observe patients in a group, to take advantage of cues from the behaviors of individual patients and redirect the dance, to provide encouragement to the participants, and to encourage creativity. Goldberg and Fitzpatrick (1980) believed that a master's prepared psychiatric clinical specialist was qualified to lead movement therapy groups. Nurses need to have an understanding of the technique chosen, be able to assess the patient population with whom they are working, and to provide guidance to the patients on the movements to use.

RESEARCH QUESTIONS

Nurses can gain much information about use of movement therapies from the research that has been done in music therapy, physical therapy, and dance therapy. However, research on the use of the various movement therapies within the context of nursing is needed. Some of the areas for future research include:

1. What are the characteristics of persons who benefit most from group movement therapy sessions as opposed to the characteristics of those for whom individual sessions should be used?
2. While the majority of attention has been focused on the use of creative dance, would the use of folk dances, ballroom dances, or other dance forms produce equal or better results with particular groups of patients?

3. What is the relationship between imagery and movement therapy? Do persons who possess greater ability to image benefit more from movement therapy?

4. Van Deusen and Harlowe (1987) found that use of a movement therapy technique in persons with rheumatoid arthritis resulted in better compliance with a treatment regimen. Is this finding generalizable to patients with other conditions?

5. What are the movement therapies that would be appropriate to use with persons who are bedridden?

6. In many of the reports cited movement therapy has been combined with other interventions. Studies designs that allow for measuring the effects of these various interventions are needed.

REFERENCES

Adler, R.F., & Fisher, P. (1984). My self—through music, movement and art. *The Arts in Psychotherapy* 11:203–208.

Bartenieff, I., & Lewis, D. (1980). *Body movement: Coping with the environment.* New York: Gordon and Breach, Science Publishers.

Batzas, E. (1982). Movement therapy in the classroom. Pp. 268–276 in E. Nickerson & K. O'Laughlin eds., *Helping through action: Action-oriented therapies.* Amherst, MA: Human Resources Development Press.

Benjamin, B. (1983). The singing hospital—integrated group therapy in the black mentally ill. *South African Medical Journal* 63:897–899.

Berryman-Miller, S. (1986). Benefits of dance in the process of aging and retirement for the older adult. *Activities, Adaptation, & Aging* 9:43–51.

Boots, S., & Hogan, C. (1981). Creative movement and health. *Topics in Clinical Nursing* 3(2): 23–31.

Bumanis, A., & Yoder, J.W. (1987). Music and dance: Tools for reality orientation. *Activities, Adaptation, & Aging* 10:23–35.

Eskow, L. (1978). Drama and movement in therapy. *Physiotherapy* 64:70–73.

Feder, E., & Feder, B. (1982). The therapeutic use of dance and movement. Pp. 141–149 in E. Nickerson & K. O'Laughlin eds., *Helping through action: Action-oriented therapies.* Amherst, MA: Human Resources Development Press.

Gerhart, K. (1979). Increasing sensory and motor stimulation for patients with quadriplegia. *Physical Therapy* 59:1518–1520.

Goldberg, W., & Fitzpatrick J. (1980). Movement therapy with the aged. *Nursing Research* 29:339–346.

Grodner, S., Braff, D., Janowsky, D., & Clopton, P. (1982). Efficacy of art/movement therapy in elevating mood. *The Arts in Psychotherapy* 9:217–225.

Haxthausen, M., & Leman, R. (1987). *Body sense: Exercise for relaxation.* New York: Pantheon Books.

Hecox, B., Levine, E., & Scott, D. (1976). Dance in physical rehabilitation. *Physical Therapy* 56:919–924.

Laban, R. (1975). *Modern educational dance.* London: Macdonald and Evans LTD.

Lange, R. (1975). *The nature of dance.* London: Macdonald and Evans LTD.

Molinaro, J., Kleinfeld, M., & Lebed, S. (1986). Physical therapy and dance in the surgical management of breast cancer. *Physical Therapy* 66:967–969.

Sandel, S.L. (1978). Movement therapy with geriatric patients in a convalescent home. *Home & Community Psychiatry* 29:738–741.

Schoop, T. (1974). *Won't you join in the dance?* Palo Alto: National Press Books.

Staum, M. (1981). An analysis of movement in therapy. *Journal of Music Therapy* 18:7–24.

Toombs, M. (1968). Dance therapy. Pp. 329–344 in E. Gaston ed., *Music in Therapy.* New York: Macmillan.

Van Deusen, J., & Harlowe, D. (1987). A comparison of the ROM dance home exercise/rest program with traditional routines. *Occupational Therapy Journal of Research* 7:349–361.

Van Zandt, S., & Lorenzen, L. (1985). You're not too old to dance: creative movement and older adults. *Activities, Adaptation, & Aging* 6:121–130.

Wigman, M. (1966). *The language of dance* (trans. W. Sorell). Middletown, CT: Wesleyan University Press.

Wisher, P. (1972). Psychological contributions of dance to the adjustment of the deaf. *Rehabilitation Record* 13(3):1–4.

CHAPTER 10

POSITIONING

OVERVIEW

Positioning is an intervention frequently used by nurses in many settings. According to Fontaine and McQuillan (1989), positioning is one of the interventions most often used by nurses in critical care units. Kinney's review of nursing research in critical care nursing confirms their statement (1984). However, Fontaine and McQuillan cited evidence that 63% of nurses working in critical care units who were surveyed stated no awareness about the use of therapeutic positioning techniques in providing nursing care.

Positioning is used to promote comfort, to prevent complications such as decubitus ulcers, and to facilitate the performance of diagnostic or therapeutic procedures. When a nurse walks into a patient's room and sees that the patient has slid toward the foot of the bed, an almost automatic response occurs in that immediate attention is given to re-positioning the patient to promote comfort. Nurses assist in positioning patients for diagnostic and therapeutic procedures, such as spinal taps and chest drainage. Correct positioning not only promotes better outcomes for the procedures but also reduces discomfort. Turning and positioning critically ill and bedridden patients every two hours is a practice with a long history in nursing. Teaching patients positions that will promote better ventilation in conditions such as chronic obstructive pulmonary disease and providing information about positions that will reduce pain for persons with chronic back problems are other examples of how nurses use the intervention of positioning. Thus strong evidence exists to support positioning as an independent nursing intervention.

Another aspect of positioning is how the nurse "positions self" when interacting with patients. Sitting down to talk with patients who are in bed or in wheel chairs, maintaining a distance so as to respect the patient's space, and understanding how one's body language affects a patient are important components of patient-nurse interactions. Although these aspects of positioning are critical to nursing, they will not be included in this chapter.

Definition

Tyler (1984) defined positioning as a bodily posture assumed by patients for comfort or to facilitate the implementation of therapeutic and diagnostic procedures. Although comfort is not the prime outcome for this latter type of positioning, the nurse needs to be cognizant of comfort and try to decrease the amount of discomfort experienced. Prevention of complications is not included in Tyler's definition, but it is an important purpose for the use of certain positions and the changing of positions.

Scientific Basis

The scientific basis for the use of positioning varies depending on the purpose for which it is being used. The scientific basis for positioning to promote skin integrity, to facilitate gas exchange, to promote cerebral perfusion, and to promote comfort will be presented.

Skin Care

Positioning in relation to skin care has received considerable attention in nursing (Copeland-Fields & Hoshiko, 1989; Ebersole & Hess, 1990; Steffel et al., 1980). Turning schedules, use of assistive devices, and proper positioning are critical in the care of persons who have decreased mobility and sensation. Forces on an area of the body that are of sufficient strength and for a long enough period of time so as to obstruct blood flow will result in tissue necrosis. The pressure forces need to exceed normal capillary pressure for damage to occur; this is 14 mm Hg for venous flow and 35 mm Hg for arterial flow. Tissue damage occurs when the pressure exceeds 60 mm Hg for one hour. In persons with normal sensation and mobility, automatic position changes are made. However, persons with decreased mobility, sensation, or alertness require assistance in changing positions, and they need to be taught strategies that they can use to decrease constant pressure.

Ventilation

Hurn (1988) noted that the use of specific body positions would maximize oxygenation and ventilation even in the presence of lung pathology. In healthy persons, ventilation-perfusion ratios are increased in the dependent lung bases when the person is upright (Fontaine & McQuillan, 1989). The volume of ventilation is greater at the base of the lungs, but the perfusion ratio is greater at the apex of the lungs. The effects of various positions on ventilation have been examined. Piehl and Brown (1976) reported that patients in respiratory failure had improved paO2 after being placed in a prone position; in most instances this positioning was achieved through the use of a Circ-O-Lectric bed. A number of researchers have shown that oxygenation is increased in patients with unilateral lung problems when the patient is positioned so that the lung with no pathology is dependent (Banasik et al., 1987; Rivara et al., 1984). Utilization of gravitational pull appears to have an impact on improvement of oxygenation.

Cerebral Perfusion

Adequate cerebral tissue perfusion in patients with head injuries is an objective of many therapies used in the care of this population. Maintaining normal intracranial pressures or reducing increased pressures aids in cerebral tissue perfusion. Positioning plays a key role in the attainment of this objective. Elevating the head of the bed 30 degrees assists in decreasing intracranial pressure (Parsons & Wilson, 1984; Shalit & Umansky, 1977). However, elevating the head of the bed to a 90-degree position may increase pressure as it results in sharp flexion of the hips (Fontaine & McQuillan, 1989). Keeping the head and neck in alignment reduces interference with venous return (Mitchell & Mauss, 1978; Mitchell et al., 1981). Use of proper positioning techniques decreases tissue compromise in persons prone to increases in intracranial pressure.

Positioning for comfort is a skill most nurses possess. Proper alignment prevents pull on body structures. Unless a paralyzed arm is supported, tremendous pull on the shoulder socket and muscles occurs. Not only does proper positioning increase the patient's comfort, but it has major implications for the functioning of body systems such as the circulatory and respiratory systems. Correct positioning avoids pressure on certain areas, thus providing for adequate circulation to all body areas. Correct positioning promotes ventilation and oxygenation of the lungs.

INTERVENTION

Technique

Numerous techniques for positioning exist. Fundamentals of nursing texts contain many pages on positioning techniques to promote skin integrity, to prevent contractures, and to achieve adequate ventilation. Content in these texts addresses the various positions that are used for respiratory therapy, diagnostic tests such as lumbar punctures or barium enemas, and positions to be used postoperatively for various surgical procedures. Correct use of these and other techniques does much to promote positive patient outcomes.

Findings from research studies on positioning of patients with increased intracranial pressure (ICP) or the potential for increased intracranial pressure will be used as the basis for describing positioning for this group of patients.

Positioning in Increased ICP

Although much research is still required in the area of positioning of persons with increased or the potential for increased intracranial pressure, the studies that have been completed provide a basis for the positioning of patients to promote cerebral perfusion (Mitchell, 1986). Elevation of the head of the bed, flexion and extension of body parts, and turning schedules have been examined.

Durward and colleagues (1983) found that elevating the head of the bed 15–30 degrees resulted in the lowest intracranial pressure readings, and the cerebral perfusion and cardiac output remained stable when subjects were in this position. Elevating the head of the bed in excess of a 45-degree angle often results in increases in ICP (Mitchell et al., 1981). Although horizontal or head down positions are often listed as contraindications for persons with increased ICP, Lee (1989) reported that 20% of the patients in his study demonstrated reduction in ICP in this position. Based on findings from studies, it can be recommended that patients with or potential for increased ICP be placed in a position with the head of their bed elevated 15–30 degrees.

Positioning the patient to avoid sharp flexion of the hips will assist in maintaining the ICP within normal range. Turning the patient may result in increases in ICP, but these changes are often transient in nature (Parsons & Wilson, 1984). Maintaining the head and neck in alignment with the trunk of the body has been demonstrated to be a critical factor in preventing increases in ICP when turning and positioning patients (Mitchell et al., 1981). Using two or three persons to turn the patient and placing rolls or small pillows to keep the head and neck in alignment are needed.

USES

The preceding content has indicated ways in which positioning has been used as a nursing intervention. It is encouraging to see the body of research that is developing regarding the use of this independent nursing intervention (Fontaine & McQuillan, 1989; Mitchell, 1986; Noll & Fountain, 1990; Quaglietti et al., 1988). The use of this intervention in patients who have cardiovascular problems and for patients who are prone to spasticity because of neurological problems will be examined.

Cardiovascular Problems

Effects of positioning on the physiological status of postmyocardial infarction patients has been studied. Quaglietti and colleagues (1988) studied the effects that several types of position changes had on the rate pressure product (RPP) of persons who were recovering from an uncomplicated myocardial infarction. Findings revealed that assumption of a supine, semi-Fowler's position at 70 degrees or sitting in a chair did not significantly alter the RPP of the subjects. The investigators state that these findings are congruent with those of others who have examined positioning in persons with postmyocardial infarction.

Noll and Fountain examined the effect that a backrest position had on the mixed oxygen saturation in patients who had had coronary artery bypass surgery. The effects of three positions—head elevated 20 degrees, head elevated 40 degrees, and head flat—were studied. No significant differences were found among the oxygen saturation measurements taken for each position. The investigators concluded that the head of the bed could be elevated to a 40-degree angle to promote patient comfort. The sample used in the study included 30 subjects who were hemodynamically stable and under 70 years of age. Thus, additional studies are needed before these findings can be generalized.

Spasticity in Patients with Neurological Conditions

Proper positioning plays a key role in preventing contractures in persons who have neurological pathology (Ferido & Habel, 1986). Use of side-lying, semi-prone, and high Fowler's positions help to inhibit abnormal posturing in persons who have suffered head trauma. The prone and semi-prone positions are effective since they alter the effects of the tonic labyrinth and tonic neck reflexes (Palmer & Wyness, 1988). In persons with conditions in which spasticity may occur, rapid change in positions often results in increased muscle tone (Palmer & Wyness, 1988). Thus, slow, gentle changing of positioning is needed.

Precautions

Incorrect positioning of patients can have serious deleterious effects on them. Knowledge from research studies will guide nurses in choosing the correct position(s) to use for a patient with a particular pathology. Keeping a patient with a head injury in a flat position may precipitate increases in intracranial pressure. Likewise, patients with chronic obstructive pulmonary disease should not be placed in a recumbent position. Metzger and Therrien (1990) noted that persons with a history of atherosclerotic cardiovascular disease who are on bedrest should be positioned with the head of the bed flat when activities in which the valsalva maneuver is likely to occur will be performed. Attention to positioning of patients is also needed during diagnostic procedures, such as x-rays. Patients may be left in an untherapeutic position for protracted periods of time which may result in complications. Thus nurses can alert other health professionals to the impact that positioning has on patient outcomes

RESEARCH

Nurses have begun to examine the outcomes resulting from the use of various positions for patients having specific conditions. In some instances, myths have been dispelled. Other findings have pointed to the need for increased caution in turning and positioning patients. In almost all studies on positioning the sample sizes have been very small, preventing the generalization of findings. The following are some of the areas in which further research is necessary so as to provide a more scientific basis for the use of positioning in nursing therapeutics:

1. What are effective mechanisms for maintaining the head and neck in alignment in persons who have suffered a head injury and who have decreased levels of responsiveness? In many instances these persons are restless and move from the position in which they were positioned. This often results in the neck being bent, which interferes with venous return and leads to an increase in intracranial pressure.
2. Validation of the positioning protocols that have been developed for patients with various conditions, such as the one for trauma patients that has been proposed by Norton and Conforti (1985), is needed. Many protocols are presented in the literature, but few have been subjected to clinical trials.
3. What are assessments nurses should make to determine if the patient is in a comfortable position? Students and novices need to become more attuned to these observations.
4. Schermer (1988) reviewed the literature on the effect that position had on hemodynamic measurements. Great variation existed in the degree of head elevation used. Further studies are needed to provide more definitive direction for care. A meta-analysis of studies in this area would be useful.

REFERENCES

Banasik, J.L., Bruya, M.A., Steadman, R.E., & Demand, J.K. (1987). Effect of position on arterial oxygenation in postoperative coronary revascularization. *Heart & Lung* 16:652–657.

Copeland-Fields, L.D., & Hoshiko, B.R. (1989). Clinical validation of Braden and Bergstrom's conceptual schema of pressure sore risk factors. *Rehabilitation Nursing* 14:257–260.

Durward, Q.J., Amacher, A.L., DelMaestro, R.F., & Sibbard, W. (1983). Cerebral and cardiovascular responses in head elevation in patients with intracranial hypertension. *Journal of Neurosurgery* 59:938–944.

Ebersole, P., & Hess, P. (1990). *Toward healthy aging*. St. Louis: C.V. Mosby.

Ferido, T., & Habel, M. (1988). Spasticity in head trauma and CVA patients: etiology and management. *Journal of Neuroscience Nursing* 20:17–22.

Fontaine, D.K., & McQuillan, K. (1989). Positioning as a nursing therapy in trauma care. *Critical Care Nursing Clinics of North America* 1:105–112.

Hurn, P.D. (1988). Thoracic injuries. Pp. 449–490 in V. Cardona, P. Hurn, R. Mason, A.M. Scanlon-Schlipp, & S.W. Veise-Berry eds., *Trauma nursing from resuscitation through rehabilitation*. Philadelphia: W.B. Saunders.

Kinney, M.R. (1984). The scientific basis for critical care nursing practice: 1972 to 1982. *Heart & Lung* 13:116–123.

Lee, S. (1989). Intracranial pressure changes during positioning of patients with severe head injury. *Heart & Lung* 18:411–414.

Metzger, B.L., & Therrien, B. (1990). Effect of position on cardiovascular response during the valsalva maneuver. *Nursing Research* 39:198–202.

Mitchell, P.H. (1986). Intracranial hypertension: Influence of nursing care activities. *Nursing Clinics of North America* 21:563–576.

Mitchell, P.H., & Mauss, N.K. (1978). Relationship of patient-nurse activities to intracranial variations: A pilot study. *Nursing Research* 27:4–10.

Mitchell, P.H., Ozuna, J., & Lipe, H.P. (1981). Moving the patient in bed: Effects of turning and range of motion on intracranial pressure. *Nursing Research* 30:212–218.

Noll, M.L., & Fountain, R.L. (1990). Effects of backrest position on mixed venous oxygen saturation in patients with mechanical ventilation after coronary artery bypass surgery. *Heart & Lung* 19:243–251.

Norton, L.C., & Conforti, C.G. (1985). The effects of body position on oxygenation. *Heart & Lung* 14:45–51.

Palmer, M., & Wyness, M.A. (1988). Positioning and handling: Important considerations in the care of the severely head-injured patient. *Journal of Neuroscience Nursing* 20:42–49.

Parsons, L.C., & Wilson, M.M. (1984). Cerebrovascular status of severe closed head injured patients following passive position changes. *Nursing Research* 33:68–75.

Piehl, M.A., & Brown, R.S. (1976). Use of extreme position changes in acute respiratory failure. *Critical Care Medicine* 4:13–14.

Quaglietti, S.E., Stotts, N.A., & Lovejoy, N.C. (1988). The effect of selected positions on rate pressure product of the postmyocardial infarction patient. *Journal of Cardiovascular Nursing* 2(4):77–85.

Rivara, D., Artucio, H., Arcos, J., & Hiriart, C. (1984). Positional hypoxemia during artificial ventilation. *Critical Care Medicine* 12:436–438.

Schermer, L. (1988). Physiologic and technical variables affecting hemodynamic measurements. *Critical Care Nurse* 8(2):33–40.

Shalit, M.N., & Umansky, F. (1977). Effect of routine bedside procedures on intracranial pressure. *Israel Journal of Medical Science* 13:881–886.

Steffel, P., Schenk, E., & Walker, S. (1980). Reducing devices for pressure sores with respect to nursing care procedures. *Nursing Research* 29:228–230.

Tyler, M. (1984). The respiratory effects of body positioning and immobilization. *Respiratory Care* 29:472.

COGNITIVE INTERVENTIONS

CHAPTER 11

GUIDED IMAGERY

Kathleen Maykoski Sodergren

BACKGROUND

Imagery techniques involve the use of images or of fantasy to achieve specific health-related goals. The more sophisticated uses of imagery are in psychotherapy, but recently imagery is being used in association with interventions aimed at achieving altered states of awareness to facilitate control of the autonomic nervous system and other physiologic mechanisms. Imagery has been advocated as a means of bypassing inhibitory mechanisms so as to facilitate rapid access to the psyche, and as a means of bypassing neurological mechanisms in order to give generalized instructions to the body.

Considerable research on imagery exists in the areas of information processing, memory, and athletics. While few well-controlled studies with large numbers of subjects are available to support the use of imagery in the health fields, there is a growing body of small-scale studies and anecdotal evidence that strongly supports the use of imagery, suggesting that it has great potential as a therapeutic intervention in nursing.

Imagery can be used to enhance other forms of nursing and medical therapy. For example, imagery has been used with cancer patients in conjunction with chemotherapy or radiation therapy with the aim of improving the body's response to therapy. Imagery has been used to assist in the control of pain, in both chronic and acute situations, to augment relaxation, distraction, or hypnagogic therapies. The stressors associated with illness, such as the inability to tolerate ambiguity, high need for control, and viewing oneself as inadequate to deal with a situation, have been treated with imagery.

Definition

Imagery is defined as the formation of a mental representation of an object that is usually only perceived through the senses. Images can have visual, auditory, olfactory, gustatory, and/or tactile-proprioceptive qualities. They can vary in their degree of clarity and intensity. Images may be experienced in dreams, fantasies, or during states of complete awareness.

Practitioners differ greatly as to what they mean when they speak about imagery and in what they advocate in the way of treatment. Most of the major differences are due to the philosophic and theoretical systems on which their practice is based; imagery is used by those from a strict psychoanalytic background, cognitive behaviorists, those with a bent toward Eastern medicine, and those from a traditional orientation toward Western medicine but who are sensitive to the mind-body connection. There will be some attempt here to represent each of these views and to give some examples as to how different methods might be used by nurses in a variety of practice settings.

Scientific Basis

Horowitz (1978) provides a conceptual framework from which to organize some of the knowledge about thought basic to a discussion of imagery. Although this framework may not be consistent with that underlying all the different views of imagery, it is useful for the present purpose. There are three modalities in which meaning is represented in thought: the enactive, the lexical, and the imagic modes.

Motor response memories are represented in enactive thought. When enactive thought is stimulated, for example, in thinking about reaching for some object across the table, it is reflected in mild tensing of muscle groups, momentary gestures, and slight changes in facial expression, in this instance, a tensing of the muscles in the shoulder and arm. Enactive thinking is believed to give rise to nonverbal behavior, which at times will belie messages given in verbal communication. When we tell a lie our hands will often cover our mouths. Control in the enactive mode is thought to lie primarily in the limbic system and in the cortical motor areas of the brain. Control of the emotions is ascribed to the limbic system, and emotion is readily manifested through the tensing of facial muscles. Schwartz (1976) has described distinct facial muscle tensing patterns reliably detected by electromyography that can be associated with several specific emotions. The enactive mode can be accessed by way of the imagic mode. Images may be connected with emotions, which trigger enactive thought, revealing itself in observable behavior.

In the lexical mode, words and grammar are used in thinking about objects. In its pure form, lexical thought is absent in both the images and the subvocalization of the words. It is lexical thought that makes it possible to communicate clearly and logically. Lexical thought enables us to think in multiple languages and to represent ideas in the form of mathematical formulas. Lexical thinking involves sequential processing of information; that is, the cognitive sequencing of information is somewhat fixed and cause-effect thinking dominates. It is believed that the control for lexical thinking is primarily in the left hemisphere of the brain. There is evidence of lexical thinking associated with directed imagery and in secondary process regulation, which are somewhat dependent on verbalization. The left hemisphere appears to be more sensitive to perceiving negative emotion.

In the imagic mode, persons perceive and continue to process perceptual information. Processing is in the form of dreams, fantasies, and images. Spatial information is processed in this mode as well as melody and other purely sensory experiences. The imagic mode is used in primary process thinking which is both primitive and direct. Imagic thought is controlled primarily through right hemisphere activity. It is closely tied to emotion, especially to positive emotion, and by accessing the imagic mode, emotions can be re-experienced and transformed.

All stimuli enter the mind by way of the senses in the form of images and are transformed there into the enactive, lexical, or imagic modes. In ordinary, conscious thought, the three modes function together and are indistinguishable. All are equally important to cognitive functioning. Persons may call upon the various modes of thought for various purposes, for example in using lexical thought for mathematics, but ordinarily they cannot be separated totally from one another. For example, images of food may intrude on the mathematician. Individuals differ in their tendency to use a particular mode of thought. An athlete may better develop enactive thought, a physicist imagic thought, and a music critic lexical thought. There are individual differences in the ability to elicit visual or auditory images. Some persons report they are unable to experience a visual image even when suggestions are quite graphic in their detail.

Kunzendorf (1981) studied individual differences in imagery abilities and the ability to control skin temperature. He found that prevalence of imagery scores correlated significantly with skin temperature control, whereas there was no relationship between vividness of imagery and control. This suggests that processing of mental images is facilitated in those who frequently use visual, auditory, and tactile-proprioceptive images, and that better imagers may have better control of centrifugal fibers in the autonomic nervous system that direct automatic body processes. Horowitz (1981) suggests that in using imagery techniques, the professional causes an alteration in the regulation of the flow of information in the patient, causing the patient to develop new controls and insight into the way he or she has depicted experience in the past.

If individuals can use imagery to understand and control their own patterns of thinking, to access and more deeply experience emotion, and to control aspects of autonomic functioning, they have a powerful tool to use in the promotion of health.

INTERVENTION

Techniques

The nurse has a unique access to patients at times when they are in need of assistance with dealing with the effects of illness or with aspects of its treatment. There are a variety of techniques described in the literature that are useful to the nurse and are adaptable to various levels of skill the nurse may have. When the patient experiences stress, it is often because of the absence of a skill that is needed to respond to a particular stressor, or, if the skill is present, the patient does not think of using it in the situation at hand. Many of the imagery techniques are aimed at the latter situation and are designed to give the patient insight concerning the nature of the problem so that the proper response can be selected. Other techniques are designed to assist patients to work out a solution in a symbolic way, giving them practice so they can try the new skill in the real-life situation. Most of these approaches to intervention make the assumption that the patient has the ability to fantasize or form images. For patients who do not have this ability, imagery is not an appropriate intervention for short-term problems such as in handling momentary pain. For those patients with chronic or prolonged problems, the patient may wish to try to develop an ability to form images. There are suggestions later in this chapter to assist in such cases.

Guided Affective Imagery

Leuner (1977) developed Guided Affective Imagery (GAI) in an attempt to eliminate the problems associated with studying random and unpredictable fantasies. The technique evolved from the work of Schultz and Luthe (1959) on autogenic training. Their program for inducing the autogenic state required training the subject in relaxation and in image induction. It took from six months to two years for the subject to be able to reach the autogenic state and to elicit fantasies. There were very few subjects who were able to reach this state or who persisted in training this long. Leuner (1977) discovered that by making relaxation suggestions, the therapist could immediately assist the individual to use the imagination technique. The initial images, while usually vague, assisted the individual to relax more deeply, achieving an altered state of consciousness in which the images are deep and colorful. Leuner's technique required the presence of a therapist who assisted in inducing the hypnagogic state, in offering protection, and in intervening to affect the flow of images. The therapist was to have an understanding of symbolism and of the patient's history to assist in the interpretation of symbols, with the goal being that the subject would gain insight into their meaning. The therapist would then help the patient to act on these symbols to restructure the imaginative field, a necessary condition for change.

Leuner (1978) developed 12 standard motifs to be used in guided imagery in which the patient is likely to experience some symbolic conflict and on which the patient can act within the context of the imagined situation. The standard motifs were constructed at three levels designed to bring the client into increasingly difficult conflict situations appropriate for a therapist at the beginning, intermediate, or advanced levels of training. At the beginning level, the therapist might suggest starting the imagery in a meadow, beside a brook, at the foot of a mountain, beside a house, or at the edge of a woods. As the patient begins to describe the surroundings, the therapist leads the patient to describe the situation more fully and to bring conflicts into focus. At this level, the therapist attempts to guide the patient toward reconciliation with hostile figures who appear or toward pacification of these figures by feeding or enriching them.

In most nursing situations, patients are deluged with conflict as they respond to the limitations an illness or its treatment places on their daily lives and the lives of their families and co-workers. The beginning level described by Leuner is appropriate for the nurse who has been educated in the basic principles underlying psychiatric nursing practice. The nurse has the communication skills to guide a patient in exploring an imaginary situation and to help the patient identify how the conflict in the imaginary situation mirrors that in the actual situation. An example from the practice of a nurse working in a maternal-child setting illustrates how the nurse used this imagery technique to assist a patient to gain insight and to determine a course of action to reduce her stress in dealing with infertility.

A 40-year-old woman who had undergone several years of treatment for infertility was depressed and experiencing her situation as hopeless. She was asked to place herself in a meadow. The grass was brown and had been cut. There were small hills in the meadow. On the left was a woods, in front of her at some distance there was a fence and a farm house. She was unable to describe anything to her right or behind her. It was fall. The leaves were brown and falling from the trees. There were no flowers, no birds, only the sound of a soft wind. The sky was grey, but it was not raining.

The woman was asked to walk across the field to the house. At first, although she continued to walk, the house always appeared in the distance, never becoming any closer. The woman was then asked to approach the woods but not to enter. She was told to wait and that someone would come out of the woods and meet her there. Finally a small boy came out of the woods crying uncontrollably. The woman tried to quiet him but was unable to. This caused her to experience considerable distress. At this point she began crying and reported that she and her husband had been having considerable conflict over their decision to have a child. Her husband did not want children as he did not want to be "tied down." She reported regarding this attitude as childish and felt her husband did not want to make any personal sacrifice and would never "grow." The woman was asked if she saw the crying child as representing her husband. She said it was and that she felt too much anger to try and appease him.

She was then asked to imagine something she could do to get him to grow. She then saw a bear come out of the woods. She began to attack the bear with the intention of killing it to get meat to feed the child. The bear began to overwhelm her when the child ran to her defense. He then grew large and the bear turned into a toy which the man gave her and which she then threw into the woods.

At this the woman felt considerably relieved and began speaking as if there was a future for her even if they should never have a child. The woman related feeling desperate as she was nearing menopause and was more concerned with losing the opportunity to have a child sometime in the future than she was despondent because she was infertile. The woman subsequently decided to terminate fertility treatment. The characteristics of the meadow scene reflected the woman's view that she was infertile and in the "autumn" of her life. The bear represented her powerful urge for motherhood. During following sessions, the meadow changed to summer as the woman began to view her life as warm and comfortable, and she gained optimism about the future.

Leuner indicates that there should be a high degree of association between the motif selected and the suspected area of conflict, as the therapist wishes to bring the core of the conflict into focus. In one instance, Leuner describes a patient with a severe cardiac neurosis who was unable to express strong aggressive feelings. With this patient, he suggested a lion motif. The patient was asked to become a lion and to encounter an adversary, in this case a customer. The lion meekly laid at the customer's feet and turned into a small dog. Leuner treated the man for several months before the lion was able to confront his adversary, chasing him away.

The pleasant atmosphere of the meadow makes a good motif for beginning the fantasy. It is easy to incorporate the other motifs as well, one can imagine the brook flowing through the meadow or a mountain in the distance. As was true with the woman discussed previously, depressed persons will imagine the mountain, a symbol of aspirations, as too high to climb, or very low. The motif of the house is thought to represent one's personality. Viewing the house from within while going from room to room may be revealing. Often there are persons within the house who must be dealt with. When the woods figures in the motif, Leuner suggests not allowing the patient to enter it but to allow figures to emerge and be dealt with. Threatening figures are easier to deal with in the light.

Table 11.1
Steps In the Guided Affective Imagery Technique

1. Ask patient to assume a comfortable position, preferably reclining with eyes closed
2. Make suggestions to induce relaxation
3. Reinforce relaxation by suggesting peaceful images
4. Suggest deeper relaxation
5. Suggest motif
6. Assist patient to elaborate on the description of the setting
7. Attempt to provoke conflict within the motif
8. Have patient reconcile conflict symbolically
9. Take patient out of the fantasy situation
10. Discuss the patient's interpretation of the symbolism and conflict resolution
11. Ask patient to comment on insights and interpretations the therapist may have made

Assisting the patient to develop the fantasy situation requires some courage for most nurses who have no experience with such interventions. Often practicing with a friend and experimenting with helping the friend to describe all the details of the scene such as the colors and smells, the feeling of the sun or a breeze on the skin, will help the nurse relax and enjoy this alternative way of helping someone understand and deal with his or her situation. A summary of the steps of the guided affective imagery technique are presented in Table 11.1.

The Chakra System of Imagery

In the Eastern view of the human as an energy system, it becomes the role of the individual's consciousness to balance energy forces within the body creating harmony and increasing consciousness. The person has seven energy centers called chakras within the body. Energy is concentrated in these centers and energy flows through them and out to the rest of the body. It is these channels that are tapped in acupuncture. All illness, physical or emotional, is believed to result from an interruption in the flow of energy through the energy system.

Each of the energy centers has its own function and symbolic meaning. The base center is located at the base of the spine and is concerned with basic survival. The energy located here is used for creative activity and regenerative activity. The spleen center is located between the naval and the pubis and is the center for purification and digestion and sexual passion. The solar plexus center is immediately above the naval and is concerned with power and emotion and overcoming the effects of stress. The heart center is concerned with unconditional love and compassion. It controls factors that determine immunity. The throat center is concerned with expression of the integrated self and metabolic, neuromuscular functions. The brow center is concerned with heightened consciousness, intuition, and supranormal powers. It operates above the limits of the senses. The crown center is located at the top of the head and is concerned with the relationship between the soul and cosmic consciousness, cosmic energy, or God. It is these same energy centers that are a focus in the interventions of therapeutic touch (see Chapter 20).

Gallegos (1983) developed a visualization method in which the patient is assisted to achieve a state of relaxation. He suggests the patient imagine being a seed that has been in the ground for the winter. He takes the seed through the process of growth proceeding from early spring to summer flowering and fall beauty. This image assists the patient to achieve deeper relaxation. The patient is then asked to focus on each chakra, beginning with the crown center and proceeding to the base center. At each center the patient imagines the center, and the feelings associated with that center, as some animal that embodies the feelings the patient associates with that center. The patient has a conversation with the animal where the animal is asked to reveal its name and say anything else it wishes to reveal to the client at this time. Once the animals have revealed themselves, the nurse guides the patient to bring out two animals at a time, introduce them, and observe the nature of their interaction. If there is conflict between the animals, the patient and the nurse help the animals to settle the conflict or to alter conditions in such a way that they can live in harmony. Occasionally one or both of the animals must change, even transform itself into another animal. The animals must decide which of them is to grow or change. The patient is asked to "become" each of the animals, in turn, to gain the animal's perspective. Because the animals are projected images, there is a bypassing of the inhibitions, and through the animal's conversations, the patient gains insight as to the nature of the conflicts within. In having to maintain harmony between the animals, the individual learns to maintain harmony between the energy centers, and so promotes physical and emotional health. The patient often experiences guidance, support, and a feeling of warmth from the conversation and advice that flow from these inner centers. Gallegos reports that the animals that arise from each center are characteristic of the function of the center. For example, the power animal might be a panther or an untamed stallion, and the emotional animal might be caged, or particularly spirited.

Gallegos' use of animal imagery, while it comes from a distinct philosophic background, is similar to the Dual Imagery described by Shorr (1978). Shorr believes that inner conflicts are represented by the symbolic conflict created when two forces come together in opposition in the form of images. The conflict cannot be resolved without pain and loss. In the conversation between opposing forces, the individual comes to an awareness of conflict. While the conflict in the case of the chakras is inner conflict, Shorr suggests there is a need to examine conflict between the self and outside forces and persons. Dual imagery may be useful in this regard. For example, the heart animal of the patient might talk to the consciousness animal of her husband. Or the power animal of the tornado victim might confront the tornado.

When bringing two images together, there is a risk of conflict, but in projected form, it is easier to resolve conflict in a way that produces optimum growth. The author has used imagery in conjunction with the practice of therapeutic touch. Patients are asked to visualize bringing energy in the form of "bright light" into themselves through the crown center. They then bring the warm bright light progressively through each chakra from the bow to the base center, in an attempt to balance their own energy and bring about self-healing. Patients who are ill are often unable to overcome blocks in the flow of energy within themselves. The healer, in the case of therapeutic touch, assists in overcoming these blocks in energy flow so that the patient can engage in self-healing.

Visualization to Promote Relaxation

An adaptation of imagery techniques may be used to induce a state of altered consciousness before the nurse suggests ways that the patient might operate on the fantasy to bring about physical changes. The nurse suggests that the patient imagine being in a place he or she would find relaxing. A relaxing image is highly individual because the same image, such as floating on a lake or sitting on the side of a mountain, may relax one person and cause another intense anxiety. The scene should be one that the patient has actually experienced previously and found to be relaxing.

Scenes commonly used to induce relaxation include sitting on a hillside watching a sunset, lying in a field watching clouds float by, sitting on a warm beach watching the sea, sitting by a fire on a snowy evening, and floating through water or through space.

The nurse encourages the patient to experience the scene with all the senses, clarifying the image while relaxing the body. Suggestions for relaxation, such as are described in Chapter 6, should follow until the nurse judges that the patient is relaxed. The nurse then suggests that the patient allow an image to form that represents the illness. Physiologically accurate representations are not desirable. In a relaxed state, the patient should be able to elicit a symbolic representation of the illness that captures its meaning from the patient's perspective. If the patient is unable to do this, the nurse might suggest the patient visualize it as an animal. Pressuring a patient to bring forth a vision when he or she cannot will create anxiety, so if the patient indicates an inability to proceed, the nurse should make continued relaxation suggestions and make a second attempt at another time.

When the illness has been visualized, the patient is encouraged to imagine some inner force that would effectively act on the vision. For example:

> A 60-year-old man with cancer of the lung who had been relaxing in a garden imagined his lungs to be a maze formed by hedges. He was unable to get out of the maze as it was blocked by giant mole hills with fierce giant moles peering out at him. He imagined his treatment as giving him tremendous power to leap over the mole hills and to gain enough height that he could see over the hedges, noting the design and enabling him to get out of the maze.

When the patient is experiencing an undesirable symptom such as pain or nausea or a craving, such as for food or cigarettes, the patient is encouraged to remove the undesirable feeling and put it in a place where it is accessible but where it is not within the area of experience. As an alternative, the patient might remove only the feeling itself. Rosenberg (1982) suggests using an image of a fog or a light rain to induce anesthesia. The fog is inhaled, numbing sensation in the nose, respiratory tract, and wherever the patient moves it, before bringing it to the area of pain or nausea. The rain lightly touches and numbs the skin of an unaffected area and is gradually moved to the area of pain.

Korn (1983) suggests a technique for assisting the patient to develop "glove anesthesia." The patient images the hand being immersed in freezing cold water and becoming numb. The hand is first placed over some unaffected area and the anesthesia is transferred to this area. When the patient is able to do this successfully, the hand is placed over the area of pain and the numbness is transferred. To successfully use a kinesthetic image, the patient in chronic pain usually has to have had experience with using other forms of imagery, such as visual or auditory imagery. With practice, some patients become very adept at transferring anesthesia from a hand to a painful area. It is evident that developing such a skill takes a good deal of time, so this technique could not be used in situations when there is no time to practice before the painful circumstance. When pain is severe, it may be sufficiently distracting that, even if the patient has developed skill in the technique, a "coach" might have to be present to assist in directing the attention while using the technique. In childbirth, this coach may be the husband. In the clinic during a procedure, it may be the nurse. Some patients use a tape recording in which the coach slowly goes through each step of the procedure. Because the "glove anesthesia" technique requires considerable practice to be effective, many patients get discouraged with it. Highlighting signs of success, such as noting the patient was able to make the hand cold to touch or able to enduce enough anesthesia in the hand or unaffected area to feel no pinprick, will encourage the patient to persist in trying to develop a skill that may take several weeks of effort.

Group Therapy

Imagery is used primarily with individuals but there are several clinicians who report having used it with groups. Leuner asks group members to lie on their backs in a circle with their heads in the center. He uses music to promote imagery and imagination. In some instances the clinician suggests the topic and group members contribute to developing a group fantasy. Individuals then discuss the meaning of the fantasy to themselves in the group setting, with assistance and support being offered by the group members. In other instances the group decides on a topic for the fantasy and the group leader allows them to guide the experience themselves.

Madden (1982) describes the fantasies developed by groups of obese women who have successfully lost weight and groups who have remained obese. She used a procedure called fantasy chaining to elicit the group fantasies.

The fantasies revealed how these women viewed themselves and others. Madden describes three themes that emerged from group fantasy chaining: the revulsion vision, the survival vision, and the insulation vision. In the revulsion vision, subjects viewed themselves as outcasts who are considered ugly by others. They view that they must constantly battle the harassment and oppression of others who control their social world. In the survival vision, subjects see the world in black and white, those who are fit and healthy and those who are fat and dying. Their battles are directed toward staying alive. In the insulation vision, subjects see themselves as protected by layers of fat and their struggle is to remain secure.

By identifying the extent to which individuals share in the fantasy vision of the group, Madden believes intervention can be structured. It is suggested that fantasy, itself, could provide the setting to be used to restructure the vision. The group might confront the conflict in the fantasy setting, removing impediments to their freedom to be the person they want to be, or to gain the control they wish to possess.

Shorr (1978) suggests several methods that can be used effectively with groups. One method is his "finish the sentence" approach in which the group leader begins the discussion with an unfinished sentence, such as "I cannot give you _____," "I have to prove _____," or "If I could, I would _____." It is sometimes effective for the group leader to suggest that the group members imagine they are a particular one of the members when finishing the sentence. The group leader might suggest a fantasy, such as going on a trip to a deserted island, and have each member imagine what would occur on the trip and how each other member would behave.

Gallegos' animal imagery might also be effective in a group setting. Each member might imagine a conversation or confrontation between one of their chakra animals and one of another group member.

Group methods give members feedback as to how they are seen by other people, which is an important part of forming one's view of oneself. Shorr cautions that in instances in which a person feels sexually inadequate, mixed sex groups are initially quite difficult. In a climate where acceptance of the other is expected, this difficulty associated with self-exposure can be somewhat reduced.

In group settings, inducing imagery by exposing the group to a common odor will often trigger images from the past. In medical settings, the odor of rubbing alcohol or hospital disinfectant may trigger memories of early experiences in that setting. Baking bread or peanut butter often trigger warm memories of childhood. The smell of burning leaves will often trigger fond memories of childhood play. Childhood memories may be used to explore the way a person viewed his or her situation, friends and family, common feelings of rejection, and relationships with caring or uncaring parents.

Measurement of Effectiveness

There are few controlled studies of the effectiveness of imagery techniques, and almost no replicated studies. It may be that this is a consequence of the inability to truly control the independent variable in therapeutic settings. Most clinicians using imagery methods have used case studies that are designed to illustrate the change in a poorly defined, dependent variable such as insight, anxiety, healthy changes in behavior, or conflict resolution. There are a number of self-report measures that have been used and on which there is reliability data.

White et al. (1977) reviewed measures of the vividness of mental imagery, types of imaginal ability, and imagery control. Standardized tests that measure vividness of imagery in seven sensory modalities were evaluated, including several that measure visual imagery alone, visual imagery with eyes open and eyes closed, and vividness of imaginal and daydream processes and attention–curiosity processes. In addition, preferred mode of imagery, particularly visualization–verbalization, was measured. Validity and reliability data and social desirability data from the tests that they reviewed are provided.

Several physiologic measures have been found to correlate with imagery. These include regularity of respiration and alpha frequency of the electroencephalogram (White et al., 1977). Schwartz (1976) studied electromyogram (EMG) changes resulting from elicitation of specific emotional states with imagery, and reports consistent facial muscle EMG patterns associated with six emotions.

There are nonstandardized measures of imagery variables as well. Shorr (1978) examined the meaning of several hundred responses to an imagined situation. From commonalities in the responses, he was able to determine that there was a consistency in the meaning of these situations across individuals. One example is the situation in which the person is asked to imagine viewing three closed doors. He or she is instructed to open each door, in turn, and to describe what is seen behind the door. After describing whatever is behind the doors, the person is to imagine being that object or person, and to "finish the sentences" that the therapist presents (I wish that I was _____. I am _____. I feel _____., etc.). Shorr determined that the middle door represented the area of sexuality or relationships with significant persons. The left door represented a major current conflict, and the right door a possible resolution of that conflict.

The measurements of the effectiveness of visualization used by Simonton et al. (1978) were positively correlated with attitude and length of life after treatment.

It is clear that the study of imagery as a therapeutic technique is in its early stages. For the clinician, it is suggested that if imagery is used to bring about some desired outcome, the clinician keep detailed records that will help in the demonstration of the conditions under which imagery is effective or ineffective in the clinical setting.

USES

The situations in which imagery has been used in health care settings are varied, and the technique to be selected is based on the outcome the nurse desires. When the nurse wishes to assist the patient to control physiologic functions, techniques involving deep relaxation and the symbolic representation of physiologic control mechanisms are used. When patient insight and strengthening of personal resources to withstand stress are desired outcomes, symbolic representation of conflict and its resolution are used. The ability of the patient to use imagination techniques and the willingness of the patient to be guided in these techniques, as well as to practice them, will determine their success. Several uses for imagery are discussed briefly here.

Pain

Imagery techniques have been used in the rehabilitation of patients with chronic pain. One purpose of imagery in this setting has been to restructure patients' cognitive appraisal of their situations, relieving discouragement and hopelessness, changing the expectation that pain will continue, increasing energy, and shifting the focus of life away from pain. Korn (1983) reports using imagery as a part of a multimodal treatment program. He hypothesized that possible reasons imagery is successful in relieving pain is that it may interfere with the processing of pain information or that imagery might enhance secretion of endorphins, thereby relieving pain. Korn suggests using imagery to create a place of safety leading to a reduction of anxiety and stress. When this level of imagery is mastered, patients are guided to imagine some mechanism they can operate that will "shut off" the pain. Because pain is primarily a kinesthetic experience, competing kinesthetic images have been found to be difficult to invoke. Visual or auditory images are more readily used by those in chronic pain.

McCaffery (1979) suggests that imagery may be used to assist patients to remove themselves from the pain through relaxation and through analgesia. Patients may remove themselves from the situation simply by taking imaginary vacations, experiencing themselves fishing, lying on the beach, hiking, reliving the relaxing and pleasant feelings associated with these experiences. She cautions that the patient should not relive experiences that have caused pain in the past as this association might intensify the pain of the moment rather than relieve it.

Pleasant imagery alone appears to be ineffective in bringing about the relief of pain. Geden et al. (1984) compared five cognitive strategies designed to reduce the simulated pain of labor. They found that only when the subject mentally operated on the pain sensation, transforming it to an alternative sensation, did subjects report pain relief. In another study, Geden et al. (1989) explored the combination of music and imagery for the relief of simulated labor pain. They found that only subjects using their own imagery in combination with music reported a decrease in pain.

Ballard and Madsen (1988), in a simulated pain situation, found that subjects who focused on images external to their experience (an outward journey in a spacecraft) experienced less pain than subjects who focused on images internal to their experience (limbs feeling warm and heavy; blowing away the pain). Raft et al. (1986) indicate the content of the image is important. They found that when the subject generated a number of pleasant images, and the therapist selected one which was free from past emotional conflict and which came from a successful period in the patient's life, it was more effective in bringing about pain relief. Since emotion is a major factor in pain perception, imagery which enhances positive emotion and promotes energy should be superior to that which induces arousal by focusing on conflict, safety, withdrawal, or sensation.

Rehabilitation

Korn (1983) reports two case studies in which patients with neurological insults were treated with imagery. A girl with a closed head injury used imagery to relearn swallowing mechanisms and motor skills, and a man relearned sitting balance, speech, and memory using imagery after suffering a cerebrovascular accident. If Horowitz's (1978) model is used, one might hypothesize that imagery facilitates the entry into enactive thought, bypassing disrupted mechanisms usually used in processing such information. These case studies do not provide sufficient evidence from which to draw generalized conclusions, but the findings are reasonable. Korn suggests that through imagery, the individual re-experiences the psychomotor task, activating sensory and neuromuscular mechanisms similar to those invoked when carrying out the task originally. This is consistent with findings derived from research on imagery use by athletes. It has been shown that to benefit from mental practice, the athlete must be familiar with the task and intersperse mental rehearsal throughout the entire period of learning a skill. When imagining motor tasks, it is more effective to imagine experiencing the actual activities than to imagine observing the activity as an outsider. Visual imagery is most effective when applied from the perspective of the actor. Turner et al. (1982) report that mental practice in skill acquisition is transferrable bilaterally; that is, subjects who practice imagining the activity show more competent performance when the physical performance is changed from the dominant to nondominant hand. They found it was the degree of control of the image achieved through practice and not the vividness of the image that was important. There is much known about development of motor and proprioceptive skills that may be transferrable to the rehabilitation setting, but it is not known how the loss of regulatory mechanisms through injury and disease affects the processing of information through the imagic mode.

Relaxation

The use of guided imagery techniques in conjunction with relaxation techniques facilitates the induction of the relaxed state. Those who can control images are able to reach the relaxed state more quickly, achieve deeper relaxation, and remain in a relaxed state for longer periods. The outcomes associated with the relaxation response, such as decrease in muscle tension, decrease in anxiety, and decrease in symptomatology associated with stress, are augmented with using guided imagery with relaxation techniques.

One patient who was anxious about wearing an oxygen mask, as she had been extremely dyspneic when wearing one earlier, was able to imagine wearing the mask and feeling a cool breeze wafting over her as she laid on the beach. The feeling of relaxation she experienced enabled her to try the mask without anxiety.

Malignancy

In studying differences between cancer patients and control subjects, LeShan (1959) showed that those who developed malignancies had psychological profiles with the following characteristics: (1) inability to express anger and resentment or to forgive, (2) tension related to the loss of a parent, and (3) feelings of hopelessness and inability to cope. Simonton and Simonton (1975), while treating cancer patients in a radiology practice, noticed an increase in remissions for cancer patients who were enthusiastic about their treatment and who had positive beliefs about its efficacy. In comparing these two poles of hopelessness and enthusiasm in the patient with cancer, and in examining the relationship between stress and the immune system, Simonton and Simonton developed a technique using imagery in conjunction with relaxation therapy for the treatment of cancer. It should be noted that Simonton and Simonton used imagery in conjunction with other medical treatments in subjects who were somewhat self-selected, that is who persisted with training in the use of imagery. Simonton et al. (1978) report that of 159 medically incurable patients treated with imagery, survival time was double that of the national norm. In the Simonton method, individuals are taught to use relaxation techniques and to visualize the cancer symbolically, for example as rats running around the body or as rotten fruit hanging on a tree. They are then asked to visualize the treatment (chemotherapy, radiation) or their own body attacking the cancer, for example as large cats eating up the rats or a fierce wind blowing the rotten fruit from the tree. In subjects who imagine the treatment as ineffectual, such as a bird pecking at the fruit, there is an attempt to strengthen the image—changing the bird into a bear who devours the fruit, for example. Hall (1983) reports using imagery with children with cancer to strengthen feelings of attachment and parental protection, to increase the efficacy of immune mechanisms, and to decrease symptoms that interfere with the quality of life. Rosenberg (1982) and Margolis (1982) report successfully using imagery in conjunction with hypnosis with cancer patients to reduce pain and discomfort, strengthen the self-image, strengthen coping skills, alleviate fear, and deepen relaxation.

Imagery has been useful for relieving unpleasant symptoms associated with chemotherapy. Lyles et al. (1982) found that guided imagery in combination with relaxation training relieved anticipatory nausea and vomiting. Frank (1985) found that a combination of music and imagery reduced anxiety and the self-reported duration of vomiting in patients receiving chemotherapy. Since anxiety is related to anticipatory symptoms and might have a carryover effect on post-chemotherapy symptoms, imagery that promotes distraction and relaxation may be beneficial for chemotherapy patients. It should be noted that all patients do not benefit from distraction techniques. Many people have a need to monitor their symptoms, even unpleasant ones, and anxiety is actually created by attempts to interfere with this monitoring activity.

Depression

Smith (1982) advocates using imagery in the treatment of hopelessness. She characterizes hopelessness as a sense of apathy, passivity, futility, and lessened will to live, a giving up on life. This state follows a pessimistic view of life, and is accompanied by a restriction in the ability to imagine. In a study of college students exposed to imagery techniques in a workshop, there was no significant change demonstrated in hopelessness scores, but behavioral changes were observed after the study, suggesting an improvement in communication skills and a reduction in stress. Margolis (1982) reports case studies supporting the effectiveness of imagery in depression and helplessness.

Phobias

Singer and Pope (1978) report that imagery is useful in systematic desensitization in the treatment of phobias. Because the fear generated by the phobic object is a consequence of the symbolism of that object, imagery is a useful medium from which to test the consequences of approaching the phobic object without danger prior to the actual contact with it. Through imagery techniques the meaning of the phobic object to the individual may be ascertained and changed or confronted in some symbolic way.

Lang (1979) advocates assisting the patient to focus on stimulus properties of the image, such as the details of the scene, rather than on response properties, such as feeling warm or feeling the heart racing. Patients are asked to imagine the phobic situation in its least threatening form, master it without arousal, and then proceed to a little more threatening form with each trial. In cancer chemotherapy patients with anticipatory symptoms, for example, one might begin by selecting the home situation where the patient is getting dressed prior to leaving for the clinic. After a state of deep relaxation is induced, the patient is asked to elaborate on the sensory details in that setting until he can do so without arousal or nausea. The nurse then assists the patient to image progressively more anxiety-provoking situations such as getting in the car, walking into the clinic, and finally receiving the injection. The patient must deal with each of them until he can do so without arousal. It usually takes only about three or four sessions until the patient is able to endure the phobia-producing situation without arousal.

Psychotherapy

Imagery is used in psychotherapy for many purposes. It is helpful in exploring repressed ideas, because fantasy bypasses the normal censorship. Therapists who have used imagery have found it particularly helpful in periods when there is little forward movement. When patients have difficulty expressing something in words, they might be able to describe an image that captures the experience in such a way that both patient and therapist gain insight. Imagery may also be used to detect areas where motivation is blocked. Leuner (1977) has developed a series of scenarios to be used in Guided Affective Imagery that are especially useful in this regard. Fantasy has been used effectively with schizophrenics to broaden their available symbolism, but the nurse is cautioned that this requires a good deal of expertise in the psychotherapeutic process. Ettin (1982) suggests using imagery to establish connectedness with the patient and to improve client–therapist communication. Twente et al. (1978) used eidetic therapy with psychiatric patients in insight-oriented inpatient and outpatient settings and in both individual and group therapy. They found patients were able to identify areas of conflict very rapidly and gained insight into common thinking patterns. They were able to locate and treat specific events that had been traumatic during the patient's development. Twente et al. describe a treatment program where patients are trained to use eidetic therapy techniques, including practice exercises and record keeping. They were assisted in the interpretation of symptoms by the therapist. The patients were reported to develop self-reliance, were able to identify areas in which they needed therapy, and were more motivated than subjects not receiving eidetic therapy.

Surgery

Guided imagery has been used to facilitate recovery from surgery. Leja (1989) found a decrease in postsurgical depression in elderly patients who mentally rehearsed images of the home environment. Holden-Lund (1988) had postoperative patients imagine a journey through the body to the wound site and picture healing the wound. She found treated subjects had lower urinary cortisol levels, lower state anxiety, and less erythema at the wound site than a comparison group.

Problem Solving

Imagery has been used to assist patients in problem-solving situations. In one instance, four patients hospitalized with multiple sclerosis, who had marked decreases from their former ability to perform activities of daily living, were asked to use proprioceptive imagery to anticipate problems they would encounter when going home from the hospital and completing the necessary activities of one day at home. Until this point the patients saw no difficulties in going home and anticipated no changes in their routine from before hospitalization. In imagining the movements of getting in and out of the car, the house, the kitchen, and the bathroom, the patients were able to visualize specific difficulties and determine solutions for the problems that they would encounter. Several patients found the experience traumatic or emotionally draining as they said they had been overly optimistic. All were grateful for the imagery experience and later reported the solutions they had imagined were helpful when coping at home.

Some of the uses of imagery in health-related situations are summarized in Table 11.2.

Precautions

The lack of replicated, controlled studies concerning the effectiveness of imagery in producing specific outcomes means that clinicians must rely on experience, both their own and that of their colleagues, to suggest areas of precaution in practice. The major guideline is to produce no harm to the patient, whether physical or psychological.

Table 11.2
Suggested Uses of Imagery

Condition	Source
Conflict resolution	Leuner (1978)
Crisis intervention	Leuner (1978)
Phobias	Singer & Pope (1978), Lang (1979)
Depression	Korn (1983), Margolis (1982), Twente et al. (1978), Leja (1989)
Hopelessness	Margolis (1982)
Cancer	Hall (1983), LeShan (1959), Simonton et al. (1978), Lyles (1982), Frank (1985)
Improve immune function	Hall (1982), Simonton et al. (1978)
Pain	Korn (1983), McCaffery (1979), Rosenberg (1982), Ballard (1988), Geden et al. (1984, 1989)
Obesity	Madden (1982), Singer & Pope (1978)
Strengthen coping skills	Hall (1983), Korn (1983)
Rehabilitation	Korn (1983)
Cardiac neurosis	Leuner (1977)
Nausea	Rosenberg (1982), Lyles et al. (1982), Frank (1985)
Anxiety	Korn (1983), Rosenberg (1982), Frank (1985)
Childbirth	McCaffery (1979), Geden et al. (1983, 1989)
Hypnotherapy	Hall (1983), Margolis (1982), Rosenberg (1982)
Group therapy	Shorr (1978)
Psychotherapy	Ettin (1982), Leuner (1978), Shorr (1978), Twente et al. (1978)
Sleep	McCaffery (1979)

The person in actual control of the imagery is the patient. There are many patients who do not wish to use imagery because they fear lack of control, they do not think they have the ability, or because they believe it is wrong to allow the imagination to wander freely. Since there are many therapies available to the nurse, an attitude of "let's try it and see if it works" or casual suggestions as to how to proceed will remove pressure from the situation, permitting the relaxation necessary for this therapy to be effective.

When imagery is used to augment some other therapy, such as in the case of chemotherapy in patients with cancer, it is important to emphasize the interrelationship of the two approaches. When a treatment such as chemotherapy has undesirable side effects, patients will sometimes look at alternative therapies as an excuse to discontinue the undesired treatment. The nurse must caution the patient concerning the importance of both treatment regimens.

Another precaution in using imagery is that the nurse should attempt to predict the physiologic effects of the treatment and make a judgment as to the desirability of these effects on the individual patient. For some patients, the effects of deep relaxation, such as slowing of the heart rate, are not desired. Other physical effects must also be anticipated. For example, when inducing "glove anesthesia," hand temperature is often lowered. This may be an undesirable effect in certain patients with circulatory problems.

It is unclear to this author if using imagery with psychotic patients is harmful. Several references (Ettin, 1982; Twente et al., 1978) report using imagery with psychotics without negative effects. McCaffery (1979), however, cautions against using this therapy with these patients. This author would advise that as it is the patient who has control of the image, it would appear that imagery would not be dangerous for such patients, but that only nurses with considerable experience with psychotic patients and with guided imagery should proceed with its use and should attempt to assist the patient to alter the image.

The nurse with little knowledge of psychotherapy should use caution in helping patients interpret symbolic material. One guideline is to determine the level of feeling or emotion which is being conveyed by the patient and to respond to the patient at this same level or a level only slightly deeper. When the patient is expressing emotion, a superficial response to the level of feeling expressed or response to a much deeper level of feeling than that actually expressed can be nontherapeutic. In instances where the conflict expressed by the patient is not interpretable or is not responsive to the nurse's intervention, the patient can be referred to a competent psychotherapist. In most instances, the nurse will find that patients are capable of using imagery to strengthen their own coping skills, and the nurse needs only to suggest how imagery can be used and gently guide their progress.

RESEARCH QUESTIONS

The major questions concerning imagery as an intervention in nursing can be summarized in one larger question: Under what conditions do particular imagery procedures produce what outcomes? Subquestions might include:

1. What are the characteristics of the image?
2. Must the image be of a specific degree of vividness?
3. What characteristics are necessary in the imager that can bring about visual, auditory, and kinesthetic images?
4. What kinds of images are effective in bringing about specific outcomes such as pain relief or improved immunologic function?
5. Are some types of images better than others?
6. Can outcomes be measured objectively?
7. What kinds of images promote relaxation?
8. Do imagery and relaxation techniques have interaction effects?

Practitioners have a responsibility to keep accurate records describing the interventions they use with such specificity that relevant variables can be identified and that the interventions can be replicated. Records must be specific as to both the desired and the unanticipated outcomes of the interventions. Researchers have a responsibility to define clearly the dependent and independent variables and to make their studies replicable. In the area of imagery there is a great deal to be learned that will benefit the patient and the practitioner of the future.

REFERENCES

Ballard, S., & Madsen, R. (1988). *Differentiating the effect of two types of imagery on pain response as mediated by self-consciousness, a personality trait.* Unpublished Master's paper. University of Minnesota, Minneapolis.

Ettin, M.F. (1982). Imagery in client-therapist communications. *American Journal of Psychoanalysis* 42:229–237.

Frank, J.M. (1985). The effects of music therapy and guided visual imagery on chemotherapy induced nausea and vomiting. *Oncology Nursing Forum* 12:47–52.

Gallegos, E.S. (1983). Animal imagery, the chakra system and psychotherapy. *Journal of Transpersonal Psychology* 15:125–136.

Geden, E.A., Beck, N., Hauge, G., & Pohlman, S. (1989). Self-report and psychophysiological effects of five pain-coping strategies. *Nursing Research* 33:260–265.

Geden, E.A., Lower, M., Beattie, S., & Beck, N. (1989). Effects of music and imagery on physiologic and self-report of analogued labor pain. *Nursing Research* 38:37–41.

Hall, M.D. (1983). Using relaxation imagery with children with malignancies: A developmental perspective. *American Journal of Clinical Hypnosis* 25:143–149.

Holden-Lund, C. (1988). Effects of relaxation with guided imagery on surgical stress and wound healing. *Research in Nursing and Health* 11:235–244.

Horowitz, M.J. (1988). *Image formation and cognition.* New York: Appleton-Century-Crofts.

Korn, E.R. (1983). The use of altered states of consciousness and imagery in physical and pain rehabilitation. *Journal of Mental Imagery* 7:25–34.

Kunzendorf, R.G. (1981). Individual differences in imagery and autonomic control. *Journal of Mental Imagery* 5:47–60.

Lang, P.J. (1979). A bio-informational theory of emotional imagery. *Psychophysiology* 16:495–512.

Leja, A.M. (1989). Using guided imagery to combat postsurgical depression. *Journal of Gerontological Nursing* 15:7–11.

LeShan, L. (1959). Psychological states as factors in the development of malignant disease: A critical review. *Journal of the National Cancer Institute* 22:1–18.

Leuner, H. (1977). Guided affective imagery: An account of its development. *Journal of Mental Imagery* 1:73–92.

____. (1978). Basic principles and therapeutic efficacy of guided affective imagery. Pp. 125–166 in J. Singer & K. Pope eds., *The power of human imagination.* New York: Plenum Press.

Lyles, J.N., Burish, T.G., Krozely, M.G., & Oldham, R.K. (1982). Efficacy of relaxation training and guided imagery in reducing the aversiveness of cancer chemotherapy. *Journal of Consulting and Clinical Psychology* 50:509–524.

Madden, M.J. (1982). *The symbolic world of obesity: A study of the rhetorical vision of obese women.* Doctoral dissertation. University of Minnesota, Minneapolis, MN.

Margolis, C.G. (1982). Hypnotic imagery with cancer patients. *American Journal of Clinical Hypnosis* 25:128–134.

McCaffery, M. (1979). *Nursing management of the patient with pain.* Philadelphia: J.B. Lippincott.

Raft, D., Smith, R.H., & Warred, N. (1986). Selection of imagery in the relief of chronic and acute clinical pain. *Journal of Psychosomatic Research* 30:481–488.

Rosenberg, S.W. (1982). Hypnosis in cancer care: Imagery to enhance the control of the physiological and psychological "side effects" of cancer therapy. *American Journal of Clinical Hypnosis* 25:122–127.

Schultz, J.H., & Luthe, W. (1959). *Autogenic therapy: A psychophysiologic approach in psychotherapy.* New York: Grune & Stratton.

Schwartz, G.E. (1976). Facial muscle patterning to affective imagery in depressed and nondepressed subjects. *Science* 192:489–491.

Shorr, J.E. (1978). Clinical use of categories of therapeutic imagery. Pp. 95–122 in J. Singer, & K. Pope eds., *The power of human imagination.* New York: Plenum Press.

Simonton, O.C., & Simonton, S.S. (1975). Belief system and management of the emotional aspects of malignancy. *Journal of Transpersonal Psychology* 7:24–47.

Simonton, O.C., Simonton, S.S., & Creighton, J.L. (1978). *Getting well again.* New York: Bantam Books.

Singer, J.L., & Pope, K.S. (1978). *The power of human imagination.* New York: Plenum Press.

Smith, D. (1982). Guided imagination as an intervention in hopelessness. *Journal of Psychiatric Nursing and Mental Health Services* 20:29–32.

Turner, P.E., Kohl, R.M., & Morris, L.W. (1982). Individual differences in skilled performance following imagery of bilateral skill. *Perceptual and Motor Skills* 55:771–780.

Twente, G.E., Turner, D., & Haney, J. (1978). Eidetics in the hospital setting and private practice: A report on eidetic therapy procedures employed with sixty-nine patients. *Journal of Mental Imagery* 2:275–290.

White, K., Sheehan, W., & Ashton, R. (1977). Imagery assessment: A survey of self-report measures. *Journal of Mental Imagery* 1:145–170.

CHAPTER 12

DECISIONAL CONTROL

(Note: Material in this chapter is based on content provided by A. Marilyn Sime for the first edition.)

BACKGROUND

The quest for personal control is prevalent in Western cultures (Moch, 1988). Empowering patients is frequently stated as a goal of nursing. Nurses often have assumed that providing patients with opportunities for making decisions regarding their care will result in stress reduction and promote self-care. Few studies, however, have explored decisional control and its implications for nursing practice. This chapter will document studies that have been done and provide content that will guide nurses in giving control to patients who desire it.

Definition

Personal control has been used in referring to a variety of types of control. Averill (1973) distinguished three types of personal control: behavioral control, cognitive control, and decisional control. Behavioral control relates to the performance of a direct action on the environment. The person engages in direct action that can change the event in some way or control when the event is encountered. Cognitive control includes obtaining and interpreting information and developing a cognitive plan of action. Specifically, cognitive control is the processing or use of information in such a way that a potential threat is objectively evaluated or appraised. The intervention of sensation information which is presented in Chapter 19 is an example of a cognitive control strategy. Decisional control, according to Averill (1973), is the choosing or contributing to choice of alternative courses of action. The individual may choose from among a number of options that are available. Decisional control and volitional control are used interchangeably.

Scientific Basis

Zimbardo (1969) was one of the first persons to study personal control. He studied persons' responses in situations in which external controls of behavior were removed, thus shifting control of behavior to internal constraints. Deindividuation was the term Zimbardo attached to this process. The person has the opportunity to engage in behaviors that are "freed from obligations, liabilities, and restrictions imposed by guilt, shame, and fear" (Zimbardo, 1969:248). These behaviors may, at times, be antisocial actions. This view of decisional control resulting from removal of external constraints to behavior suggests that too many response choices may lead to emotional, impulsive, and irrational behaviors.

Subjects in a study by Lewis and Blanchard (1971) were given the choice of whether they wished to give or receive an electric shock in a sham learning experiment. Three levels of choice were possible. High-choice subjects had complete freedom to be the giver or receiver. All chose to be the giver of the shock to the learner. In the middle-choice group, it was suggested to some that they be the giver and to others that they be the receivers, but all were given the choice of either role. In the no-choice group, subjects were assigned to be givers or receivers. Results demonstrated that perception of freedom of choice depended upon the role assumed or assigned. Those in the role of giver, the more desirable role, reported more freedom of choice even if they were assigned to the role. Averill (1973), in a discussion of the study, concluded that persons experience choice when they are acting according to their beliefs or doing that with which they agree.

Langer and Rodin (1976) studied the effects of enhanced choice and responsibility on nursing home residents. Subjects in the experimental group were told that they could decide such things as how to arrange their rooms, activities in which they wished to engage, and what night to attend a movie. They also were given an opportunity to accept (all did) or reject having a plant, the type of plant, and the care the plant needed. The comparison group was told about the staff's responsibility to them and which night they were to attend the movie. They were given a plant but were told that the staff would care for it. Assessments made after three weeks revealed that subjects in the experimental group were more alert, engaged in more activities, and had a greater sense of well-being than subjects in the comparison group. A follow-up assessment at 18 months (Rodin & Langer, 1977) documented that subjects in the control group continued to be more happy, alert, and active than subjects in the comparison group.

Kallio (1979) conducted a study on effects of decisional control in patients in a critical care unit. He reasoned that if the stresses of the critical care unit resulted in learned helplessness, a prediction consistent with Seligman's theory of learned helplessness (1975), the provision of elements of decisional control should result in the reduction of stress responses. Subjects in the control group received a taped orientation message about the unit, equipment, and staff. No information on decisional control was provided. Subjects in the experimental group were provided with a taped message that described decisional control opportunities that would be available to them. These included how they wished to display their cards, letters, flowers, and plant; when they wished to sit in the chair or walk; when they wished to have their bath; and if they wished to watch television or listen to the radio. Subjects who were provided with the opportunity for decisional control reported less fatigue, anxiety, anger, and depression than did subjects in the control group. They also perceived a statistically significant increase in the amount of control that they had over daily activities.

In two studies on control in hospitalized patients, Dennis (1987, 1990) found that patients want to know, understand, and be given information on diagnostic tests, therapies, and surgeries they will have and what these mean to their daily living. Dennis (1987) concluded "that patients did want to have control over the people and events that had an impact on their well-being and quality of life while they were in the hospital" (p. 154). However, she found that not all patients wished to have control or to have control over all events.

INTERVENTION

Findings from the above studies revealed that the scope of activities given to patients for them to make decisions about were quite narrow in scope. Caution is needed, however, to insure that the activities chosen are ones for which the patient can have control.

Technique

The work of Zimbardo (1969) suggests that choice options be limited in number. Options provided by Kallio (1979) were quite circumscribed. Kallio discussed only decisions related to display of greeting cards, placement of flowers, time of ambulation and bath, and choices regarding reading materials, radio, and television programming. Instructions indicated that patients were free to make decisions related to these areas; they were not forced to do so. The opportunity for decisional control was provided, not required.

Options provided by Kallio (1979) were personally meaningful to the patients. Decisional options need to be presented very explicitly and clearly. A part of the Kallio (1979) message was:

> ...you may wish to have your cards from your friends or family displayed on the wall so you can see them better. Or you may want them arranged on the window ledge or even kept in a drawer. You may take care of your cards however you desire. [p. 95]

This kind of clarity and explicitness is critical for the decisional control opportunity to have meaning for the patient and for the patient to actually perceive that the opportunity is a reality.

Nurses need to give attention to the nature of the options that will be provided to the patient. What are areas in which the patient can have control? Boeing and Mongera (1989) listed the following as nursing interventions that can give more control to patients in critical care units:

> Allowing patient and family to establish times to visit.
> Providing the patient control over lighting, television, etc.
> Providing a choice on diversional activities.
> Establishing a method for communication that is effective for the patient and family.

Once these have been identified and presented to the patient, the staff must be consistent in providing these options to the patient. Fuchs (1987) noted that recording these care decisions in the plan of care and staff members respecting and following the plan is important.

Measurement of Effectiveness

Most measures of outcomes for decisional control have involved mood states, behavioral activity, and perception of control. Observer reports and self-reports, such as the Profile of Mood States, have been used in measuring mood states. Engagement in activities such as reading, visiting, and sitting alone has been used to measure behavioral activities (Langer & Rodin, 1976). A rating scale has been used to measure the patient's perception of control (Kallio, 1979).

The nurse using the intervention of decisional control will need to identify specific outcomes desired with patients for whom it is being used. Those desired outcomes will vary depending on the condition of the patient and the presence of situational constraints.

USES

Decisional control has been shown to be an effective intervention with elderly in nursing homes (Langer & Rodin, 1976; Schulz, 1976) and patients in critical care units (Kallio, 1979). In addition, Dennis (1987, 1990) demonstrated that hospitalized patients desired to make decisions regarding diagnosis, treatment, and surgery. Fuchs (1987) suggested that decisional control would be beneficial in combating powerlessness in patients in renal failure.

Although minimal research has been done on the use of decisional control, it appears that vulnerable populations would benefit from being provided with the opportunity to make decisions on various aspects of care and the environment.

Precautions

As has been noted in previous sections, adequate assessment of patients is needed to determine if a person wants to make decisions. Patients need to have the freedom to accept or reject the opportunity. Moch (1988) discusses the personal control/uncontrol balance that persons may desire. She proposes that nurses need to be attentive to a patient's letting go of control over a situation. Also, the number of options provided should be limited so as not to overwhelm the patient.

A second area in which care is needed is that the decisional control options must be realistic and actually available to the patient. For example, a patient may be offered the opportunity to select when he/she would like to eat. However, this may not be a feasible option in the hospital or nursing home. Patients may become depressed or feel more helpless as a result.

RESEARCH

As was indicated, few studies have been done on the intervention of decisional control. Dennis (1987, 1990) has provided some perspectives on control in hospitalized patients. However, several types of control were addressed. Areas in which additional research is needed include:

1. What are the characteristics of persons who would benefit from decisional control and those of persons for whom it should not be used? Assessment instruments to do this also are needed.
2. Most research on decisional control has involved situations presumed to be stressful. It is unclear whether the research results to date represent a main effect of choice or an interaction effect of stress and choice.
3. How do the outcomes from decisional control compare with the use of behavioral or cognitive control interventions?

REFERENCES

Averill, J.R. (1973). Personal control over aversive stimuli and its relationship to stress. *Psychological Bulletin* 80:286–303.

Boeing, M.H., & Mongera, C.O. (1989). Powerlessness in critical care patients. *Dimensions of Critical Care Nursing* 8:274–279.

Dennis, K.E. (1987). Dimensions of client control. *Nursing Research* 36:151–156.

____. (1990). Patient's control and the information imperative: Clarification and confirmation. *Nursing Research* 39:162–166.

Fuchs, J. (1987). Use of decisional control to combat powerlessness. *ANNA* 14(1):11–13, 56.

Kallio, J.T. (1979). *The relationship among perceived control, mood state, and perception of nursing care for a control-induced and comparison group of patients in the critical care setting.* Unpublished Master's thesis, University of Minnesota, Minneapolis, MN.

Langer, E.J., & Rodin, J. (1976). The effects of choice and enhanced personal responsibility for the aged: A field experiment in an institutional setting. *Journal of Personality and Social Psychology* 34:191–196.

Lewis, P., & Blanchard, E.B. (1971). Perception of choice and locus of control. *Psychological Reports* 28:67–70.

Moch, S.D. (1988). Towards a personal control/uncontrol balance. *Journal of Advanced Nursing* 13: 119–123.

Rodin, J., & Langer, E.J. (1977). Long-term effects of a control-relevant intervention with the institutionalized aged. *Journal of Personality and Social Psychology* 35:897–902.

Schulz, R. (1976). Effects of control and predictability on the physical and psychological well-being of the institutionalized aged. *Journal of Personality and Social Psychology* 33:563–573.

Seligman, M.E. (1975). *Helplessness: On depression, development, and death.* San Francisco: W. H. Freeman and Company.

Zimbardo, P.G. (1969). The human choice: Individuation, reason, and order versus deindividuation, impulse, and class. In D. Levine ed., *Nebraska symposium on motivation: 1969.* Lincoln: University of Nebraska Press.

CHAPTER 13

JOURNAL

BACKGROUND

Journals have been used extensively by persons throughout history. Libraries abound with volumes of personal journals; countless other journals are found in drawers and attics. The journals of explorers such as Marco Polo provide us with a vivid picture not only of the places visited but also reactions to the new culture encountered. *Markings* by Dag Hammarskjold (1964), former Secretary General of the United Nations, reveals his inner struggle and growth and has had an impact on succeeding generations.

A review of nursing literature revealed little documentation on the use of journals as a nursing intervention. Logs and journals have been used as a teaching strategy by nurse educators. They have been used in ascertaining ethical decision-making (Crisham, personal communication, 1984), increasing staff sensitivity to the dying patient (Burkhalter, 1975), keeping the instructor abreast of care provided to community health patients, and helping students deal with fears and concerns generated in caring for patients with psychiatric disorders. Although minimal data were found for the use of journals as a nursing intervention, it is the author's belief that journaling is a viable and useful strategy for nurses to use with a variety of patient populations. Progoff (1975) contended that keeping a journal enables persons to draw on their inherent resources and strengthen their inner capacities. Thus, journals promote independence, which is a goal of many nursing models. This chapter will provide a basis for using journals for specific patient conditions. It is anticipated that the reader will identify other populations for whom journals would be an appropriate intervention. A graduate nursing student who used the journal as an intervention with young persons who had chronic neurological conditions remarked:

> It is a creative intervention for the client and includes the client in all phases of the process.
> Of course, research will need to be done in this area to prove its worth. [Stenglein, 1984:22]

Definition

What differentiates a journal from a diary? According to Baldwin (1977), a diary is a more formal pattern of daily entries and merely a record of observations and experiences. A journal, on the other hand, is a tool for recording the process of one's life (Baldwin, 1977). Diaries are more superficial, recording facts and events. Journals contain experiences and activities but also incorporate the person's reflections and the impact these events have on the person's total life. The interplay between the conscious and the unconscious characterizes journal entries.

Baldwin (1977) enumerated three assumptions she believed implicit in the journal process. They are:

1. A person is capable of having a relationship with one's own mind.
2. This relationship will be intelligent and essentially benevolent. Journal writing is asking the mind to reveal that which is waiting for attention in the unconscious.
3. This activity is valid and essential for a person's well-being.

Scientific Basis

Different results occur when the thought process is written than when it is spoken (Baldwin, 1977). Journal recording requires coordination among memory, muscular movements, and feedback from sight and sound (if the entries are subsequently read). Writing necessitates a slower process than talking, allowing for reflection on the content that has been written.

Ira Progoff, a psychologist from the Jungian school, has been foremost in developing a systematized method for journal keeping. *At a Journal Workshop* (1975) provides the basis for the use of the Intensive Journal format and guidance in its use. He views this transpsychological approach as, "providing active techniques that enable the individual to draw upon his inherent resources for becoming a whole person" [p. 9]. Through the use of the techniques prescribed, the person discovers capabilities that he did not know he possessed. Progoff (1975) stated:

> The *Intensive Journal* process and its procedures for the person's work provide an instrument and a method by which we can develop interior capacities strong enough to be relied upon in meeting trials of our life. It gives us a means of private and personal discipline with which to develop our inner muscles. When we rely upon these, we are indeed self-reliant because these inner capacities are ourselves. [p.15]

Through journal recording persons are able to connect themselves with the continuity, the inner thread, of their lives and thus enhance integration and wholeness. Awareness of this continuity occurs as the person reflects on specific events and periods, records them, and then carries out a dialogue linking past and present events and reactions to them.

Journals can be helpful during times of change precipitated by circumstances external to the person. Reviewing how one handled previous changes may offer suggestions on how to handle the present situation. Reflection on journal entries also may suggest changes that a person should make (Simons, 1978). Knowing oneself better may pave the way for establishing new goals in life. Baldwin (1977) stated that in keeping a journal, the person assumes responsibility for his/her own growth and possesses the power to deal with life. The journal record also may suggest to the person when assistance from others is needed.

Keeping a journal is particularly beneficial during times of conflict and difficulty; it also is useful during relaxed periods when deepening is desired (Progoff, 1975). Developmental points, such as adolescence, middle age, and retirement, are specific times when journals have been an effective intervention.

INTERVENTION

Many techniques exist for journal recording. Baldwin (1977) described flow writing. This is merely writing down thoughts that occur and elaborating on these. The *Intensive Journal* of Progoff (1975) is a systematic manner for dividing and recording entries and dialoguing with and between specific sections. Simons' (1978) technique is similar to Progoff's method, but it contains fewer sections. The technique proposed by Progoff will be presented in this chapter along with modifications that would facilitate its use as a nursing intervention.

Technique

Progoff (1975) saw the primary purpose in using journals as helping the person establish and strengthen personal integrity. Journals kept in a manner that did not help the person grow or that were narrow in focus were viewed by Progoff as being more detrimental than beneficial. The method used for the *Intensive Journal* grew out of data he gathered from studying lives of creative persons. A structure was established for the workbook that enables the person to reflect and carry forward the process of growth that is occurring

Table 13.1
Sections in the *Intensive Journal Workbook* (Progoff, 1975)

Life/Time Dimension
    Life history log
    Steppingstones
    Intersections
    Roads taken and not taken
    Now: the open moment

Dialogue Dimension
    Dialogue with persons
    Dialogue with work
    Dialogue with society
    Dialogue with events
    Dialogue with the body

Depth Dimension
    Dream log
    Dream enlargements
    Twilight imagery log
    Imagery extensions
    Inner Wisdom Dialogue

Period Log

Daily Log

in his/her life. Exercises were devised to assist persons in exploring the contents of their lives through use of the various sections of the *Intensive Journal*. An entry in one section evokes memories related to other sections. Thus, the person moves between and among the various sections.

The majority of persons are introduced to the *Intensive Journal* at workshops conducted by Progoff and his associates. A workbook, which is divided into sections, is used to guide the process. During the workshop instructions on the use of the workbook are presented and persons begin to make entries into many of the sections.

Table 13.1 presents the 19 sections of Progoff's *Intensive Journal* (1975). These miniprocesses fit into three clusters: Life/Time Dimension, Dialogue Dimension, and Depth Dimension. Each has a specific place in helping the person explore his/her life, become more self-reliant, and grow. In addition, a period log and a daily log are used.

The first dimension, Life/Time, focuses on the continuity of the person's life. It is central to the rest of the journal in that all experiences occur in a time frame. Included in these miniprocesses are all phenomena that relate to the progression of experiences and cumulatively form one's life history. According to Progoff (1975):

> Working in our life history is progressive. Its cumulative effect is to draw our life into focus so that we have a basis for making decisions that are pressing at the moment, and also to give us a perspective of the pattern and context of our life as a whole. [p. 98]

The sections of the Life/Time Dimension include Life History Log, Steppingstones, Intersections, Roads Taken and Not Taken, and Now: The Open Moment. Facts of one's past life are included in the Life

History Log. These are recorded without judgment or censorship. In Steppingstones, the person records the significant points of movement from life's beginning to the present. The section Intersections explores moments of choice and why certain decisions were made. Unlived possibilities can be explored in the section of Roads Taken and Not Taken. Now: The Open Moment section provides the person with opportunity to decide how he will proceed in the future based on the knowledge gained about self in the use of the journal process.

Sections included in the Dialogue Dimension are Dialogue with Persons, Dialogue with Work, Dialogue with Society, Dialogue with Events, and Dialogue with the Body. The purpose of these sections is to help the person bring diverse life areas into relation to each other. In the Dialogue with Persons section, the aim is to draw forth the potential relationships with various persons present. This is a very important aspect of one's life. By reflecting on one's work in Dialogue with Work, the person gains insight into works that are possible and evolves tangible ways for accomplishing them that will enhance growth as a total person. Steppingstones in the development of one's body are described in the Dialogue with Body section. Recognition of the fullness and continuity of the body is an expected outcome. Events that have had a meaningful impact on one's life and occurrences that are outside self but have an inner importance are recorded in the section Dialogue with Events. The purpose of the Dialogue with Society section is to help the person integrate a relationship with the larger aspect of humanity. Dialogues with one's culture or nation are recorded.

Five sections, Dream Log, Dream Enlargements, Twilight Imagery Log, Imagery Extensions, and Inner Wisdom Dialogue, compose the Depth Dimension. In the Depth Dimension sections the person moves from the purely personal to the deeper than personal areas of life. Considerable attention is paid to dreams as they reflect the tensions and anxieties of life. Past dreams that can be recalled are written down in the Dream Log. These are reflected upon in the Dream Enlargement Section; the dreams are re-entered so that they can be continued to conclusion. The Twilight Imagery Log and Imagery Extensions sections are similar to the two dream sections; in Twilight Imagery, images generated when the person is sitting quietly are recorded and then later expanded upon. One of the key sections of the entire process is the Inner Wisdom Dialogue Section; it is the culmination of the process. The person seeks to establish a dialogue relationship with possibilities of spiritual contact and a larger awareness that reflect the depth of one's inner wisdom.

Two sections of the Intensive Journal that are not part of the three dimensions described above are the Period Log and the Daily Log. These two sections are worked on first. Entries for the Period Log come from sitting quietly and focusing on one's present life and the images that are generated. These are then recorded in a brief fashion unless something is very poignant. A checklist of things to be recorded includes physical aspects of one's life that are important, events relating to social or political issues, and any events or occurrences that were extremely meaningful. The importance at this time is to record the events and feelings in a nonjudgmental fashion. Later, these are re-read and serve as the basis for entries in other sections.

The Daily Log provides the person with the opportunity to record events and reactions as they happen. Recording the event when it is fresh in one's memory allows for feelings and subtle features to be written down. Progoff (1975) noted that as much as possible the focus should be on the essence of the experience. Too often persons list the event but do not relate the accompanying mental images or emotional feelings. Again, the entries are made in a nonjudgmental manner.

Writing thoughts and feelings may be therapeutic in and of itself. A critical element of journal writing is re-reading the entry after recording it. The reading may be done silently or aloud. Progoff (1975) found that reading aloud made a stronger impact on the person than silent reading. One also may return to past entries and read these to help in gaining insight into one's present life.

The method of Progoff entails much interaction between and among the sections. The person uses the material in the sections to become more aware of his/her total being and this serves as an impetus for growth. Because of the many sections and specific functions for each, a neophyte may feel overwhelmed. It is suggested that the nurse select those sections that would be most appropriate for the patient at this particular

Table 13.2

Important Points to Remember in Keeping a Journal

1. Be brief—only write as much as necessary to get your point across.
2. Do not worry about spelling, grammar, or sentences.
3. It is not a lot of work—the more you use it, the easier it will become.
4. Start with the period section, and always focus on the now of your life.
5. Write in the daily log everyday or at least three times a week.
6. You must make at least one positive statement about yourself, your strengths or your abilities in every entry.
7. Review your daily log at least every week, and rewrite all the positive comments you have made about yourself since your last entry.
8. Record all of your feelings about your body and then concentrate on ways of changing your attitudes and ways of coping with and accepting your condition—keep a proper perspective; your body and your condition are only a small part of you.
9. If you stop writing for awhile, do not give up—Start again.
10. Your journal is private; it is only for your eyes; be honest with yourself.
11. Do not analyze too much—by re-reading your entries you will get the feedback you need to help you grow.

Source: From E. Stenglein (1984). *Help yourself grow.* Unpublished manuscript, University of Minnesota, School of Nursing, Minneapolis, MN. Used with permission.

time. Use of the Daily and Period Logs would usually be very helpful. Stenglein (1984) added the Dialogue with Body section to the Daily and Period Logs in working with persons with physical disabilities. The directions she developed for keeping a journal are given in Table 13.2. In addition to daily entries, Simons (1978) advocated using dialogues with people, body, work, dreams, important moments, feelings, and unfinished plans.

Simons (1978) presented a number of techniques that were helpful to persons beginning the journal process. Constructing a clock and asking the self what time it is in one's life is one strategy. The person answers questions such as is it too late or too soon for specific activities. Identifying time needed for activities or persons is another variation of responding to a clock. Developing a road map is another technique. The person indicates life goals and the routes and detours actually taken, along with the feelings that accompanied these choices. Plans for the future can be mapped out. Death and rebirth is a third technique described by Simons. Persons list five things that are dying in their lives and five that are being born. One from each list is selected and expanded on, including feelings, hindrances, and helps.

Recording

Many types of books exist for recording journal entries. A loose-leaf notebook has an advantage over the bound book as it allows for pages to be added, removed, or placed side by side for comparison and contrast. Notebooks are relatively inexpensive. Whatever type of book is used, it should be used solely for making journal entries.

Some people like to use different colored pens for various types of entries. Because reference to past entries is important in the use of journals, the entries should be made in ink as pencil fades over time.

Time to Write

When persons begin to use a journal, making daily entries is important. Simons (1978) noted that fidelity is needed for the journal experience to be therapeutic. Setting aside 15 to 30 minutes at a particular time each day is helpful for establishing the habit. Some persons find it useful to carry their notebook with them so entries can be made at various times of the day. Progoff stressed the importance of a quiet atmosphere for reflecting and writing. Journal writing should be the servant and not the master (Simons, 1978). After writing has become a habit, entries can be made when the need is felt, which may or may not be on a daily basis.

Private Versus Group

Progoff uses workshops for teaching his *Intensive Journal* process. At points, persons volunteer to read portions of their entry sections aloud. Guided journal support groups were suggested by Baldwin (1977) as a way to assist persons beginning to use journals. These meet once or twice a month. Journal entries may also be used as the basis for therapy sessions. Sharing journal entries, however, should always be on a volunteer basis. When teaching this intervention to a patient, the nurse stresses the privacy of the entries and that the person does not have to share the recorded matter with anyone unless he or she chooses to do so.

Measurement of Effectiveness

It is difficult to measure the effectiveness of journals because the intended outcomes may appear long after the intervention was taught. Depending on the intent of the intervention, outcomes could be established, however, that will provide the nurse with information on whether or not there is movement toward the goal. Handling major life changes without undue anxiety, improvement in self-esteem as measured by more positive statements about self or improvement on self-esteem scales, and self-statements about improved feelings of well-being are some indicators that can be used for measuring progress. Indices for determining overall well-being could also be used.

USES

Journals can be useful in a variety of situations. Areas for use of journals include persons undergoing or facing a change, persons with low self-esteem, persons desiring improved well-being, as a diagnostic tool, and as an adjunct to psychotherapy. The first four uses will be detailed.

Change

Numerous anecdotal references can be found that document beneficial effects of journal use during times of change. Losses due to death, separation, or chronic illnesses require changes. Keeping a journal may assist the person to uncover feelings associated with the loss and to identify ways to adapt to the change. Simons (1978) noted that journals were an effective intervention at turning points in one's life, including securing a new position, going away to college, getting married, and retiring from work. Journals help to prepare the person for the inner changes needed to accompany external life changes (Baldwin, 1977). Journals provide a person with internal and external support systems during periods of change. A nurse who was working with persons who had AIDS found journaling to be beneficial for this population.

Self-Esteem

According to Simons (1978), keeping a journal provides a person with a clearer sense of self. For persons who are experiencing a change in their body, that is, paralysis from a spinal cord injury, a journal may help them identify personal resources that can be used for building a future that at first had appeared bleak. A form of journal recording is used in the intervention of thought-stopping; the person records when negative thoughts occur and the associated events and feelings. The person is instructed to generate positive thoughts about self. Stenglein (1984) had patients with physical disabilities converse with their body; at the end of the conversation, they were to record one positive fact about their body. These recordings then helped persons to use their strengths in adapting to and living with their disability.

Well-Being

Health promotion and prevention of illness are often cited as outcomes of nursing actions. Journals can be used effectively in helping patients become more self-reliant and achieve a higher health status. Progoff (1975) believed that previously untapped knowledge is activated through the journal process. Keeping a journal provides the person with a way of responding independently to one's own growth from one's own viewpoint and seeing self as healthy and evolving (Baldwin, 1977). Interaction with the various journal sections promotes a more integrated self. Runions (1984) instructed the mother of a seriously ill adolescent to keep a journal. The intervention proved to be very helpful to the mother; it assisted her in handling the information being provided and in coping with the crisis.

Diagnostic Tool

Kolkmeier (1982) incorporated use of journals into the biofeedback training of persons with hypertension. Patients were asked to record their reactions to stressful situations, practice of relaxation, and general feeling of well-being or presence of symptoms. These recordings served as the basis for discussion with the nurse at clinic visits. Keeping a journal helps the person detect problems; persons often know something is wrong long before they know what it is that is bothering them (Baldwin, 1977). Sharing these feelings and findings may help uncover the underlying problem. Murray (1985) utilized the diary for studying the occurrence of symptoms in persons with psychological problems. Numerous other studies have documented the effectiveness of diaries in promoting adherence to therapeutic regimens (Verbrugge, 1980).

Precautions

Journals are not for everyone (Simons, 1978). The nurse can provide the patient with information about the journal process, but if the person is not attentive to keeping the journal, other interventions need to be considered. Fear that others will find and read the entries deters some persons from keeping a journal. For journaling to be truly effective, there is need for it to be private; nurses should not pressure patients to share entries. Journals should be prescribed with caution for persons who tend to be extremely introspective. Close monitoring of this group of patients will detect if journal recording is intensifying introspection and withdrawal. Simons (1978) noted that the journal may be useful in healing memories and helping the person become less introspective.

Nurses need to have an understanding of journals and knowledge of the particular form being used. Continued guidance and follow-up are necessary after the technique has been explained. Because little research has been done on the use of journals, careful attention to the effects on the patient and the attainment of outcomes is essential.

RESEARCH QUESTIONS

The formal use of journals as a nursing intervention has received minimal attention in the literature. This chapter has suggested some patient conditions for which it seems to be an appropriate intervention. Systematic investigations are needed to determine if the journal is an effective intervention. The following are only a few of the many questions for which definitive data are needed:

1. What technique(s) is practical and effective for use in clinical practice? Progoff's method is well developed, but its complexity makes it rather impractical for use in limited time frames or for persons under extreme stress.
2. What are the characteristics of persons who benefit most from journals? What are the characteristics of persons for whom journals should not be prescribed. McKinney (1982) found that 43% of students he studied were enthusiastic about keeping a journal.
3. Does the use of journals aid persons in accepting chronic illness or disability?
4. Does group teaching and use foster daily journal writing? Does use of groups improve the outcomes obtained?

REFERENCES

Baldwin, C. (1977). *One to one*. New York: M. Evans and Co.

Burkhalter, P. (1975). Fostering staff sensitivity to the dying patient. *Supervisor Nurse* 6(4):54–59.

Hammarskjold, D. (1964). *Markings*. London: Faber & Faber.

Kolkmeier, L. (1982). Biofeedback-relaxation therapy for hypertension. *Topics in Clinical Nursing* 3(4):69–74.

McKinney, F. (1982). Free writing as therapy. Pp. 60–65 in E. Nickerson & K. O'Laughlin eds., *Helping through action: action-oriented therapies*. Amherst, MA: Human Resources Development Press.

Murray, J. (1985). The use of health diaries in the field of psychiatric illness in general practice. *Psychological Medicine* 15:827–840.

Progoff, I. (1975). *At a journal workshop*. New York: Dialogue House Library.

Runions, J. (1984). The diary: a self-directed approach to coping with stress. *Canadian Nurse* 80(5):24–28.

Simons, G. (1978). *Keeping your personal journal*. New York: Paulist Press.

Stenglein, E. (1984). *Help yourself use a journal*. Unpublished manuscript, University of Minnesota, School of Nursing, Minneapolis.

Verbrugge, L. (1980). Health diaries. *Medical Care* 13:73–95.

CHAPTER 14

REMINISCENCE

BACKGROUND

"Mrs. Johnson is living in the past. That's all she wants to talk about. If only we could get her to think about what she has to do today." Such statements often are made by nurses, other health professionals, and family members concerning elderly persons. Until recently, elders' engagement in reflecting on and talking about the past has been viewed negatively (Coleman, 1986). Reminiscing about the past, however, can assist the person in making the adaptations necessary for meaningful living. Reminiscence is an intervention used to achieve specific outcomes.

Talking about past accomplishments is an integral aspect of tribal societies. It is their medium for transmitting the history and traditions of their culture to future generations. Everyone reminisces, but this is not always done in as orderly a fashion as is done in life histories (McMordie & Blom, 1979). Reminiscing begins at about age ten and continues throughout life (Havighurst & Glasser, 1972).

Whereas reminiscing has been used largely as an intervention with the elderly, it also has been used with younger persons who have conditions in which death is imminent. Chubon (1980) found life review to be beneficial in working with younger persons who have end-stage renal disease. As nurses become more familiar with reminiscence and use it, other populations and conditions for which it is appropriate may be identified.

Definition

Two terms, life review and reminiscence, have been used interchangeably when referring to the process of reflecting on one's past life. Burnside (1990) differentiates between the two interventions. Reminiscence is supportive with the aim being not to increase anxiety; life decisions and life-style are reinforced. In contrast, the intent of life review is to uncover past events; it involves recalling the past and working through the feelings associated with life events. Anxiety may be increased during this process. Despite clear delineations between these two interventions, many persons continue to use the two terms interchangeably.

Butler (1963) defined life review as:

> A naturally occurring, universal mental process characterized by the progressive return to consciousness of past experiences, and particularly, the resurgence of unresolved conflicts; simultaneously, and normally, these reviewed experiences and conflicts can be surveyed and integrated. [p. 66]

This definition points out the therapeutic usefulness of reviewing one's past life. Life review, according to Lewis and Butler (1974), is a universal mental process brought about by the realization that life is waning and death is approaching.

Less precise definitions were found for reminiscence. King (1982) defined it as "memory that has been filtered through time and altered by the person's other life experiences" (p. 22). Reminiscence has been viewed by many as simply the process of recalling past life experiences. Reminiscence, in this chapter, is defined as a planned strategy to help persons recall past events, feelings, and thoughts.

McMahon and Rhudick (1964) identified three types of reminiscence: Glorifies the past and berates the present, storytelling, and life review. The person who glorifies the past often has difficulties adjusting to the present life situation. In storytelling about the past, the person is bitter about neither the past nor the present, but merely recounts episodes that have happened. Life review tends to be used by those who feel guilt or remorse about the past and need to justify their lives. It provides for the completion of unfinished business. Merriman (1989) cites a number of types of reminiscence including recreational and therapeutic reminiscence (Clements, 1982). Recreational reminiscence is light and fun; it is that which persons do when sitting around and recalling the "good old days." In contrast, therapeutic reminiscing is work and it may be painful.

Scientific Basis

Reminiscence is an adaptive strategy that helps the person compensate for the many losses currently being experienced and for past inadequacies (Ryden, 1981). Erikson's (1950) final developmental stage is that of ego integrity versus despair. In this stage the person accepts his life cycle as something that had to occur and in which no substitutions are permitted. Unless this occurs the person despairs and becomes depressed. According to Ryden (1981), reminiscence is a natural healing process. It is a part of the letting go, a realization that the past is past and that what happened during life was all right. Ebersole (1976a) contended that until persons have dealt with feelings about the past, they are unable to deal with the present.

Reminiscing helps the person maintain self-esteem. Recalling past accomplishments helps elderly persons gain pride about what they have done in life (Matteson & Munsat, 1982). Boylin et al. (1976) found a significant correlation between frequency of reminiscing and scores on a measure of ego adjustment in a group of institutionalized elderly males. Using a group process for reminiscence, Hala (1975) found participants took more interest in personal hygiene and had an improved self-concept. The findings of McMahon and Rhudick (1964) are in agreement with this; they found that veterans who reminisced were better adjusted and had a higher self-esteem and self-identity than those who did not reminisce as much. Beadleson-Baird and Lara (1988) reported that use of reminiscence decreased anxiety and depression in acutely ill geriatric patients.

Reminiscence may assist persons in using their creative potential for furthering personality integration (Postema, 1971). Reviewing the past suggests to the patient and the nurse how the individual previously has solved problems and approached situations; these data may be helpful to the person in dealing with present concerns. Pincus (1970) noted that reminiscing helps the elderly cope with the stresses inherent in advancing age.

Persons who seem to be focusing on the past may be struggling with developmental tasks associated with ego integrity (Ryden, 1981). Both the positive and the negative aspects of the person's past need to be explored. Reminiscence allows the person an opportunity to resolve conflicts in the past and to rid the self of guilt associated with them.

The studies done on the use of reminiscence with elderly persons suggest that it is an effective strategy in assisting persons to adapt to their present life situation and to continue to grow and be productive. Less evidence is available to support its use with other populations, but findings from its use with elderly persons suggest that it should be explored as useful for patients who are facing death or life crises.

INTERVENTION

Technique

Reminiscence has been used on an individual basis and with groups. More studies have been done on its use in groups than on an individual basis. It is difficult to determine if the effects obtained resulted from being part of a group or from the use of reminiscence. However, use of reminiscence in a group has much merit. Both approaches will be presented with indications for when each would be the most appropriate to use. Simple reminiscence will be differentiated from life review.

Individual

A time is established with the patient, and the time and length of each session is adhered to. The nurse is seated next to the patient so that both are comfortable. Being a good listener is important, especially when the same content seems to be repeated at each session and sometimes several times during a session. Repetitive content cues the nurse to further explore this area. It may mean that the person has not completed dealing with this content; unresolved conflict or guilt concerning the episode may exist.

Verbally supporting recall of past events and asking open-ended questions are ways in which the nurse can stimulate the patient to explore the past. Expression of both positive and negative feelings is encouraged, with the nurse empathizing and acknowledging both (Ryden, 1981). If the nurse does not feel competent in handling the negative feelings that are being expressed, referrals to clergy or psychiatric clinical specialists are made.

The patient may wish to record events and memories recalled. These serve as a legacy to family and friends. Other patients may wish to incorporate pictures and mementos along with the written material. Wax (1983) found that poetry was an excellent mode for helping aged deaf recall their past and express feelings about events and memories. She began the session by reading Robert Frost's poem, "The Road Not Taken." Poems written by the group fit into four groupings: memories; loss, change, and bereavement; awareness of changing status and roles; and present experiences. Merriman (1989) found that the structure of reminiscence comprised four components: selection, immersion, withdrawal, and closure.

The number of sessions needed that specifically address reminiscence will vary from patient to patient. The nurse may find that initially several sessions a week are most therapeutic, but reducing these to once a week or less is possible as time progresses. Informing family members about the value of recalling the past and serving as the listener may assist families in helping elderly members. Because of the negative connotations associated with "living in the past," family members may often discourage reflections on past events.

An advantage of one-to-one sessions is that a relationship is established between the nurse and the patient (McMordie & Blom, 1979). Individual sessions require less planning and coordinating than is required for group sessions. One-to-one is best for persons with short attention spans as the length of sessions can be tailored to fit with this deficit. Persons who are very withdrawn may, at first, respond better in individual sessions.

Group

Groups frequently are used for reminiscing. One-hour sessions held once a week are common. Lappe (1987) used reminiscence with groups for a 10-week period; significant improvement in self-esteem scores occurred. It is important that the time and place be established before the group is begun. If either is changed after the group is initiated, patients may become confused or upset.

Authors differed in the number of participants they believed should compose a reminiscence group. McMordie and Blom (1979) believed that a group should comprise four to eight members. This size group could incorporate one or two patients with cognitive impairments. Ebersole (1976a) recommended groups of seven to ten members. If patients tend to be more disoriented or agitated, a smaller number is best so that individual problems can be addressed.

According to McMordie and Blom (1979), elderly do best in structured situations. They held group meetings once a week for ten weeks and used the theme of progression through life. The first session focused on childhood with succeeding sessions progressing to the present. Themes such as holidays, seasons, sports, or ethnic events can be used for specific sessions. Group membership should be stable over time to promote cohesiveness (Ebersole, 1976a). Group consensus is used if another person wishes to join the group.

Running a reminiscence group requires special skills to keep the group on target, particularly if a number of the members have deficits that prevent them from giving full attention to the topic. Ebersole (1976b) presented suggestions for handling some of the problems encountered in reminiscence groups. When repetitive content persists, the leader can ask for elaboration on it or events that are related to the topic. Assuring everyone that each person will have his or her time to speak helps prevent simultaneous monologues. Sometimes members of a group do not begin to express their feelings until the group has met several times; strategies to encourage members to participate are needed. A planned topic for each session helps to prevent this. Provisions to decrease the problems arising from deficits need to be made. These include the reduction of outside noises so that persons can hear and having members speak loudly enough so that those with hearing deficits can feel like full participants.

Lewis and Butler (1974) used a variety of strategies in life-review psychotherapy sessions with individuals. Methods that were effective in eliciting memories and that were also enjoyable for the patient included developing written or taped autobiographies; making pilgrimages to past events in person or through correspondence; attending reunions; doing a genealogy; referring to scrapbooks, photo albums, and old letters; and summing up one's life work. The latter technique is particularly appropriate for persons who do not have children or have little contact with their children.

Sherman (1987) incorporated relaxation techniques into their life review sessions. After the relaxation component, participants were directed to silently focus on something that they felt good about or enjoyed; attention was directed to the pleasant feelings experienced while focusing on this experience. These feelings were shared. The group then turned to stages of the life cycle and reviewed aspects of the various stages.

Measurement of Effectiveness

A variety of methods has been used to determine the effectiveness of reminiscence. Increases in self-esteem and ego integrity were commonly used measures. Lewis (1971) developed a Q-sort that measured the person's present self-concept and the person's view of self in the past. Gibson (1980) used Hoffmeister's Self-Esteem Questionnaire to measure changes in self-esteem in adult male alcoholics who participated in group reminiscence. Improvement in personal appearance is another criterion that could be used to measure improvement in self-esteem.

Self-report and observations by the therapists and staff were used by Matteson and Munsat (1982) to determine the effectiveness of group reminiscence sessions. A form for observing social interactions could be developed and used to determine if changes from prereminiscence sessions occurred.

Serenity and lessening of depression were other variables that were reported to be positively affected by engaging in reminiscence. Lappe (1987) used the Zung Depression Scale to measure changes in the mood of elderly who participated in reminiscence groups. Life satisfaction (Sherman, 1987) and happiness (Rattenbury & Stones, 1989) are other measures that have been used as indicators of the effectiveness of reminiscence.

USES

This chapter has primarily addressed the use of reminiscence with the elderly. Table 14.1 lists populations and conditions for which reminiscence has been used. Elderly who are making major life adjustments such as moving find reminiscence to be helpful. Ebersole (1976a) noted that reminiscence helped persons close chapters in their lives and live more fully in the present. Coleman (1986) identified reminiscence as being useful in preventing mental deterioration in the elderly.

Although adjustments may need to be made for elderly with deficits, they should be included in reminiscence sessions. Settings that provide room for wheelchairs and beds should be chosen so that persons with mobility problems can be included. Adaptations may be necessary if elderly with hearing or visual problems are part of the group.

Chubon (1980) used reminiscence for persons with end-stage renal disease; the majority of the patients were on dialysis. Another younger population with whom reminiscence has been used is alcoholics (Chubon, 1980). Life review helped this group gain a better picture of their self-worth.

Precautions

Reminiscence is not an appropriate intervention for all elderly persons. According to Ryden (1981), those who are primarily focusing on the present may be in an extended stage of generativity (Erikson's eight

Table 14.1
Uses of Reminiscence

End-stage renal disease (Chubon, 1980)

Alcoholics (Gibson, 1980)

Elderly
    Depression (Lappe, 1987)
    Making changes (Ebersole, 1976b)
    Deafness (Wax, 1983)
    Improved cognitive functioning (Coleman, 1986)
    Adaptation to aging (Beadleson-Baird & Lara, 1988)
    Improved ego-integrity (Oleson, 1989)

---

stages), and are concentrating on ways to be productive; turning their attention to the past would be disruptive. An accurate and thorough assessment of patients will help determine whether they are in the generativity versus stagnation stage or the ego integrity versus despair stage.

Some persons may use reminiscence to avoid reality and the present situation (King, 1982). Living almost exclusively in the past can lead to despair. Reminiscence may also make the person feel more lonely and isolated (McMordie & Blom, 1979). Extra support and attention is required to help persons cope with these uncomfortable feelings. It is difficult to use reminiscence with persons who have receptive aphasia because they are not able to follow instructions. A one-to-one session using mementos and photos may be helpful in working with this population. Burnside (1990) cautioned that nurses should proceed slowly in using reminiscence with persons who have paranoid tendencies as asking questions about their past may increase their suspiciousness.

The energy level of the elderly person needs to be assessed (Burnside, 1990). Fatigue may interfere with the enjoyment a person should obtain from reminiscing. Likewise, the nurse must assess for the presence of any discomfort resulting from reminiscence.

RESEARCH QUESTIONS

Nurses have used reminiscence as a nursing intervention not only with the elderly but also with other patient populations. The intervention offers much promise in helping persons adapt to changes in their lives. Burnside (1990), Kovach (1990), and Merriman (1989) provide excellent reviews of the use of reminiscence and problems present in the research that has been conducted. Notably, the lack of specificity in describing the technique that was used in a study is a common problem. Merriman states that the use of different techniques, even though they are described as reminiscence, may account for the discrepancies in results that have been reported.

The following are areas in which research is needed so that more certainty can be had in when to use reminiscence and with whom to use it.

1. What are valid and reliable instruments that can be used to measure the effectiveness of reminiscence for specific problems? Tools that are specifically suited for use in busy clinical areas are lacking. Also, a number of the measures that have been used do not have validity and reliability established for their use with elderly populations.
2. Are there other patient populations/conditions for which reminiscence would be an appropriate intervention?
3. When reminiscence groups are used, which effects are due to the use of reminiscence and which result from the group process?

4. What is the ideal number of persons to be included in a reminiscence group? What are other structural variables surrounding the use of reminiscence groups that affect the outcome?
5. In which situations is life review rather than reminiscence more effective?

REFERENCES

Beadleson-Baird, M., & Lara, L.L. (1988). Reminiscing: Nursing actions for the acutely ill geriatric patient. *Issues in Mental Health Nursing* 9:83–94.

Boylin, W., Gordon, S., & Nehrke, M. (1976). Reminiscing and ego integrity in institutionalized elderly males. *The Gerontologist* 16:118–124.

Burnside, I. (1990). Reminiscence: An independent nursing intervention for the elderly. *Issues in Mental Health Nursing* 11:33–48.

Butler, R. (1963). The life review: An interpretation of reminiscence in the aged. *Psychiatry* 26:65–76.

Chubon, S. (1980). A novel approach to the process of life review. *Journal of Gerontological Nursing* 6:543–546.

Coleman, P. (1986). Issues in the therapeutic use of reminiscence with elderly people. Pp. 41–64 in I. Hanley & M. Gilhooly eds., *Psychological therapies for the elderly*. New York: New York University Press.

Ebersole, P. (1976a). Reminiscing and group psychotherapy with the aged. Pp. 214–230 in I. Burnside ed., *Nursing and the aged*. New York: McGraw Hill.

_____. (1976b). Problems of group reminiscing with the institutionalized aged. *Journal of Gerontological Nursing* 2:23–27.

Erikson, E. (1950). *Childhood and society*. New York: Norton.

Gibson, D. (1980). Reminiscence, self-esteem, and self-other satisfaction in adult male alcoholics. *JPN and Mental Health Services* 18(3):7–11.

Hala, M. (1975). Reminiscing group therapy project. *Journal of Gerontology* 27:245–253.

Havighurst, R., & Glasser, R. (1972). An exploratory study of reminiscence. *Journal of Gerontology* 27:245–253.

King, K. (1982). Reminiscing psychotherapy with aging people. *JPN and Mental Health Services* 20(2):20–25.

Kovach, C.R. (1990). Promise and problems in reminiscence research. *Journal of Gerontological Nursing,* 16(4):10–14.

Lappe, J.M. (1987). Reminiscing: The life review therapy. *Journal of Gerontological Nursing* 13:12–16.

Lewis, C. (1971). Reminiscing and self-concept in old age. *Journal of Gerontology* 26:240–243.

Lewis, M., & Butler, R. (1974). Life-review therapy. *Geriatrics* 29(11):165–173.

Matteson, M., & Munsat, E. (1982). Group reminiscing therapy with elderly clients. *Issues in Mental Health Nursing* 4:177–189.

McMahon, A., & Rhudick, P. (1964). Reminiscing: Adaptational significance in the aged. *Archives of General Psychiatry* 10:292–298.

McMordie, R., & Blom, S. (1979). Life review therapy: Psychotherapy for the elderly. *Perspectives in Psychiatric Care* 27:162–166.

Merriman, S.B. (1989). The structure of simple reminiscence. *The Gerontologist* 29:761–767.

Oleson, M. (1989). Legacies, reminiscence, and ego-integrity. *Nurse Educator* 14(6):6–7.

Pincus, A. (1970). Reminiscing in aging and its implications for social work practice. *Social Work* 15(3):47–53.

Postema, L. (1971). Reminiscence, time orientation, and self-concept in aged men. *Dissertation Abstracts International* 31:6880–1B.

Rattenbury, C., & Stones, M.J. (1989). A controlled evaluation of reminiscence and current topics discussion groups in a nursing home context. *The Gerontologist* 29:768–771.

Ryden, M. (1981). Nursing intervention in support of reminiscence. *Journal of Gerontological Nursing* 7:461–463.

Sherman, E. (1987). Reminiscence groups for community elderly. *The Gerontologist* 27:569–572.

Wax, T. (1983). Poetry efforts by aged deaf: Expression of life cycle experience. *The Gerontologist* 23:462–466.

CHAPTER **15**

YOGA

Miriam Cameron, PhD., R.N.

BACKGROUND

Millions of people practice Yoga for effective stress management, weight regulation, and physical fitness no matter what their age or physical condition (Uma et al., 1989). Nursing's holistic perspective fits well with the Yoga philosophy. Because Yoga marshals the strength of body and mind, nursing writers describe it as an important aid in health and healing (Goodwin, 1984; Hider, 1983; Nathaniels, 1984; Prakasamma & Bhaduri, 1984; Starre, 1989). This chapter provides an overview of Yoga and how nurses can use it as an independent nursing intervention.

Definition

Yoga, an ancient Hindu discipline meaning union or joining together, aims to increase control of the body, mind, and spirit in order to integrate them and bring them into harmony with the Universal Spirit (Singh et al., 1990). Although the major types of Yoga employ different techniques, they are designed to achieve this unifying aim. Yoga consists of eight stages (Table 15.1). Ideally, these stages lead to inner and outer beauty, a calm mind, the ability to concentrate, a high state of health, and self-realization (Maehta, 1990). Stages pertinent to nursing involve universal and individual ethical guidelines, postures, breathing, and meditation.

Table 15.1
The Stages of Yoga

1. Universal ethical guidelines
2. Individual ethical guidelines
3. Postures
4. Rhythmic control of the breath
5. Withdrawal and emancipation of the mind from the domination of the senses and exterior objects
6. Concentration
7. Meditation
8. A state of super-consciousness brought about by profound meditation in which the individual becomes one with the Universal Spirit

Source: From B.K.S. Iyengar. (1979). *Light On Yoga*. New York: Schocken Books.

Universal and Individual Ethical Guidelines

Yoga may be practiced within or without a religion. Yogis, people for whom Yoga is a way of life, have found that a certain philosophical understanding makes Yoga more successful. This ethical foundation aims at inhibition of ego-consciousness, held to be the underlying basis of unhappiness, pain, and most diseases. Yogis follow five universal ethical guidelines: nonviolence, truth, non-stealing, continence, and non-coveting. They adhere to five individual ethical guidelines: purity, contentment, austerity, study of the self, and dedication to the Universal Spirit. The Yogic ideal is to be gentle, loving, free from anger, and helpful to other people (Samskrti & Veda, 1985).

These ethical guidelines include teachings about nutrition, which is thought to play a vital role in achieving the Yogic ideal. Yoga views the body as a precision instrument designed to function at its peak on small amounts of high-quality food. The body is able to cope with most microorganisms as long as it is in a pure, clean, healthy state with an ability to call upon its defense agents as needed. Yoga suggests getting the most possible sustenance, called prana or life-force, from foods that provide energy instead of taking it away. For most Yogis, a well-balanced vegetarian diet provides the most life-force and does not require violence to animals, fish, and poultry. Yogic teachings are consistent with sound nutritional principles (Hittleman, 1988).

Postures

Yoga uses carefully designed postures to methodically massage the body. Done in sequence, the postures produce passive, prolonged, gentle stretching of specific groups of muscles, tendons, and ligaments (Brownstein & Dembert, 1989). Although many of the hundreds of postures require astonishing dexterity and years of practice, one only needs to perform a few simple postures to achieve results. Yoga doesn't encourage anything unnatural or harmful. Every posture is designed for the development of human potential (Christensen, 1987).

Breathing

Yoga teaches that breathing directly affects well-being and determines to a great extent the length and quality of life. Present in all forms of nourishment, life-force is most accessible and constant in air. The more life-force in one's body, the more alive one is. People who breathe in a rapid, erratic fashion develop nervous bodies and minds and they shorten their lives. Slow, rhythmic breathing through the nose lessens anxieties and causes an increase in the ability to concentrate (Hittleman, 1988).

Meditation

Yogic meditation is a profound state of quietude and relaxation in which one temporarily withdraws from the external environment in order to develop awareness of the inner self. Yoga teaches that through meditation one gradually perceives the Universal Spirit, the source of existence, and becomes integrated with this spirit. With elevated consciousness, one becomes increasingly free of the confining limitations of ego and experiences true joy and peace. By meditating regularly, one becomes more alive and aware in daily life. At first, the experience of letting go may be confined to times of meditation. Gradually, this feeling carries over into everyday activities and relaxation becomes a way of life (Hittleman, 1988).

Scientific Basis

For centuries, Yogic institutions in India have made health claims, published in obscure journals or books (Goyeche et al., 1982). Recently, researchers studying Yoga have published their work in mainstream journals. This research has been conducted primarily in India, although studies have been done in the United States, Australia, Japan, the United Kingdom, and other countries.

Published research involving Yoga often has used small samples, focused on short periods of time, and involved subjective judgments (Brownstein & Dembert, 1989; Muralidhara & Ranganathan, 1982;

Nagarathna & Nagendra, 1985). Based on personal experiences of instructors, Yogic techniques are not standardized (Walia et al., 1989). Because the studies have tested various Yogic techniques, findings are difficult to compare. However, nearly all of this research indicates the efficacy of Yoga. Many of these studies are pertinent to nurses.

Findings indicate a relationship between Yoga and improvement in the heart, blood, and blood vessels (Mohan et al., 1986; Muralidhara & Ranganathan, 1982). Yoga induced a state of blood hypocoagulability (Chohan et al., 1984). In persons with hypertension, Yoga lowered blood pressure and need for medications (Brownstein & Dembert, 1989; Chaudhary et al., 1988; Sundar et al., 1984).

Studies have found that the practice of Yoga vitalizes neuroendocrine/metabolic/immune processes (Chohan et al., 1984). Yoga produced a hypometabolic state and stabilized the autonomic nervous system (Contaldo, 1987; Raju et al., 1986; Sacks et al., 1986). For diabetics, blood sugar levels and use of medications dropped, acute complications diminished, and a feeling of well-being increased. Yoga appeared to improve utilization of insulin by reducing stress, instilling a sense of discipline, and changing the hormonal/biochemical profile (Sahay, 1986).

Many researchers have reported a relationship between Yoga and improved respiratory functions. Persons with asthma, pleural effusion, severe chronic airway obstruction, and chronic obstructive pulmonary disease (COPD) used Yoga to control attacks. As their symptoms decreased, they needed less medications. By relaxing muscles and mind, Yoga appeared to reduce psychological overactivity, emotional instability, and efferent vagal discharge (Goyechne et al., 1982; Kulpati et al., 1982; Makwana et al., 1988; Miles, 1964; Nagarathna & Nagendra, 1985; Nagendra & Nagarathna, 1986; Prakasamma & Bhaduri, 1984; Schuster, 1987; Singh, 1987a, b; Singh et al., 1990; Tandon, 1978).

In various studies, the practice of Yoga led to a high state of physical fitness. Practitioners regulated their weight. They increased their body flexibility and muscular efficiency (Pansare et al., 1989; Selvamurthy et al., 1988; Udupa & Singh, 1972). Their tolerance to cold improved (Benson et al., 1982; Selvamurthy et al., 1988).

Researchers have reported that Yoga improves psychological functioning. Persons who engaged in Yoga showed greater tolerance to stress, less mental fatigue, increased intellectual performance, and improved memory (Selvamurthy et al., 1988; Udupa & Singh, 1972). Children with mild to severe mental retardation demonstrated improvement in IQ and social adaptation. Their joints loosened, muscles relaxed, and locomotor skills improved. They gained control over breathing and the mind, facilitating psychomotor coordination, concentration, and memory (Uma et al., 1989).

Yoga appears to rehabilitate the vital organs and endocrine glands by consuming little energy and producing maximal efficiency. Improvement in posture, breathing, and circulation creates an environment promoting self-regulation, healing, and well-being (Blumenthal et al., 1989; Muralidhara & Ranganathan, 1982). Because of Yoga's holistic nature, new research methodologies may be needed to adequately determine its scientific basis.

INTERVENTION

Technique

The only effective way to learn Yoga, an experiential discipline, is to practice it (Christensen, 1987). Although qualified teachers provide the best instruction, nurses can use illustrated books to learn Yoga themselves and teach it to clients (Christensen, 1987; Hittleman, 1988; Maehta, 1990; Samskrti & Veda, 1985). Whether working with a Yoga instructor and/or using a book, nurses need to adapt Yoga to their own and clients' individual needs.

Nurses may use Yoga alone or with other interventions. They may select one Yogic technique or combine techniques. Nurses are using Yogic techniques when they suggest that clients stretch to reduce stiffness or take deep breaths to decrease anxiety.

Table 15.2
Directions for Chest Expansion Posture

1. Stand in a relaxed posture, spine straight, arms at sides, feet close together. Gracefully bring hands up to touch chest, arms high, palms facing downward.
2. Slowly straighten arms at chest level outward in front. Feel elbows stretching.
3. Slowly bring arms behind the back, keeping them high at shoulder level. Feel shoulders stretching. Lower arms slightly and interlace fingers behind the back.
4. With fingers interlaced behind the back, very slowly and gently bend backward. Keep arms high. Look upward. Hold without motion for a count of 10.
5. With fingers interlaced behind the back, very slowly and gently bend forward, bringing arms high over back. Neck muscles are relaxed. Forehead points toward knees. Knees do not bend. Feel spine stretching gently. Hold without motion for a count of 20.
6. Slowly straighten to upright position. Unclasp hands. Relax.
7. Repeat the posture twice.

Source: From R.L. Hittleman. (1988). *Richard Hittleman's Yoga 28 Day Exercise Plan.* New York: Bantam Books.

Nutrition

Yoga recommends living on a minimum of food, eating what is light, agreeable, and fully nourishing. To obtain the most life-force, Yogis eat food in its natural state as much as possible. Primarily vegetarians, they eat little or no meat, fish, or poultry, which are considered to require more life-force for digestion than they impart. Yogis eat few different kinds of foods at each meal so that the body can quickly and completely utilize food. They avoid refined sugar products, coffee, alcoholic beverages, and an overabundance of high protein preparations, which they view as artificial stimulants that deplete their life-force (Hittleman, 1988).

Postures

Yoga suggests doing Yogic postures in a quiet, well-ventilated area, wearing clothing that allows for freedom of movement. Any time of day is fine except within 90 minutes of eating. Yogis perform the postures slowly and deliberately without strain to preclude pain and injury and promote musculoskeletal flexibility. They seek to move gracefully and rhythmically with brief holding periods, being relaxed and balanced at all times. Focusing on the posture, they temporarily suspend thinking. If the mind wanders, they bring it back gently and firmly (Hittleman, 1988; Iyengar, 1979). Table 15.2 describes a Yogic posture.

Breathing

Yogic breathing involves subjective, inner focusing on the breath, excluding external stimuli. Breathing primarily through the nose, Yogis attempt to utilize the lungs in their entirety and extract the most life-force

Table 15.3
Directions for Complete Breath

1. Sit in a comfortable position with back straight.
2. Exhale deeply, contract abdomen.
3. Inhale slowly, distend abdomen.
4. Continue inhalation, expand chest.
5. Continue inhalation, raise shoulders.
6. Retain breath for count of 5.
7. Exhale deeply, relax shoulders and chest, contract abdomen.
8. Perform 10 times, pausing between repetitions whenever necessary.

Source: From R.L. Hittleman. (1988). *Richard Hittleman's Yoga 28 Day Exercise Plan.* New York: Bantam Books.

Table 15.4
Directions for Yogic Meditation on the Breath

1. Sit in a comfortable position with back straight.
2. Gently close eyes.
3. Breath slowly and rhythmically through nose.
4. Focus on breathing. Listen to how it sounds. Feel the air go in and out of the nostrils. Become aware of the gentle rise and fall of the abdomen.
5. If the mind wanders away, bring it back to the breath.
6. Stay in this position for 10–15 minutes.

Source: From H. Kent. (1985). *Yoga for the disabled.* Wellingborough, NY: Thorsons Publishing Group.

possible. Many Yogic breathing techniques are available (Brownstein & Dembert, 1989). Table 15.3 describes a Yogic breathing technique.

Meditation

To focus and calm the mind, Yogic meditation concentrates on a repeated sound (mantra), a scene, a concept, an object, or the breath. One can experiment to discover which technique works best. Meditation can be practiced whenever one needs renewal (Hittleman, 1988). Table 15.4 describes a Yogic meditation technique.

Measurement of Effectiveness

People who faithfully use Yoga claim that they experience improved physical, mental, and spiritual health no matter what their age or physical condition. Their musculoskeletal flexibility increases and they have better balance. Their weight becomes regulated and redistributed. They feel more physical and mental relaxation. They experience greater emotional control, mental clarity, improved concentration, and a positive mental outlook (Brownstein & Dembert, 1989; Iyengar, 1979). Use of appropriate Yogic techniques can lead to improvement in specific health problems.

USES

Conditions

Anyone can practice Yoga. Children, elderly people, pregnant women, persons with AIDS, and disabled individuals have experienced its benefits (Kent, 1985; Starre, 1989). To promote wellness, many researchers suggest that Yoga be popularized among persons who don't have serious health problems (Muralidhara & Ranganathan, 1982).

Nursing literature describes nurses who do Yoga themselves (Goodwin, 1984; Starre, 1989) and they successfully teach Yoga to people who have had strokes (Nathaniels, 1984), people with visual impairment (Hider, 1983), and people with pleural effusion (Prakasamma & Bhaduri, 1984). Yoga is used as a therapy adjunct or alternative in fields such as aviation in which side effects from medications can cause problems (Brownstein & Dembert, 1989). Some substance abuse programs combine Yoga and the Twelve Steps of Alcoholics Anonymous. Table 15.5 describes some additional uses of Yoga not previously discussed in this chapter. Many Yoga books contain specific techniques to deal with every conceivable situation (Iyengar, 1979).

Table 15.5
Some Additional Conditions for Which Yoga Has Been Used

Anxiety (Goyeche et al., 1982)
Arthritis (Hittleman, 1988)
Back pain (Nespor, 1989)
Disabilities (Kent, 1985)
Ethical problems (Iyengar, 1979)
Expectoration of mucus (Goyeche et al., 1982)
Leprosy (Appa Rao et al., 1982)
Personal discipline (Wilson, 1985)
Suppressed emotions (Sharma & Agnihotri, 1982)

Precautions

Before recommending Yoga to clients, nurses need to become knowledgeable about it so they can successfully adapt Yoga to their own and clients' individual needs. By doing careful and ongoing nursing assessments, nurses can determine if and when the practice of Yoga is beneficial to clients. Nurses need to encourage clients to seek their own inner wisdom when practicing Yoga. Although nurses and other instructors can point the way, clients must learn to trust their own intuition so that Yoga will benefit them (Sharma & Agnihotri, 1982; Starre, 1989; Udupa & Singh, 1972).

Most health problems develop over time and Yoga won't alleviate them immediately. Minor problems may respond quickly but serious problems require sustained, patient practice. Yoga advocates gradual change. One receives the full benefit of Yoga according to one's own needs (Hittleman, 1988; Starre, 1989). The most benefits occur from regular practice and a combination of Yogic ethical guidelines, nutrition, postures, breathing, and meditation (Sharma & Agnihotri, 1982).

Published complications of Yoga are rare. Yogic breathing exacerbated one man's asthma (Tamarin et al., 1988). Another man's practice of shoulder stands and headstands for 15–20 minutes a day may have been a factor in his development of early glaucomatous optic disk changes and visual field loss (Rice & Allen, 1985). Sharma and Agnihotri (1982) warn that persons with latent or manifest psychopathology may experience acute disorganizational states during the practice of Yoga. They may feel overwhelmed by emotionally charged material coming to mind.

The few reports about complications do not indicate if the persons involved were adequately trained and supervised in Yoga. These people may have been overzealous in their use of Yogic techniques (Brownstein & Dembert, 1989). Most complications may be avoided by following the Yogic principles of gentleness, moderation, noncompetition, and nonmaleficence.

RESEARCH QUESTIONS

Although nursing writers view Yoga as an effective, natural, independent nursing intervention, nursing literature provides little guidance for applying Yoga in nursing practice. Few nursing studies using Yoga have been reported. The apparent efficacy of Yoga calls for more nursing research involving Yoga. Some questions that need to be answered are:

1. Which claims of Yogic practice are accurate and why?
2. Because of Yoga's holistic nature, what research methodologies are needed to study the effectiveness of Yoga as a nursing intervention?

3. What are the characteristics of a person who practices Yoga regularly compared with a person who does not practice Yoga or stops practicing Yoga?
4. How can nurses adapt Yoga for increased use in long-term care, mental health and addictions nursing, pain management, care of persons with respiratory difficulties, health promotion, post-operative care, rehabilitation nursing, and other areas of nursing practice?
5. What changes, if any, does the regular practice of Yoga make in the immune system?

REFERENCES

Appa Rao, A.V.N., Krishna, D.R., Ramanakar, T.V., & Prabhakar, M.C. (1982). "Jala Neti" a yoga technique for nasal comfort and hygiene in leprosy patients. *Leprosy in India* 54(4):691–694.

Benson, H., Lehmann, J.W., Malhotra, M.S., Goldman, R.F., Hopkins, J., & Epstein, M.D. (1982). Body temperature changes during the practice of g Tum-mo yoga. *Nature* 295(5846):234–236.

Blumenthal, J.A., Emery, C.F., Madden, D.J., George, L.K., Coleman, R.E., Riddle, M.W., McKee, D.C., Reasoner, J., & Williams, R.S. (1989). Cardiovascular and behavioral effects of aerobic exercise training in healthy older men and women. *Journal of Gerontology* 44(5):147–157.

Brownstein, A.H., and Dembert, M.L. (1989). Treatment of essential hypertension with yoga relaxation therapy in a USAF aviator. *Aviation, Space, and Environmental Medicine* 60(7):684–687.

Chaudhary, A.K., Bhatnagar, H.N.S., Bhatnagar, L.K., & Chaudhary, K. (1988). Comparative study of the effect of drugs and relaxation exercise (Yoga Shavasan) in hypertension. *Journal of the Association of Physicians of India* 36(12):721–723.

Chohan, I.S., Nayar, H.S., Thomas, P., & Geetha, N.S. (1984). Influence of yoga on blood coagulation. *Thrombosis and Haemostasis* 51(2):196–197.

Christensen, A. (1987). *The American Yoga Association Beginner's Manual.* New York: Simon & Schuster.

Contaldo, F. (1987). Yoga or fiber? Thermodynamics in the vegetarian. *JAMA* 257(10):1330.

Goodwin, S. (1984). Step by step. *Nursing Times* 80(1):50–51.

Goyeche, J.R.M., Abo, Y., & Ikemi, Y. (1982). Asthma: The yoga perspective. *Journal of Asthma* 19(3):189–201.

Hider, J. (1983). Yoga for the visually handicapped. *Nursing Mirror* 156(10):18–21.

Hittleman, R.L. (1988). *Richard Hittleman's Yoga 28 Day Exercise Plan.* New York: Bantam Books.

Iyengar, B.K.S. (1979). *Light on Yoga.* New York: Schocken Books.

Kent, H. (1985). *Yoga for the Disabled.* Wellingborough, NY: Thorsons Publishing Group.

Kulpati, D.D.S., Kamath, R.K., & Chauhan, M.R. (1982). The influence of physical conditioning by yogasanas and breathing exercises in patients of chronic obstructive lung disease. *Journal of the Association of Physicians of India* 30(12):865–868.

Maehta, S. (1990). *Yoga: The Iyengar Way.* New York: Harper & Row.

Makwana, K., Khirwadkar, N., & Gupta, H.C. (1988). Effect of short term yoga practice on ventilatory function tests. *Indian Journal of Physiology and Pharmacology* 32(3):202–208.

Miles, W.R. (1964). Oxygen consumption during three yoga-type breathing patterns. *Journal of Applied Physiology* 19:75–82.

Mohan, M., Saravanane, C., Surange, S.G., Thombre, D.P., & Chakrabarty, A.S. (1986). Effect of yoga type breathing on heart rate and cardiac axis of normal subjects. *Indian Journal of Physiology and Pharmacology* 30(4):334–340.

Muralidhara, D.V., and Ranganathan, K.V. (1982). Effect of yoga practice on cardiac recovery index. *Indian Journal of Physiology and Pharmacology* 26(4):279–283.

Nagarathna, R., & Nagendra, H.S. (1985). Yoga for bronchial asthma. *British Medical Journal* 291:1077–1079.

Nagendra, H.R., & Nagarathna, R. (1986). An integrated approach of yoga therapy for bronchial asthma. *Journal of Asthma* 23(3):123–137.

Nathaniels, E. (1984). Yoga for all. *Nursing Times* 80(1):52–54.

Nespor, K. (1989). Psychosomatics of back pain and the use of Yoga. *International Journal of Psychosomatics* 36(1–4):72–78.

Pansare, M.S., Kulkarni, A.N., & Pendse, U.B. (1989). Effect of yogic training on serum LDH levels. *The Journal of Sports Medicine and Physical Fitness* 29(2):177–178.

Prakasamma, M., & Bhaduri, A. (1984). A study of yoga as a nursing intervention in the care of patients with pleural effusion. *Journal of Advanced Nursing* 9:127–133.

Raju, P.S., Kumar, K.A., Reddy, S.S., Madhavi, S., Gnanakumari, K., Bhaskaracharyulu, C., Reddy, M.V., Annapurna, N., Reddy, M.E., Girijakumari, D., Sahay, B.K., & Murthy, K.J.R. (1986). Effect of yoga on exercise tolerance in normal healthy volunteers. *Indian Journal of Physiology and Pharmacology* 30(2):121–132.

Rice, R., & Allen, R.C. (1985). Yoga in glaucoma. *American Journal of Ophthalmology* 100(5):738–739.

Sacks, F.M., Ornish, D., Kass, E., & McLanahan, S. (1986). Dietary intake, the first law of thermodynamics, and the properties of yoga. *JAMA* 255(9):1136.

Sahay, B.K. (1986). Yoga and diabetes. *Journal of the Association of Physicians of India* 34(9):645–648.

Samskrti & Veda. (1985). *Hatha Yoga. Manual I, 2nd ed.* Honesdale, PA: The Himalayan International Institute.

Schuster, D.F. (1987). Yoga for asthma. *Medical Self-Care* 42:44–49, 54, 59.

Selvamurthy, W., Ray, U.S., Hegde, K.S., & Sharma, R.P. (1988). Physiological responses to cold in men after six months' practice of yoga exercises. *International Journal of Biometeorology* 32:188–193.

Sharma, I., & Agnihotri, S.S. (1982). Yoga therapy in psychiatric disorders. *Indian Journal of Medical Sciences* 36(7–8):138–141.

Singh, V. (1987a). Effect of respiratory exercises on asthma. *Journal of Asthma* 24(6):355–359.

____. (1987b). Kunjal: A nonspecific protective factor in management of bronchial asthma. *Journal of Asthma* 24(3):183–186.

Singh, V., Wisniewski, A., Britton, J., & Tattersfield, A. (1990). Effect of yoga breathing exercises (pranayama) on airway reactivity in subjects with asthma. *The Lancet* 335(8702):1381–1383.

Starre, B.A. (1989). Yoga: Progressing toward high level wellness. *Health Values* 13(3):48–52.

Sundar, S., Agrawal, S.K., Singh, V.P., Bhattacharya, S.K., Udupa, K.N., & Vaish, S.K. (1984). Role of yoga in management of essential hypertension. *Acta Cardiologica* 39(3):203–208.

Tamarin, F.M., Conetta, R., Brandstetter, R.D., & Chadow, H. (1988). Increased muscle enzyme activity after yoga breathing during an exacerbation of asthma. *Thorax* 43:731–732.

Tandon, M.K. (1978). Adjunct treatment with yoga in chronic severe airways obstruction. Thorax 33(4):514–517.

Udupa, K.N., & Singh, R.H. (1972). The scientific basis of yoga. *JAMA* 220(10):1365.

Uma, K., Nagendra, H.R., Nagarathna, R., Vaidehi, S., & Seethalakshmi, R. (1989). The integrated approach of yoga. *Journal of Mental Deficiency Research* 33(5):415–421.

Walia, I.J., Mehra, P., Grover, P., Earnest, C., Verma, S.K., & Sanjeev. (1989). Health status of nurses and Yoga. *The Nursing Journal of India* 80(11):287–290.

Wilson, S.R. (1985). Therapeutic processes in a yoga ashram. *American Journal of Psychotherapy* 39(2):253–262.

CHAPTER 16

VALIDATION THERAPY

Lois Taft

BACKGROUND

Validation is a therapeutic approach for interacting with disoriented elderly individuals. The goals of validation therapy are to help relieve anxiety, maintain dignity, and prevent further deterioration and withdrawal. The validation worker focuses on accepting a person's emotional reality and validating feelings rather than insisting on the accuracy of facts and orientation to present reality.

Validation therapy was originated by Naomi Feil, based on her experience as a social worker in the Montefiore Home for the Aged in Cleveland, Ohio. A lifetime of experience provided the basis for Feil's insight into the meaning of confusion in old age and strategies to restore self-worth. Feil grew up in the Montefiore Home where her father, a psychologist, and her mother, a social worker, pioneered services for the elderly in the 1940s (Feil, 1985). Feil specialized in group work with the aged at Columbia University in New York and graduated in 1956 with a Master's in Social Work.

In the early sixties, reality orientation was receiving attention as a new psychiatric technique to bring confused elderly individuals back to reality. Feil returned to the Montefiore Home in 1963, began group work with confused elderly residents, and tried to reorient them to reality. By 1965, she had abandoned the goals of reality orientation and began to explore other forms of group therapy (Feil, 1967). By 1967 she refocused therapeutic interactions on validating and supporting the residents' feelings in whatever time or location was real to them. The treatment she developed was initially known as validation/fantasy therapy; but currently it is generally referred to simply as validation therapy. Feil is now the executive director of the Validation Training Institute in Cleveland, Ohio. She has published a manual on applying validation techniques (Feil, 1982), written film scripts which demonstrate validation in individual and group settings (Feil, 1972, 1978, 1980), and conducted numerous validation workshops throughout the United States and Canada.

Definition

Validation therapy is "the process of communicating with disoriented elderly persons by validating and supporting their feelings in whatever time or location is real to them, even though this may not correspond to our 'here and now' reality" (Jones, 1985:20). Validation is not new as a communication technique. Therapeutic communication skills require the recognition of both feeling and content components in a transaction. Clarifying and reflecting feelings are strategies that are integral to therapeutic communication and the establishment of a therapeutic relationship. Validation embodies the therapeutic use of self in the caring professions. According to Feil (1985), "validation is a combination of empathy, touch, eye contact, mirroring body movements, matching voice and rhythms, picking up cues about feelings and putting them into words, accepting without judging, and genuine total listening" (pp. 91–92).

At a validation workshop in 1987, Feil used the following example to illustrate the application of validation techniques. A woman in her late fifties arrived at a nursing home to visit her 85-year-old mother. The old woman looked up from her chair, smiled at her daughter, and said "Mama." The younger woman was exasperated by her mother's display of craziness and responded by saying, " I'm not your mother. I'm your daughter. Your mother died a long time ago." This kind of communication produces frustration and pain. According to validation therapy, there is wisdom in the old woman's behavior. She has retreated to the world of love, security, and dependence that she experienced as a child. Her eyesight isn't good. The daughter reminds her of her mother. Both are people she loves. Instead of insisting on "reality," the daughter could respond to her mother's emotional reality by reflecting, "I bet you miss your mother very much." Further communication could be facilitated by encouraging reminiscence. The daughter could respond, "Tell me about your mother." Either response builds trust and communicates empathy.

Scientific Basis

Theoretical Support

Feil has proposed that her work extends Erikson's theory of developmental stages (Erikson, 1963). Erikson identified eight stages of development throughout the life-span and described a psychological conflict at each stage. The developmental crisis of old age focuses on ego integrity versus despair. According to Feil, older adults who are unable to achieve integrity may choose to retreat to the past to resolve old conflicts. The old-old (persons 85 years and older), confronting despair, may choose confusion to express repressed emotions. Despair may be avoided by expressing old unresolved feelings. Feil identified this last life stage as resolution versus vegetation (Feil, 1985). Validation promotes resolution.

Assumptions underlying validation therapy are that: (1) all behavior has meaning, (2) early learned emotional memories replace rational thinking in the disoriented old-old, and (3) retreat to the past is purposeful (Feil, 1982). Purposes of validation therapy include resolving old conflicts, reliving past pleasures, restimulating sensory memories, and retreating from painful feelings of uselessness and loneliness. Validation allows unresolved feelings to be expressed and restores dignity and self-worth through acceptance.

Humanistic principles of person-centered therapy as developed by Rogers (1951) also support validation therapy (Babins, 1986, 1988). Person-centered therapy focuses on the internal world of the client and emphasizes the dignity of each individual and his/her right to be unique. The role of the therapist is to be accessible to the client and to convey an attitude of genuineness, empathy, and unconditional positive regard. In validation therapy, empathy is used to tune in to the world of the disoriented old person. Validation requires a nonjudgmental attitude which recognizes each person as unique and conveys respect and acceptance.

Research

Minimal research has been conducted on the effectiveness of validation therapy. Feil has reported positive clinical experiences but has not substantiated clinical impressions with research.

Several attempts have been made to compare the effectiveness of validation groups versus reality orientation groups with disoriented elderly residents in institutional settings (Babins, 1985; Peoples, 1982; Robb et al., 1986). In each of these studies, however, serious methodological problems were encountered. Because of the nature of the intervention, only very small sample sizes were used in each study. Other limitations included attrition of participants and differences in the control and experimental groups, as well as questions regarding the sensitivity, reliability, and validity of the research instruments.

In response to validation therapy, Babins (1985) reported improvements in verbal and nonverbal communication skills and a slowing of mental deterioration, while at the same time noting an increase in irritability on a social behavior scale. Peoples (1982) reported qualitative improvements in communication skills and responsiveness and a decrease in aggressive behavior for participants in the validation group. Further withdrawal was reported as a response to reality orientation.

Mental status, morale, and social behavior were variables studied by Robb et al. (1986). Post-tests documented decline in all three variables in the reality orientation group. Improvements in morale and mental status were noted in the validation group; however, the differences between the pretests and post-tests for each group proved statistically nonsignificant. Further research is necessary before any conclusions can be drawn from the results of these studies. Robb et al. (1986) proposed that "conceptual generality represents a potential solution to the problem of obtaining valid results from studies that lack methodological rigor because they focus on human behavior in complex health care environments" (p. 113). Conceptual generality is explained as the accumulation of similar findings in different studies with different subjects, situational factors, and other variations in study procedures. Such aggregate results lead to greater confidence in conclusions regarding the merit of clinical interventions.

Another appropriate mechanism for evaluating the impact of validation therapy is the use of qualitative research methodologies. Zachow (1984) reported a case study in which she used validation therapy on an individual basis as one intervention to establish rapport with an extremely withdrawn, disruptive nursing home resident. The staff documented the following changes in the resident's behavior. The quantity and volume of verbal agitation was reduced, including decreased perseveration. There was an increase in alertness and the resident began to focus on people and activity in her environment. The resident was able to feed herself more frequently and was more coherent in verbal communication. Nighttime sleep patterns improved, and the use of prn Thorazine decreased by 50%. Such observations support validation therapy as a promising intervention for interacting with disoriented, elderly individuals.

INTERVENTION

Techniques

Validation can be used on an individual basis or as a focus for group work with disoriented elderly residents. In validation groups, it is important that individuals are in a group with others at a similar stage of disorientation. In addition, validation strategies are designed according to the stage of disorientation.

Individual Therapy

Stage One. This stage is labeled mild confusion (Jones, 1985) or malorientation (Feil, 1982). Individuals in stage one are oriented to person, place, and time. They desperately cling to present reality. These individuals are verbal and generally ambulatory. Their eyes are clear and focused. Their coping strategies include denial and blaming. Disorientation in this group revolves around old conflicts that were never faced and never resolved. These conflicts may be expressed in disguised forms that are generally labeled as symptoms of confusion. An example of an individual in the first stage of disorientation will be used to illustrate basic helping skills in validation therapy. The example is drawn from material presented by Feil at a validation workshop in 1987.

An 87-year-old woman in a nursing home angrily complains that big drops of water are falling from the ceiling onto her bed. The first step is to determine if, in fact, the roof leaks. However, once it has been verified that the roof does not leak, the validation worker does not argue the truth of the facts. The technique for the validation worker is to explore the person's experience. This can be done by asking who, what, when, where, and how questions.

Validation Worker: When do the drops of water fall from the ceiling?
Resident: Whenever I try to fall asleep I see drops of water form on the ceiling and splash on my bed.
Validation Worker: What color are they?
Resident: They're blue—the color of my baby's eyes.

Feil relates that if we could read this woman's life story, we might discover that she had a daughter who drowned at age three. The woman had bottled up this loss, and the accompanying guilt, during her whole life. Now, as the losses of old age accumulate, old unresolved losses erupt. This old unresolved loss expresses itself as water dripping from the ceiling, keeping her awake.

As caregivers, we rarely know with what unresolved conflicts individuals are struggling. But, by using validation techniques, it is possible to accept the reality of their feelings, to actively listen, and to empathize. The goal of validation is not to psychoanalyze. Usually it's too late to gain insight. The validation worker doesn't laugh, doesn't lie, doesn't argue, and doesn't offer a solution. This last rule may be most difficult for nurses who always want to fix things. For example, to solve the problem of the water dripping from the ceiling, the nurse may suggest the resident should move to another room. However, if the move occurs, the nurse may soon discover that water leaks from the ceiling in that room too. After all, the problem is not a leaky roof, it is a child who drowned 60 years ago. No move will ever fix that; but if the validation worker listens, explores, and cares, the water may not drip from the ceiling so often.

At this stage, feelings of loss are validated by listening and exploring the individual's experience. Other types of questions that can be used include: polarity questions (When is it the worst?), life review questions (What happened before...?), and questions that invite the resident to imagine an opposite situation (What would it be like if...?). Touch is used only if the person is ready. Persons in this stage retreat from intimate relationships and are threatened by feelings.

Stage Two. When physical and social losses accumulate and an individual gives up trying to hold on to reality, they enter stage two—time confusion. In this stage, individuals lose track of present time and retreat inward. They lose adult controls. They lose communication skills. They create unique word forms from past memories—a process identified as word doodling (Feil, 1986). They use pronouns without specific references. They use symbols to represent people and events remembered from the past. They create their own inner reality. Individuals in stage two can sometimes be recognized by unfocused, downcast eyes; a low, wavering voice; relaxed muscles; and frequent wandering.

Questions similar to those used in stage one are used to explore the person's experience in stage two. In this stage, feelings are expressed either verbally or nonverbally and the validation worker explores and accepts all feelings that are expressed. Touch and eye contact are basic helping skills at this stage. Feil (1986) summarizes the following techniques that restore dignity to the time-confused:

1. Use nonthreatening factual questions (Examples: who, what, when, where).
2. Use a vague pronoun when the meaning is not clear (Examples: he, it, someone).
3. Repeat a key word.
4. Use direct eye contact and a clear, low nurturing voice.
5. Use touch.
6. Reflect the person's feelings.
7. Link behavior with universal human needs and feelings. The person in stage two expresses these feelings in words, through symbols, with movements, and through behavior. The validation worker explores these universal feelings and expresses them out loud. In this way the emotional reality experienced by the individual is validated.

Stage Three. Many of the characteristics of individuals in stage two and three are similar, but greater withdrawal is apparent in the individual in stage three, repetitive motion. Communication skills and speech may be lost. Repetitive sounds and repetitive movements may be used to stimulate, reassure, and help resolve feelings. These individuals generally have profound sensory losses and use what Feil refers to as "kinesthetic memory" or motion to trigger emotions, give pleasure, and control anxiety. These individuals have resigned themselves to isolation and self-stimulation.

Individuals in stage three are more difficult to reach. They do not respond unless stimulated through a combination of nurturing touch and voice-tone and direct eye contact. They respond well to music and rhythms. It may be possible to reach an individual in stage three by mirroring their body movements. Another technique that may work with persons in stage three is attempting to link behavior with the feelings that person is experiencing. It is generally necessary to use trial and error. If you hit the right feelings, the person may respond with a nod, with eye contact, or with words. It may be possible to restore some speech, some rational thinking, and some social interaction through a genuine validating relationship.

Stage Four. This stage is labeled vegetation and occurs when the individual completely shuts out the outside world and gives up the struggle to live. Feil reports minimal evidence of response to validation techniques once an individual reaches this level of disorientation.

Group Therapy

Validation therapy may be useful in group work with disoriented elderly individuals. Those in the second stage of disorientation are most responsive to group work. Individuals in stage one may assist in a leadership role, but they generally feel threatened if they are included as a group member. Validation groups with 5–10 members generally meet for 20 minutes to an hour once or twice a week.

Robb et al. (1986) described validation groups as labor-intensive and, therefore, expensive; but Feil reported positive outcomes. Disoriented persons in stages two and three have minimal energy for one-to-one conversations. However, "groups trigger memories of family roles, of former social group roles, of social controls. People begin to listen. Speech improves. They care about others as they model the nurturing validation worker... and they validate each other" (Feil, 1982:62).

In validation groups, roles are assigned to each member based on former social roles. Examples of such roles include a welcomer to greet each member, a hostess to pass out refreshments, a song leader, or a chair arranger.

Universal feelings such as anger, separation, or loss provide the focus of discussion. The validation worker is active and moves from one group member to another. For example, the leader might approach a group member, use touch and eye contact to focus attention, and comment, "Mrs. Johnson misses her mother. What do you do when you miss your mother?" Feil emphasizes the importance of using last names to trigger respect.

The goal in validation groups is not to reorient, but simply to help the group members feel better. Music and rhythm are important parts of the group session and refreshments are served to conclude the meeting.

Summary

The goal of validation therapy is to relieve anxiety, maintain dignity, and prevent further deterioration and withdrawal. Through the use of validation techniques, it may also be possible to reduce the need for chemical and physical restraints. In an individualized nursing care plan, it may be possible to replace a sedative with a nursing order such as: Sing Rock-a-bye Baby with Mrs. Johnson three times a day. Rationale: It helps her remember the good times when she was raising her family of eight children. It validates her maternal love and pride in her accomplishments, and it raises her spirits to sing.

Feil (1984) summarized the basic principles of validation therapy in eight guidelines for communicating with confused elderly patients:

1. Establish a rapport with direct eye contact.
2. Listen with genuine, full attention.
3. Use touch.
4. Do not confront the patient with "the truth."
5. Express the emotional need of the person aloud, thereby affirming the person's right to feel and to express feelings.

6. With the disoriented elderly person who uses personally constructed, non-dictionary words, repeat the word, emphasizing the key words in their sentences.
7. Respond to and attempt to interpret the patient's physical actions when feelings can't be expressed with words.
8. Accept the disoriented patient's need to substitute present time and people for those of the past. [pp. 131–132]

Measurement of Effectiveness

A variety of patient outcomes have been reported in relation to validation therapy. Robb et al. (1986) measured changes in mental status, morale, and social behavior using research tools with established reliability and validity. The Mental Status Questionnaire (MSQ) developed by Fishback (1977) was used to measure mental status. The Philadelphia Geriatric Center Morale Scale (PGCMS), developed by Lawton (1975), was used to measure morale. Social behavior was measured by the Minimal Social Behavior Scale (MSBS) developed by Farina, Arenberg, and Guskin (1957). The researchers reported a number of problems encountered in the use of these tools. Mobility deficits interfered with the use of the MSBS, and problems verifying the accuracy of answers on the MSQ made it difficult to score. Such problems underscore the importance of developing and testing appropriate research instruments for use in frail elderly populations.

Behavioral, emotional, and functional outcomes of validation therapy need to be documented. Behavioral outcomes include social behavior such as alertness, responsiveness, and the number of social interactions. Problematic behaviors such as verbal agitation and aggressive behavior can also be monitored.

Patterns of ambulating, eating, and speaking can be documented to determine the impact of validation techniques on functional abilities. However, it is important to maintain realistic expectations. If the goal of validation is to reduce anxiety and maintain dignity, emotional responses may be the most significant variables to measure. Scales that measure depression, morale, and anxiety, as well as measures of affect such as smiling or crying, are some indicators that can be used for measuring progress. Sleep patterns may also be an appropriate indicator of emotional comfort.

USES

Populations

In their classic text on confusion, Wolanin and Phillips (1981) state that confusion can be a decompensating reaction resulting from disruption of pattern and meaning. The stressors of old age, including losses, powerlessness, and rejection, can result in disorientation. According to Wolanin and Phillips, the nurse can best intervene by providing support and opportunities for meaningful social interaction. Validation therapy can be effectively used to treat individuals whose confusion results from disruption of pattern and meaning.

Feil (1985) advocates the use of validation for disoriented old people who have retreated to the past to resolve old conflicts or escape painful feelings. She points out that individuals with a dementia such as Alzheimer's disease do not choose to withdraw, and they may not respond to validation techniques. However, validation techniques have been effectively used as an intervention for clients with dementia (Bleathman & Morton, 1988; Dreher, 1988; Rader et al., 1985).

Rader, Doan, and Schwab (1985) coined the term "agenda behavior" to describe "verbal and non-verbal planning and actions that cognitively impaired persons use in an effort to fulfill their felt social, emotional, and physical needs" (p. 196). Wandering is a form of agenda behavior which may threaten the safety of the disoriented elderly person. The proposed approach in response to agenda behavior is an adaptation of validation therapy. The following steps are recommended:

1. Face the resident and make direct eye contact if this does not appear to be threatening.
2. Gently touch the resident's arm, shoulder, back, or waist if he or she does not move away.
3. Listen to what the resident is communicating verbally and nonverbally. Link this to the resident's feelings.
4. Identify the agenda, the resident's plan of action, and the emotional needs the agenda is expressing.
5. Repeat specific words or phrases from the agenda ("fix supper," "your children") or state the need or emotion ("You need to go home?", "You're worried that your family won't be fed?"). [Rader et al., 1985:198]

If these five steps are followed consistently throughout the day, agenda behavior can be diminished or eliminated. These validation techniques may be successful because "residents seem to develop consistent feelings of safety and belonging in their present environment and do not need to fantasize or actually seek a past environment to feel secure" (Rader et al., 1985:198).

Precautions

Although validation therapy provides a promising therapeutic approach for working with confused, elderly individuals, it is not an appropriate intervention in all cases of confusion. Validation therapy is not appropriate when confusion is due to acute, reversible causes. The abrupt onset of confusion, or a sudden change in the severity of confusion, should prompt the nurse to suspect physiological causes. Physical assessment and prompt medical treatment are required.

RESEARCH QUESTIONS

Long-term care of the cognitively impaired elderly is often custodial rather than therapeutic. The use of validation therapy offers the caregiver an opportunity to intervene therapeutically. Validation techniques may be useful in relieving anxiety and maintaining dignity despite the ravages of old age. The following are areas in which research investigations would provide data on the application and merit of validation therapy.

1. What are assessment strategies to use to determine the stage of disorientation?
2. What are the characteristics of persons who benefit from validation therapy?
3. What are the characteristics of persons who benefit most from one-to-one validation versus group sessions?
4. What are the behavioral, emotional, and functional patient outcomes associated with validation therapy? How long do the effects last?
5. What are the longitudinal effects of validation therapy?
6. Can validation therapy provide an alternative to the use of physical and chemical restraints?
7. Can validation techniques be effectively implemented by nonprofessional staff and/or family members?
8. What is the impact of a validation therapy program on staff morale?

REFERENCES

Babins, L. (1985). *Group approaches with the disoriented elderly: Reality orientation and validation therapies.* Unpublished Master's thesis. Montreal: McGill University.

____. (1986). A humanistic approach to old-old people: A general model. *Activities, Adaptation, and Aging,* 3–4(8): 57–63.

____. (1988). Conceptual analysis of validation therapy. *International Journal of Aging and Human Development* 26:161–168.

Bleathman, C., & Morton, I. (1988). Validation therapy with the demented elderly. *Journal of Advanced Nursing* 13:511–514.

Dreher, B.B. (1988). Breaking up rigid attitudes. *Journal of Applied Gerontology* 7:121–124.

Erikson, E. (1963). *Childhood and society.* New York: W.W. Norton.

Farina, A., Arenberg, D., & Guskin, S. (1957). A scale for measuring minimal social behavior. *Journal of Consulting Psychology* 21:265–268.

Feil, E. (producer). (1972). *The Tuesday group* (film). Cleveland: Edward Feil Publications.

____. (producer). (1978). *Looking for yesterday* (film). Cleveland: Edward Feil Productions.

____. (producer). (1980). *The more we get together* (film). Cleveland: Edward Feil Productions.

Feil, N. (1967). Group therapy in a home for the aged. *Gerontologist* 7:192–195.

____. (1982). *Validation: The Feil method.* (film). Cleveland: Edward Feil Productions.

____. (1984). Communicating with the confused elderly patient. *Geriatrics* 39:131–132.

____. (1985). Resolution: The final life task. *Journal of Humanistic Psychology* 25:91–105.

____. (1986). Validation therapy for the time-confused. *Geriatric Care* 18(2):1–2.

Fishback, D.B. (1977). Mental status questionnaire for organic brain syndrome, with a new visual counting test. *Journal of the American Geriatrics Society* 24:167–170.

Jones, G. (1985). Validation therapy: A companion to reality orientation. *The Canadian Nurse* 81(3):20–23.

Lawton, M.P. (1975). The Philadelphia Geriatric Center morale scale: A revision. *Journal of Gerontology* 30:80–89.

Peoples, M. (1982). *Validation therapy versus reality orientation as treatment for disoriented institutionalized elderly.* Unpublished Master's thesis. Akron, OH: University of Akron.

Rader, J., Doan, J., and Schwab, M. (1985). How to decrease wandering, a form of agenda behavior. *Geriatric Nursing* 6:196–199.

Robb, S.S., Stegman, C.E., and Wolanin, M.O. (1986). No research versus research with compromised results: A study of validation therapy. *Nursing Research* 35:113–118.

Rogers, C.R. (1951). *Client-centered therapy: Its current practice, implications, and theory.* Boston: Houghton Mifflin.

Wolanin, M.O., and Phillips, L. (1981). *Confusion: Prevention and care.* St. Louis: C.V. Mosby.

Zachow, K.M. (1984). Helen, can you hear me? *Journal of Gerontological Nursing* 10(8):18–22.

CHAPTER 17

CONTRACTING

BACKGROUND

Patient compliance with or adherence to prescribed regimens and health practices is a major concern of health professionals. Considerable attention has been focused on ways to increase adherence (Becker & Maiman, 1980; Haynes et al., 1980; Swain & Steckel, 1981). Although providing the patient with information may help to improve adherence, education in and of itself is not sufficient. In fact, Swain and Steckel (1981) reported a higher drop out rate for persons with hypertension who had been in the patient education group than for those in the routine clinic visit group. Involving the patient in the plan of care and making the person more responsible for the outcomes of care have been found to increase adherence to health practices and regimens (Steckel, 1982; Zangari & Duffy, 1980).

Contracting is an intervention in which the patient is intimately involved in both the development and execution of the plan of care. Lewis and Minnich (1977) contended that a contract was effective in increasing compliance because it clarified the specific responsibilities of both the health care professional and the patient for achieving an agreed upon goal. The responsibility for attaining the outcome is transferred from the health care professional to the patient. Hayes and Davis (1980) stated that contracting is a strategy that has the potential for increasing congruence in values and priorities between the patient and the health professionals, leading to a mutually acceptable plan of care.

A goal of nursing is to empower the person and assist him/her to move toward independence. Contracting helps persons become integrally involved in their care. This is often accomplished in a stepwise progression. Patient involvement in the plan helps assure that the patient has the necessary knowledge about the regimen.

Many references to the use of contracting as a nursing intervention can be found in the literature. Contracting has been used in a variety of settings with diverse patient populations. Perhaps its widest use has been with patients with psychiatric problems. Although many studies on the effectiveness of contracting are found in other disciplines, few studies have tested its effectiveness within the context of nursing (Boehm, 1989).

Definition

Webster defined a contract as "a binding agreement between two or more persons or parties." According to Zangari and Duffy (1980), contracting rests on the premise that the nurse and patient are equal partners, but that each has different responsibilities for achieving the agreed upon goal. A contract explicitly details the expectations, outcomes, and responsibilities for each party. Contracts can be either written or verbal. Only written contracts will be addressed.

Contingency contracting is a specific form of contracting. Steckel (1982) defined it as:

> Identifying the desired behavior in measureable terms that are observable and acceptable to all parties involved. Contingency contracting also provides for an exchange of some form of reinforcement in return for performance of behaviors. [p. 33]

The element that differentiates contingency contracts from other types of patient contracts is reinforcement. A reinforcer is directly related to the behavior and may be positive or negative. A positive reinforcer, when presented, increases the probability of the response it follows. When a negative reinforcer is removed, the response is increased.

Treatment contracts are another type of contract that have been used in nursing (Boehm, 1989; Loomis, 1985). Loomis defined a treatment contract as

> an openly negotiated, clearly stated, written set of mutual expectations that indicates what the nurses and client can expect of each other regarding the client's treatment (or health care). [p. 9]

The purpose of treatment contracts is to provide the nurse and the client with clear expectations about the agreed upon goals and the responsibilities each has in moving toward these goals. Loomis (1985) delineated four types of treatment contracts: Care, social control, relationship, and structural change.

This chapter will focus on contingency contracts. Table 17.1 provides definitions of many of the terms that are part of contingency contracting.

Scientific Basis

Contingency contracting has its roots in operant conditioning which is based on the work of Skinner (Janz & Hartman, 1984). Contingency contracts are related to behavior modification. A premise of behavior modification is that the performance of a behavior depends on the consequences of that behavior. Kazdin (1980) stated that behavior change occurs only when the consequences contingent upon the performance of that behavior are altered. Positive or negative reinforcers can be used to bring about changes in behavior.

Classical conditioning, also called respondent conditioning, is one type of learning used by behavioral theorists. Pavlov's investigations explored classical conditioning. A specific stimulus, also called a conditioned stimulus, automatically evokes a response. Some stimuli in the person's environment elicit reflex responses; the person does not have control over these; for example, salivating when food is smelled. In classical conditioning a person is taught to respond to a neutral stimulus. A conditioned stimulus is paired with an unconditioned stimulus, which eventually results in the unconditioned stimulus singly eliciting the desired response.

Operant, or instrumental conditioning, is a second type of behavioral learning. The majority of human behaviors are voluntary and not reflexive. Voluntary behaviors are emitted spontaneously and are primarily controlled by their consequences. If behaviors can be controlled by changing their consequences, they are termed operants (Skinner, 1953). These can be increased or decreased by changing the events that follow them.

An overlap exists between classical and operant conditioning. It is now known that humans can control some of their reflex responses such as heart rate and blood pressure. Also, operant behaviors can be controlled by antecedent stimuli and not by just the consequences. Cues antecedent to the behavior may key the person to respond in a particular manner. These cues act as the stimulus for the response to occur. According to Steckel (1982), most human behaviors are learned through a combination of respondent and operant conditioning.

Reinforcement theory provides the basis for contingency contracts. Positive reinforcement results in an increase in the incidence of a behavior when it is followed closely by a favorable consequence.

Table 17.1
Definition of Terms Used in Contingency Contracting

Behavior
An observable and measureable response or action.

Chaining
A complex behavior is developed by focusing on the individual components of the behavior; this is done in a backward fashion.

Contingency
The relationship that exists between a behavior (the response targeted for change) and the activities (consequences) that follow behavior; events preceding a behavior are also part of the contingency.

Fading
Gradually removing the reinforcement given to the person.

Negative Reinforcer
An aversive event or stimulus that, when terminated, causes the frequency of the preceding response to increase.

Positive Reinforcer
An event that, when introduced, increases the likelihood of occurrence of the response it follows.

Reinforcement
An increase in the frequency of a response when it is immediately followed by a specific consequence.

Shaping
A gradual process of developing a new behavior through reinforcement of successive approximations working toward the overall desired terminal response.

Stimulus
A measureable event that may affect a behavior.

Target Behavior
The behavior that is to be changed during a behavior modification program.

Token
An object serving as a generalized conditioned reinforcer; it is often exchanged for backup reinforcers and it derives its value from them.

Reinforcers are determined by the effect they have on a behavior. The Premack Principle also is used in reinforcement. Kazdin (1980) defined it as any pair of responses or activities in which individuals freely engage; the one occurring most frequently will reinforce the less frequently occurring activity or response.

Reinforcers are unique for each person. Observing the person's behavior and determining what activities occur in relation to each other is one way to identify reinforcers. The terms "reward" and "reinforcer" are often used interchangeably. However, the two terms are distinct and should not be used interchangeably. A reward is a pleasant consequence that is not tied to the subsequent performance of the target behavior. Reinforcers are intimately linked to the targeted behavior. A reward may be written into the contract and be given when the goal is reached. Reinforcers are used to help achieve the goal.

Kazdin (1980) provided four suggestions for maximizing the effectiveness of positive reinforcement: Proximity of reinforcement to the event, magnitude or amount of reinforcement given, quality or type of reinforcement, and the scheduling of reinforcement. The closer the reinforcer is to the target behavior (behavior to be changed), the more likely it will produce positive results. Delayed reinforcement can be used after the target behavior is learned and the focus is sustaining the behavior. The more frequent the reinforcer or the greater its size, the greater will be the response. However, if the reinforcer is out of proportion to the magnitude of the behavior, it may mitigate against changing the behavior. Patient preference in the selection of the reinforcer helps assure that the quality or type of reinforcer will be effective. The schedule used in reinforcing the behavior can be continuous or intermittent and fixed or random. In continuous reinforcement the person is reinforced each time the behavior is performed, whereas in intermittent reinforcement the behavior may have to be executed a number of times before reinforcement occurs. When a fixed ratio of reinforcement is used, the person knows that after a specific number of performances, he will receive the reinforcer. No set pattern of reinforcement is used in the random ratio method. Random reinforcement is frequently used after the person has mastered the behavior and is being weaned from the reinforcer.

A behavior also may be decreased, but this is more difficult to accomplish than increasing a behavior. Extinction is one means used for decreasing a behavior. The reinforcer that has supported the behavior is removed resulting in a decrease in the target behavior (Kazdin, 1980). Rearranging the antecedent event also may be used to decrease a behavior.

INTERVENTION

Establishing rapport with the patient precedes initiating a contract. The rationale for the contract and the technique are explained. Cooperation of the patient, and often the family, is essential to the success of this intervention. Steps in contingency contracting consist of determining and defining the behavior along with its consequences and antecedent, planning and writing the contract, and evaluating the progress.

Technique

When discussing the problem/concern with the patient, a number of related problems may emerge. Priorities need to be established as attention is focused on one behavior at a time. The patient determines which one is the priority; if it is not deemed important by the patient, the chances for the outcome to be achieved are low. After the priority problem has been determined, goals are formulated. Frequently goals need to be broken down into smaller segments so that the behavior can be specifically defined. If this is not done, confusion and misunderstanding may result. Steckel (1982) stated that no step is too small to reinforce. She also suggested that starting with the easiest thing to change helps the person make progress toward the ultimate goal.

Shaping behaviors is the term given to breaking down the more complex behavior into smaller components. Each successive component is reinforced until the overall behavior is achieved; the behaviors form a chain.

Determination of Behavior, Consequences, and Antecedent

Behaviors are defined in very specific terms so that all parties know exactly what is being observed. Mager (1972) stated that a behavior needs to be so defined that all persons will know it if they see it. He cautioned against using "fuzzies." Breaking down complex behaviors into smaller segments helps avoid this problem.

Determination is made of the precise behavior and the context in which it occurs. This process may be the basis for the first contract that is established between the patient and the nurse. An agreement is written stating that the patient will come to the next meeting with a description of the context in which the behavior occurs and the number of times it occurs. Several methods may be used for this assessment. Counters can be used to keep track of how often a behavior occurs. This novelty of the counter may assist the patient to focus on the behavior and become more aware of its frequency. Keeping a diary is another method that may be used for assessing the extent of the behavior. An advantage of a diary is that the context of the behavior and the patient's feelings can be ascertained. A disadvantage of a diary is that the writing is often separated from the occurrence of the event and thus details may be lost. Also, the occurrences of the behavior may not be accurate. Establishing the baseline, the number of times the behavior occurs in a day or week, is necessary so that progress can be measured.

Antecedent behaviors serve as cues to the occurrence of the target behavior. Behaviors are frequently controlled by antecedents. Thoughts, feelings, places, or other persons are examples of antecedents (Steckel, 1982). Behaviors that are controlled by an antecedent are termed strong stimulus control behaviors.

Determining the consequences of the behavior is also part of the initial assessment. Observations by family members or health professionals are helpful in assisting the person to identify consequences and antecedents of the target behavior. An accurate picture of the context of the behavior assists in establishing the terms of the contract. Rearranging consequences is an effective way of changing behaviors (Steckel, 1982).

Planning and Writing the Contract

Kazdin (1980) listed five elements to be included in a contingency contract. They are:

1. The privileges each party expects to achieve from the contract are stated.
2. The chosen client behaviors are readily observable.
3. Sanctions for failure to meet the terms are explicit.
4. A bonus clause (extra privileges) can be used to reinforce compliance with the terms of the contract.
5. Provisions for monitoring progress are incorporated.

Table 17.2 shows an example of a contingency contract written for a person who wished to lose weight. Steckel (1982) suggested writing the contract on an 8.5- by 11-inch form and making a carbon copy. A copy of the contract serves as a reminder to each person of their duties in relation to the contract. Placing the contract in a prominent place is a constant reminder of the behavior to be changed. For hospitalized

Table 17.2
Example of a Written Contract

Contract

Dates of contract: September 1, 1990 to October 1, 1990

We agree to perform the following behaviors during the month of September.

If Anne refrains from eating junk food snacks from the time of her arrival home from work until bedtime, Marci will spend one hour playing tennis with her twice a week.

Reward: If this is adhered to for a month, Marci will buy tickets for both to attend the Northwest Tennis Tournament on October 15.

Penalty: If Anne eats junk food during the week, she will clean the apartment on Saturday.

Anne will keep a log of her evening eating, which will be shared with Marci on Friday evening.

Anne Johnson

Marci Maus

---

patients, placing the contract in the Kardex helps the staff to recall the specific components that need to carried out.

Reinforcer. A reinforcer is any consequence that strengthens a behavior. Reinforcers may be either positive or negative. A reward differs from a positive reinforcer in that, although it is also pleasant, it is not tied to the target behavior. When a negative reinforcer, an aversive stimulus, is removed, increases in the target behavior should result.

Reinforcers need to be related to the behavior. Ideas are obtained from patients regarding reinforcers they feel would be effective. Observing the behavior to be changed and the context in which it takes place also may suggest possible reinforcers. If the patient has difficulty in identifying possible reinforcers, a list of possible and realistic reinforcers can be formulated and shared with the patient. The final decision on the reinforcer rests with the patient. The nurse may use reinforcers as an item to negotiate with the patient, but final selection always resides with the patient. An example of a reinforcer is that every time the patient takes his medication without prompting, the nurse will visit with the patient for two minutes.

Measurement of Effectiveness

Some contracts include the time frame for when the contract will be evaluated. It is best to err on the side of giving too much time for reaching the goal rather than providing for too short a time frame. Not seeing sufficient progress may be discouraging for the patient. Even if it is not written, times for reviewing the contract need to be established and known to both parties. Flexibility in reaching a goal is needed; unforeseen circumstances may arise that affect the agreed-upon activities. Also, an unrealistic time frame may have been established initially.

Methods for keeping track of progress are used to determine if the goal has been achieved; they also can serve to motivate the patient to continue with the contract. Graphs are an easy method to use for depicting progress over time. Graphs also display the occurrence of plateaus. Providing an explanation to the patient about the possibility of plateaus before the contract begins helps decrease the discouragement associated with this seeming lack of progress. Steckel (1982) recommended reinforcing the patient for maintaining the plateau. If the plateau continues for a period of time, the elements of the contract should be reviewed. Alternate reinforcers may be needed. If the target behavior is part of a chain, previous behaviors may again need to be reinforced.

Fading is the term used to describe the weaning process from the reinforcer. A fixed ratio of reinforcement may be used at first so that the person is receiving less reinforcement but knows when it will occur. This is followed by random reinforcement; the person knows that the behavior will be reinforced on some occasions but is not certain when this will happen. When the behavior has been sustained with less and less reinforcement, no reinforcement is given. However, follow-up is needed to determine if the behavior continues.

USES

Contingency contracts have been used with diverse populations. Boehm (1989) reviewed the research that had been conducted on the use of contracting within nursing: 20 articles, with only 8 of these research-based, were found. Contracts have been used with students and teachers, children and parents, patients and staff, to alter weight in obese individuals, to control drug abuse, to eliminate smoking, and to improve compliance with therapeutic regimens (Steckel & Swain, 1977). Table 17.3 lists conditions for which contracting has been used as an intervention. Two conditions, weight loss and adherence to therapeutic regimens, will be discussed.

Table 17.3
Uses of Contracting

Acquiring health behaviors (Hayes & Davis, 1980)

Adherence to diabetes mellitus regimen (Morgan & Littel, 1988)

Compliance with medical regimens (Becker & Maiman, 1980; Etzwiler, 1973; Levendusky et al., 1983; Lowe & Lutzker, 1979)

Compliance with hypertension education (Swain & Steckel, 1981)

Coronary care unit patients (Ziemann & Dracup, 1989)

Elimination of drugs (Boudin, 1972; Hall et al., 1977)

Elimination of smoking (Neisworth, 1972)

Prevention of suicide (Twiname, 1981)

Prevent unplanned pregnancy (Van Dover, 1986)

Psychiatric patients (Loomis, 1985)

Weight reduction (Mann, 1972; Wing et al., 1981)

Weight Loss

Weight loss is a concern of many persons in our society. Countless programs for weight loss, using a variety of techniques, exist. A frequently voiced complaint of persons who have attended these programs is that after achieving their goal, they are unable to maintain the weight loss. This discourages the person from enrolling in another program and trying again. Too often programs focus only on weight loss and not on changes in behavior and life style.

Mann (1972) used contingency contracting with eight subjects who wished to lose weight. Five of the eight reached their goal; the mean weight loss was 32 pounds. The goal, however, was weight loss and not behavior change. It was not reported if the persons maintained their desired weight. Jeffrey and colleagues (1978) used three contingencies (weight loss, calories, and attendance) for three groups desiring to lose weight. Each member of the group deposited $200 before the sessions began. All three groups lost weight, with the calorie and attendance groups losing the most. Weight loss was maintained after the sessions were ended. Wing et al. (1981) compared the effects of two types of contingency contracts. Both groups deposited money with a specified amount returned at each weight loss session and in each maintenance meeting. Group one received money for weight loss during the training and for attendance during the maintenance period. Group two first attended instruction sessions and were rewarded for this. Subsequently they were rewarded for weight loss. Both groups lost significant amounts of weight. Again, weight gains occurred after the period of the contract. Wing and colleagues related that the three most successful patients continued to meet, formulate, and use contracts. All of the patients in the study liked the idea of contracts. In the studies cited, the researcher selected the contingency, which may have affected the outcome. Also, the focus was on the outcome and not on changing related behaviors.

Therapeutic Regimens

Over 50% of all Americans have some chronic illness. Many have prescribed regimens to be followed to prevent complications, reduce symptoms, and to control the progression of the pathology. Compliance with therapeutic regimens is extremely low. Swain and Steckel (1981) noted that many persons with chronic conditions are reluctant to assume an active role in their own care. Although information about the regimen is helpful, this in itself is often not sufficient to ensure that the patient will adhere to the regimen. Information may increase the person's anxiety. Contingency contracts offer a way to help persons incorporate the necessary practices into their life and to maintain them over time. The ultimate goal is a higher level of health for the person.

Steckel and Swain (1977), in a study of 115 outpatients with hypertension, found that persons with whom contingency contracts were established improved their knowledge about hypertension, kept clinic appointments, and had a decrease in diastolic blood pressure as compared to groups who received routine clinic care or routine care plus an educational program. Most noteworthy was the fact that no patients withdrew from the contract group, whereas there were dropouts from the other groups. Goals contracted for included:

Keep clinic appointment.
Earn a specific post-test score.
Lose weight.
Record daily food intake.
Read and study health-related materials.
Record daily blood pressures.
Change behavioral eating patterns.
Keep referral appointments.

These behaviors are all relevant for a person with hypertension and yet reflect the priority of the particular patient.

A therapeutic contract program (TCP) was used by Levendusky et al. (1983) for patients with chronic psychiatric conditions admitted to an inpatient psychiatric unit. Patients ranged in age from 18 to 72; more than 50% of the patients had had a previous hospitalization for their psychiatric condition. The aim of TCP was to develop internally attributed coping skills and self-perceptions of competence. Contracts were developed weekly with input from each patient and from the staff, and they reflected short-term goals for reaching the long-term goals. Mean length of hospitalization for patients using TCP was 71 days as compared with 107 days for similar patients in the hospital who received regular care. Readmissions were considerably less for this group after the TCP. Patients liked the use of contracts.

Morgan and Littel (1988) used teaching and contingency contracts with persons who had Type II diabetes mellitus to help them achieve control of their condition. Sixty subjects who were overweight participated in the study, with 30 subjects in the teaching-only group and 30 in the teaching and contracting group. The teaching and contracting were done in the persons' homes. A significant increase in knowledge about diabetes occurred in both groups, but no differences were found between the groups on weight loss, fasting blood sugar, and glycosylated hemoglobin. The authors noted that many of the previous studies in which positive results were obtained used motivated volunteers; random assignment was used in this study. Most importantly, the investigators stated that a definite relationship between adherence to the regimen and the outcomes used has not been established. Thus, persons may have been complying, but the measurements selected did not reflect their degree of compliance.

Precautions

Contingency contracts require time to carry out. Steckel and Swain (1977) stated that it took approximately 12 minutes to negotiate a contract with each patient in their study; more time may be necessary for patients to gain a clear understanding of what the contract requires. Patient acceptance is critical to the effectiveness of the process. If family or friends are to be involved, explanations also need to be given to them.

Because health professionals are accustomed to making decisions and implementing a plan of care without input from the patient, many may have difficulty in including the patient as an equal partner. Inservice education for the staff may be necessary.

RESEARCH QUESTIONS

Several reviews of the literature on contracting have been done (Boehm, 1989; Janz & Hartman, 1984). Most notable in Boehm's review was the small number of studies in which the effectiveness of contracting had been tested. Reasons for this lack of research in nursing may be that nurses have relied on studies that have been conducted in the behavioral sciences; that contracting conveys a sense of mechanistic control; and that formal testing has not been done although contracts have been used. Contracting, whether it be contingency contracts or treatment contracts, can empower patients in dealing with factors related to their health. The following are some of the areas in which nursing research on contracts is indicated:

1. Is the use of contracts more effective with younger age groups? Boehm (1989) posits this as a question for study.
2. How long should a person be maintained at a plateau level before revisions in the contract are made? Should reinforcers be used during the plateau stage?
3. Are there particular patient characteristics that suggest that contingency contracting would be an effective intervention to employ? Are there patient populations or conditions for whom contracts should not be used? Boehm (1989) notes that the majority of the research has been with persons with chronic conditions. Are contracts equally appropriate with persons in acute care settings? Ziemann and Dracup (1989) found that use of contracts with patients in coronary care units was effective in reducing anxiety and depression.
4. Are there occasions when negative reinforcers should be used as opposed to positive reinforcers? Since emphasis is placed on the positive, attention to the use of negative reinforcers has been minimal.

REFERENCES

Becker, M., & Maiman, L. (1980). Strategies for enhancing patient compliance. *Journal of Community Health* 6:113–135.

Boehm, S. (1989). Patient contracting. Pp. 143–153 in J. Fitzpatrick, R. Taunton, & J. Benoliel eds., *Annual review of nursing research*, vol. 7. New York: Springer.

Boudin, H. (1972). Contingency contracting as a therapeutic tool in the deceleration of amphetamine use. *Behavior Therapy* 3:604–608.

Etzwiler, D. (1973). The contract for health care. *Journal of the American Medical Association* 224:1973.

Hall, S., Cooper, J., Burmaster, S., & Polk, A. (1977). Contingency contracting as a therapeutic tool with methadone maintenance clients: Six single subject studies. *Behavior Research and Therapy* 15:438–441.

Hayes, W., & Davis, L. (1980). What is a health care contract? *Health Values: Achieving High Level Wellness* 4(2): 82–89.

Haynes, R., Sackett, D., & Taylor, D. (1980). How to detect changes and manage low patient compliance in chronic illness. *Geriatrics* 35:91–97.

Janz, N.K., & Hartman, P.E. (1984). Contingency contracting to enhance patient compliance: A review. *Patient Education and Counseling* 5:165–178.

Jeffrey, R., Thompson, P., & Wing, R. (1978). Effects on weight reduction of strong monetary contracts to calorie restriction or weight loss. *Behavior Research and Therapy* 16:363–369.

Kazdin, A. (1980). *Behavior modification in applied settings*. Homewood, IL: The Dorsey Press.

Levendusky, P., Berglas, S., Dooley, C., & Landau, R. (1983). Therapeutic contract program: Preliminary report on a behavioral alternative to the token economy. *Behavior Research and Therapy* 21:137–142.

Lewis, C., & Minnich, M. (1977). Contracts as a means of improving patient compliance. Pp. 69–75 in I. Barofsky ed., *Medication compliance: a behavioral management approach*. Thorofare, NJ: Charles B. Slack.

Loomis, M.E. (1985). Levels of contracting. *Journal of Psychosocial Nursing* 23(3):9–14.

Lowe, K., & Lutzker, J. (1979). Increasing compliance to a medical regimen with a juvenile diabetic. *Behavior Therapy* 10:57–64.

Mager, R. (1972). *Goal analysis*. Belmont, CA: Fearon Publishers.

Mann, R. (1972). The behavior-therapeutic use of contingency contracting to control adult behavior problem: Weight control. *Journal of Applied Behavior Analysis* 5:99–109.

Morgan, B.S., & Littell, D.H. (1988). A closer look at teaching and contingency contracting with Type II diabetes. *Patient Education and Counseling* 12:145–158.

Neisworth, J. (1972). Elimination of cigarette smoking through gradual phase-out of stimulus controls. *Behaviorally Speaking* 10:1–3.

Skinner, B. (1953). *Science and human behavior*. New York: Free Press.

Steckel, S. (1982). *Patient contracting*. Norwalk, CT: Appelton-Century-Crofts.

Steckel, S., & Swain, M. (1977). Contracting with patients to improve compliance. *Hospitals* 51(23):81–84.

Swain, M., & Steckel, S. (1981). Influencing adherence among hypertensives. *Research in Nursing and Health* 4:213–222.

Twiname, B. (1981). No-suicide contract for nurses. *Journal Psychiatric Nursing and Mental Health Services* 19(7): 11–12.

Van Dover, L. (1986). Influence of nurse-client contracting on a family knowledge and behaviors in a university student population. *Dissertation Abstracts International* 46:3787B.

Wing, R., Epstein, L., Marcus, M., & Shapira, B. (1981). Strong monetary contingencies for weight loss during treatment and maintenance. *Behavior Therapy* 12:702–710.

Zangari, M., & Duffy, P. (1980). Contracting with patients in day-to-day practice. *American Journal of Nursing* 80:451–455.

Ziemann, K.M., & Dracup, K. (1989). How well do CCU patient-nurse contracts work? *American Journal of Nursing* 89:691–692.

CHAPTER 18

MEDITATION

BACKGROUND

Since ancient times, meditation has been used by persons in many cultures. The practice of meditation frequently is viewed as a religious practice; however, recent attention has focused on its use as an intervention for relief of anxiety and anxiety-related disorders, for expanding awareness, and for improvement of well-being. Many meditation techniques exist; great differences are found in the focus of these various techniques and procedures used to achieve the desired goal. This chapter will provide an overall description of meditation, with Benson's relaxation response technique being discussed in depth.

Definition

Many definitions of meditation can be identified in the literature. West (1979) defined meditation as an exercise in which the individual focuses attention or awareness in order to dwell upon a single object. The definition proposed by Goleman and Schwartz (1976) is similar in that attention is focused on a single percept. They defined meditation as:

> The systematic and continued focusing of the attention on a single target percept—for example, a mantra or sound—or persistently holding a specific attentional set toward all percepts or mental contents as they spontaneously arise in the field of awareness. [p. 457]

Welwood's definition (1979) is broader than the previous two; he viewed meditation as a technique that allows a person to investigate the process of his/her consciousness and experiences and to discover the more basic underlying qualities of one's existence as an animate reality. Intense concentration blocks other stimuli allowing the person to become more aware of self.

The resurgence in interest in meditation has drawn largely from the Eastern religions, but meditation also has been an important aspect of the Western world and the Judaeo-Christian tradition. Records substantiate the use of meditation by Hindus in India as early as 1500 B.C. Taoists in China and Buddhists in India included meditation as an integral part of their religious life. Zen Buddhism in Japan developed a special form of meditation called Zazen, which is a sitting meditation in which a quiet awareness is maintained of whatever is presently happening. In Western cultures, monks and hermits went to the desert to meditate; meditation has remained a key element of monastic life. West (1979) noted the use of meditation in the American Indian culture, the Kung Zhu/twasi of Africa, and the Eskimos of North America. Although techniques vary considerably among these groups, the outcomes are very similar for all techniques.

Everly and Rosenfeld (1981) divided meditation techniques into four forms: mental repetition, physical repetition, problem concentration, and visual concentration. In mental repetition the person concentrates on a word or phrase, commonly called a mantra. Concentration on breathing is frequently the focus in physical repetition techniques; however, dance or other body movements can be the object of concentration. In samatha Buddhist meditation, the person watches or concentrates on the breath entering and flowing from the tip of the nostrils. Jogging also allows for concentrating on a physical activity, repetitive breathing, and the sound of one's feet hitting the ground. In problem contemplation techniques, an attempt is made to solve a problem that contains paradoxical components. Zen terms this the "koan." Visual concentration techniques are akin to imagery.

Transcendental meditation (TM), a much-publicized technique, was introduced into the United States in 1958 by Maharishi Mahesh Yogi. More than one million persons have attended classes to learn the technique (Puente, 1981). A variation of TM is Benson's relaxation response. TM has been used extensively as a means for decreasing stress and increasing awareness of self. Although public interest in meditation has lessened somewhat, its documented effectiveness in certain conditions makes it an intervention that nurses should consider using to achieve specific patient outcomes.

Scientific Basis

Studies on meditation cite effects in both the physiological and psychological realms. Lichstein (1988) reviewed the findings of studies in which meditation had been used. Not all persons who were taught the varying meditation techniques benefited from the intervention. Lichstein posed two possible explanations for the disparity in the findings: meditation may not have been the intervention that fit with a specific person's personality or the technique employed may not have been appropriate for achieving the desired outcome. Despite weaknesses in some of the study designs in which the effects of meditation were explored, there is substantial evidence showing positive results from its use. These results have occurred despite the fact that many of the studies used novice meditators. To obtain maximum effects from meditation, the person must first have mastered the technique.

Physiological effects that have been studied are primarily noted in the sympathetic portion of the autonomic nervous system with a decrease in heart rate (Hoffman et al., 1982; Wallace, 1970; West, 1979); a lowering or stabilization of the blood pressure (Benson et al., 1974b); a decrease in skin conductance and fewer spontaneous skin conductance responses (West, 1979); and a decrease in respiration rate and oxygen consumption (West, 1979). The lowering of oxygen consumption may be the result of a decrease in overall bodily activity that occurs because the person is resting. Decreases in arousal, however, frequently have not differed between subjects taught meditation and those taught to relax via other stress management techniques. According to West (1979), it is noteworthy that in most intrasubject comparisons, that is, when the same subject both meditates and performs the task set in the control condition, more significant decreases have always been found during meditation. Sugi and Akutsu (1968) found significant decreases in the respiratory rate and oxygen consumption in seasoned meditators; such changes are usually not found in persons who have practiced meditation for only a short time. Other physiological parameters in which positive effects have been shown include improved auditory and visual perception, improved fine motor coordination, increased serotonin levels, and decreased cortisol levels (Lichstein, 1988).

The following changes in electroencephalogram (EEG) activity have been found in persons who practice meditation:

1. The alpha amplitude increases at the beginning of meditation.
2. Theta activity, often intermixed with alpha, occurs later in meditation.
3. Bursts of high frequency beta of 20 to 40 cps can occur during deep meditation.
4. Alpha activity may persist, even with eyes open, after meditation has ceased (West, 1979).

These changes help to explain the expanded awareness and the high experienced by many persons who meditate.

West (1979) stated there are few theoretical reasons for meditation's effectiveness. Various explanations for its seeming effectiveness, however, have been proposed. Explanations include that of adaptive regression (Shafii, 1973) and desensitization, as meditating allows the person to deal with unfinished psychic material (Tart, 1971). Another possible hypothesis for the effectiveness of meditation is that it is a way of learning to experience without categorizing or predetermining (Goleman, 1977).

According to Everly and Rosenfeld (1981), the role of the focal device used in meditation allows the intuitive, nonegocentered mode of thought processing to dominate consciousness in place of the normally dominant analytic, egocentered mode of thought processing. When the left hemisphere of the brain is silenced (rational, analytic), the intuitive mode produces extraordinary awareness. This state is frequently called the "nirvana." A positive mood, an experience of unity, an alteration in time–space relationships, an enhanced sense of reality and meaning, and an acceptance of things that seem paradoxical are experienced in this superconscious state. A continuum is progressed through from the beginning meditation to this superconscious state.

This superconscious state differs from sleep. Metabolism decreases gradually during sleep, whereas the drop during meditation occurs during the first few minutes (Benson, 1975). Alpha waves increase during meditation but are found infrequently during sleep. Rapid eye movement activity found during sleep is not experienced during meditation. The two states, sleep and superconsciousness of meditation, are not interchangeable, although persons who meditate regularly often relate requiring less sleep than previously.

Meditation's effect on decreases in anxiety could fit into the model suggested by Brown (1977) for the basis of effects seen in progressive relaxation. Because the person is concentrating on a thought or object, other thoughts are not able to intrude. Thus, the cycle of stimulation and production of more anxiety is broken. Many meditation techniques incorporate aspects of progressive relaxation as an initial phase of the technique.

It is not just the immediate effects of meditation that are considered beneficial, but more importantly the general relation of these effects to a person's entire life that is deemed important. Through the practice of meditation, a person achieves an overall calmness.

INTERVENTION

A variety of meditation techniques are presented in the literature (Carrington, 1984; Goleman, 1977; Lichstein, 1988). Nurses wishing to explore the specifics of these techniques are referred to the listed sources. Table 18.1 lists some of the common forms of meditation described by LeShan (1974) and Lichstein (1988). Benson's relaxation response, a widely used noncultic technique, will be detailed in this chapter. Many research studies have explored the effectiveness of this technique with various patient populations. Benson notes that the physiological findings found in his laboratory were similar to those found in clinical studies in which the TM technique was used.

Technique

The relaxation response incorporates four elements; these are common in many of the other relaxation techniques. These elements are a quiet environment, a mental device, a passive attitude, and a comfortable position.

A quiet environment, which is an element of Benson's technique, eliminates outside stimuli and allows the person to concentrate on the mental device. Some persons prefer a church or chapel for meditating, but such a place is usually not readily accessible. Playing music while meditating is not advocated because it may draw the person's attention away from the internal processes. Persons should select the place they wish to use for meditation and continue to use that place. This eliminates adjusting to new surroundings and stimuli each time a person meditates.

Table 18.1
Selected Meditation Techniques

Contemplation

Person focuses on something in an active manner; no words are used.

Breathing

Person focuses on breathing. Attention is drawn to rhythm of breathing and air being drawn in and exhaled.

Bubble

Person observes own consciousness; meditates on stream of consciousness; each thought is a bubble arising into space; the content of thought is not explored.

Gaze

Person focuses attention on a visual object, often a mandala, which is a geometric design.

Theraveda Type

Person meditates on self-generated rhythms; chooses a body rhythm that occurs automatically (heart, breath) and focuses on it.

Mantra

Person assumes a comfortable position. Word or phrase is chanted or repeated over and over.

Sufi Movement

Group of people join hands and form a circle; heads, bodies, and feet are moved in and out like a flower opening; chanting is done in conjunction with movement.

Sensory Awareness

Person lies on the floor and focuses attention on all body parts and all of their dimensions.

Unstructured

Person chooses image or concept and explores nature and meaning of it and feelings about it; active exploration is done.

Safe Harbor

Person assumes comfortable position and lets consciousness drift within self; seeks safe and secure place.

Use of the mental device helps to shift the mind from logical, externally oriented thought to inner rumination. The purpose of the mental device is to preoccupy oneself with an emotionally neutral, repetitive, and monotonous stimulus (Lichstein, 1988). Unlike in TM in which the teacher gives the student a mantra, in Benson's technique each person selects his own mental device, which is used whenever the person meditates. The mental device may be a sound, word, or phrase that is repeated silently or aloud. Persons may choose to use a phrase or portion of a religious prayer or psalm. Fixation on an object also is sometimes used as the mental device.

Benson (1975) stresses that a passive attitude is the most important element in eliciting the physiological response resulting from meditation. Persons should be aware that distracting thoughts and images may occur. These should not be a cause of worry, but rather, a "let it happen" attitude should be assumed. When distractions do occur, the person is instructed to simply return to use of the mental device. Repetition of the mental device or focusing attention on one's breathing helps in overcoming distractions. Distracting thoughts do not indicate that a person is not performing the technique correctly, but rather that renewed attention to the mental device is required. Even experienced meditators encounter distractions. Preparing oneself for meditation by relaxing the body helps reduce distractions.

A comfortable position contributes to overall relaxation. Sitting in a chair that gives support to the body and yet allows for comfort is ideal. Sleep may result if the person tries to meditate in a recumbent position. Benson hypothesizes that the uncomfortable positions such as kneeling or sitting cross legged that are advocated in some techniques are intended to keep the person from falling asleep.

The specific instructions for the relaxation response include:

1. Sit quietly in a comfortable position.
2. Close your eyes.
3. Deeply relax all your muscles, beginning at your feet and progressing to your face. Remain relaxed throughout the meditation.
4. Breathe through your nose. Become aware of your breathing. As you breathe out, say the word, "one," silently to yourself. For example, breathe in . . . out, "one (or whatever mental device is being used)," in . . . out, "one." Breathe easily and naturally.
5. Continue for 10 to 20 minutes. You may open your eyes to check the time, but do not use an alarm. When you finish, sit quietly for several minutes with your eyes open. Do not stand up for a few minutes. If you need help keeping track of time, a radio alarm with music is preferred. A loud alarm will startle you and negate the restfulness achieved.
6. Do not worry whether you are successful in achieving a deep level of relaxation. Maintain a passive attitude and permit relaxation to occur at its own pace. When distracting thoughts occur, try to ignore them by not dwelling on them and return to repeating the mental device. With practice, the response should come with little effort. Practice the technique once or twice daily, but not within two hours after any meal, as the digestive processes seem to interfere with the elicitation of the relaxation response (Benson, 1975).

In the research studies that have been cited, different techniques have been used. Benson (1975) emphasized fitting the technique to the individual and make modifications as necessary. Therefore, before any teaching is initiated, an assessment of the individual is needed to determine what might be the most appropriate technique to use for a particular person or for a specific condition. This requires that a nurse have knowledge about specific meditation techniques.

The instructor's personal experience with the use of meditation techniques is ideal. Familiarity with the literature on meditation will be of assistance in selecting a specific technique to use with particular conditions.

Mastery of the technique results from daily or twice daily practice. LeShan (1974) commented that learning to meditate is hard work. Few authors provide information on the number of formal teaching sessions necessary for learning a technique; six or seven teaching sessions were recommended by Credidio (1982). Puente (1981) found that physiological responses associated with meditation did not occur after five days of practice; the Maharishi stated that persons should experience changes after this length of time. Findings in a study by Credidio (1982) revealed electromyographic (EMG) changes occurring after six instructional sessions. According to Lehrer et al. (1980), four to five weeks of daily practice are needed before significant psychophysiologic changes are noted. Puente (1981) found that individuals who had meditated for one and one-half years had the same physiological arousal levels as were found in persons who had meditated for over five years. A number of critics (West, 1979; Goleman & Schwartz, 1976) commented that because novices were used in many studies, findings may be misleading as physiological changes usually occur only after meditation has been practiced for a longer time. Thus, the effectiveness of meditation is even more convincing because positive results frequently occurred with novice meditators.

Measurement of Effectiveness

The purpose for which meditation is used will dictate the parameters to be used in evaluating its effectiveness. Commonly used measures include heart rate, blood pressure, respiratory rate, oxygen consumption, skin conductance, EEG and EMG recordings, scores on anxiety scales, and subjective reports. Benson (1975) reported that subjects practicing the relaxation response were calmer, more receptive to ideas, more patient, committed to daily exercise, drank less, and were happier overall. Although Credidio (1982) found no changes on the scores of the Eysenck Personality Inventory between persons taught meditation and persons in the control group, subjective reports indicated a positive reaction to the use of meditation. Because subjective reporting is very important in whether or not a person will continue to practice an intervention, distinguishing how the person feels about the effects of meditation is important.

Nurses in clinical areas can easily use blood pressure readings, heart rate, and respiratory rate as indicators of the effectiveness of meditation. These should not only be taken before and immediately after the practice of meditation, but also at other times during the day, with records kept to determine if changes occur over time. Because the person is resting while meditating, it would be expected that the readings would be lower after practice. It is also important that continued follow-up be done to determine if the effects persist.

USES

Meditation has not been as widely used as a stress management technique as have other techniques, but because of its simplicity it holds much promise as an intervention in conditions in which high levels of anxiety occur. Perhaps because it frequently is linked to religion, health personnel may be reluctant to prescribe it. Table 18.2 lists conditions for which meditation has been used. Use of meditation for patients with hypertension, anxiety associated with coronary care units, insomnia, and health promotion will be discussed.

Table 18.2
Conditions In Which Meditation Has Been Used

Chronic pain (Kabat-Zinn, 1982)
Coronary care units (Guzzetta, 1989; Melville, 1987)
Diagnostic procedures (Frenn et al., 1986)
Desensitization for phobias (Goldfried, 1971)
Drug abuse (Benson & Wallace, 1972; Shafii et al.,1975)
Headache (Benson et al., 1974a)
Health promotion (Kolkmeier, 1988)
Hypertension (Benson et al., 1974b; Blackwell et al., 1976)
Insomnia (Woolfolk et al., l976)
Menstrual discomfort (Loevsky, 1978)

Hypertension

Benson explored the effectiveness of the relaxation response with persons who had hypertension because of the decreases in blood pressure experienced by persons who had practiced TM. Statistically significant changes between the experimental and control groups were found in his initial study. Mean systolic pressures decreased from 146 to 137 mm Hg, and mean diastolic pressures from 93.5 to 88.9 mm Hg in subjects who were taught and who practiced Benson's technique. Blood pressure was not measured immediately after the person had meditated, but rather readings were taken at random times throughout the day. It is hypothesized that meditation counteracts the sympathetic responses of the flight–fight reaction to stressors. Other studies (Benson et al., 1974; Blackwell et al., 1976; Pollock et al., 1977) likewise found decreases in blood pressure in persons who regularly meditated. However, in the Blackwell and Pollock studies, only short-term (three-month) effects occurred. West (1980) attributes this to placebo effects showing diminishing returns with the passage of time. Influence of the instructor may have prompted the persons to practice initially, and as the distance from this lengthened, the motivation to practice decreased. Benson (1975) stated that the relaxation response in and of itself will probably not be sufficient to lower severe or moderately high blood pressures, but its continued use will enable persons to require fewer or reduced doses of antihypertensive medications. Practice of meditation could help to prevent the occurrence of hypertension.

Anxiety Associated with Coronary Care

A number of articles and several studies have explored the use of meditation with patients in coronary care units or those undergoing procedures related to coronary conditions (Frenn et al., 1986; Guzzetta, 1989; Melville, 1987; Moreno, 1987). Guzzetta studied the effects that music and the relaxation response had on various parameters of patients in coronary care units who had a myocardial infarct. Apical heart rates were lowered and peripheral temperatures were raised in subjects in these two groups as compared to subjects in a control group. Patients in these two groups also had fewer complications. Although Frenn and colleagues did not find significant differences in parameters measured between the group taught the relaxation response and the control group in persons undergoing a cardiac catheterization, more subjects who practiced the relaxation response had lower respiratory rates, blood pressure, and scores on the state anxiety than did subjects in the control group. Thus, there is some evidence to support the use of relaxation response as an intervention for patients who may have increased anxiety because of the diagnosis of cardiac pathology or the fear of undergoing diagnostic procedures.

Insomnia

Persons with high levels of stress frequently have difficulty getting to sleep or progressing through the normal sleep cycles. Interventions that seek to reduce stress levels should, therefore, improve sleep. Woolfolk and colleagues (1976) compared the effectiveness of meditation with progressive relaxation on decreasing insomnia. Significant improvement was found in both groups as compared to a control group. A follow-up at six months revealed that improvement persisted over time. Many elderly experience difficulties with sleep. This is also a population for whom sleeping medications may cause dangerous untoward effects. Meditation may be an excellent alternative for insomnia in the elderly.

Health Promotion

Kolkmeier (1988) notes that relaxation interventions are not only applicable for use to reduce anxiety associated with nursing and medical procedures, but also are useful to the person for all aspects of life. In an anecdotal account, Boerstler and Kornfeld noted that a mother, following her son's death, used meditation to adjust to her son's death and to change some things in her life style (Boerstler & Kornfeld, 1987). Meditation techniques assist the person in moving toward wholeness and balance. Incorporation of a meditation technique, such as the relaxation response, into a person's coping repertoire may prevent the occurrence of high levels of stress and its concomitant negative effects.

Precautions

Meditation is not a benign intervention. The nurse must be aware of side effects of the intervention, persons for whom it should not be used, and assessments to be made as the person practices meditation. Careful monitoring of reactions to medications is necessary. Doses may have to be decreased; Everly and Rosenfeld (1981) noted problems of overdosage in the use of insulin, sedatives, and cardiovascular medications in persons who meditated. Because of the effect meditation can have on the cardiovascular system, the blood pressure should be checked before the person begins to meditate. If it is below 90 mm Hg, meditation should not be practiced. Patients should be instructed not to meditate if light-headedness or dizziness is felt. Also, the person should not stand immediately after meditating because a hypotensive state frequently is found.

Benson (1975) notes that hallucinations can occur if the person meditates for too long at one time—this is usually for several hours at a time. Loss of reality contact is a possibility and continued assessment is needed to determine if this is occurring. Lazarus (1976) reported cases of attempted suicide, schizophrenia, and severe depression after the continued practice of meditation. Perhaps meditation should not be prescribed for some persons, but the characteristics of persons who would be harmed by it are unclear. Others, such as persons with Type A personalities, may not benefit from meditation (Everly & Rosenfeld, 1981).

RESEARCH QUESTIONS

Minimal nursing research was found that documented the effectiveness of meditation as a nursing intervention. Many nurses have, however, used various meditation techniques on an informal basis. Both formal research and reporting of clinical observations on the effects of meditation are needed. Some specific areas in which research is needed include:

1. What are the characteristics of persons who benefit from meditation? Do persons who continue to practice meditation differ significantly from those who are taught it and then abandon it?
2. Longitudinal studies are needed to determine the long-term effects of meditation as the majority of studies have only looked at the immediate effects of meditation.
3. How generalizable are the effects of meditation? Does its use affect other areas of the person's life than those for which it was taught? If the person is taught meditation as a means for decreasing hypertension, is there also an improvement in sleep and other areas?
4. Are there differences in outcomes in the use of the various meditation techniques? The majority of nursing studies have used Benson's relaxation response. However, a large number of other techniques are available.
5. Minimal data are available on the number of sessions required for teaching meditation. More research is needed. Also, study reports should incorporate more information on the teaching sessions.

REFERENCES

Benson, H. (1975). *The relaxation response.* New York: Avon.

Benson, H., Klemchuk, H., & Graham, J. (1974a). The usefulness of the relaxation response in the therapy of headache. *Headache* 14:49–52.

Benson, H., Rosner, B., Marzetta, B., & Klemchuk, H. (1974b). Decreased blood pressure in pharmacologically treated hypertensive patients who regularly elicited the relaxation response. *Lancet* i:289–291.

Benson, H., & Wallace, R. (1972). Decreased drug abuse with Transcendental Meditation: A study of 1,862 subjects. Pp. 369–376 in C. Arafonetis ed., *Drug abuse: proceedings of the international conference*. Philadelphia: Lea & Febiger.

Blackwell, B., Henenson, I. Bloomfield, S., Magenheim, H., Gartide, P., Nidich, S., Robinson, A., & Zigler, R. (1976). Transcendental meditation in hypertension, individual response patterns. *Lancet* i:223–226.

Boerstler, R.W., & Kornfeld, H.S. (1987). Meditation as a clinical intervention. *Journal of Psychosocial Nursing* 25(6): 25–32.

Brown, B. (1977). *Stress and the art of biofeedback*. New York: Bantam.

Carrington, P. (1984). Modern forms of meditation. Pp. 108–141 in R. Woolfolk & P. Lehrer eds., *Principles and practice of stress management*. New York: Guilford Press.

Credidio, S. (1982). Comparative effectiveness of patterned biofeedback vs meditation training on EMG and skin temperature changes. *Behavior Research and Therapy* 20:233–241.

Everly, G., & Rosenfeld, R. (1981). *The nature and treatment of the stress responses*. New York: Plenum Press.

Frenn, M., Fehring, R., & Kartes, S. (1986). Reducing the stress of cardiac catheterization by teaching relaxation. *Dimensions of Critical Care Nursing* 5:108–116.

Goldfried, M. (1971). Systematic desensitization as training in self control. *Journal of Consulting and Clinical Psychology* 39:228–234.

Goleman, D. (1977). *The varieties of the meditative experience*. New York: E. P. Dutton.

Goleman, D., & Schwartz, G. (1976). Meditation as an intervention in stress reactivity. *Journal of Consulting and Clinical Psychology* 44:456–466.

Guzzetta, C.E. (1989). Effects of relaxation and music therapy on patients in a coronary care unit with presumptive acute myocardial infarct. *Heart & Lung* 18:609–616.

Hoffman, J., Benson, H., Arns, P., Stainbrook, G., Landsburg, L., Young, J., & Gill, A. (1982). Reduced sympathetic nervous system responsivity associated with the relaxation response. *Science* 215:190–192.

Kabat-Zinn, J. (1982). An outpatient program in behavioral medicine for chronic pain based on the practice of mindfulness meditation. *General Hospital Psychiatry* 4:33–47.

Kolkmeier, L.G. (1988). Relaxation: opening the door to change. Pp. 195–222 in B. Dossey, L. Keegan, C. Guzzetta, & L. Kolkmeier eds., *Holistic nursing—a handbook for practice*. Rockville, MD: Aspen.

Lazarus, A. (1976). Psychiatric problems precipitated by transcendental meditation. *Psychological Reports* 39:601–602.

Lehrer, P., Schoicket, S., Carrington, P., & Woolfolk, R. (1980). Psychophysiological and cognitive responses to stressful stimuli in subjects practicing progressive relaxation and clinically standardized meditation. *Behavior Research and Therapy* 18:293–303.

LeShan, L. (1974). *How to meditate*. Boston: Little, Brown, and Company.

Lichstein, K.L. (1988). *Clinical relaxation strategies*. New York: John Wiley & Sons.

Loevsky, J. (1978). Menstruation: Alternatives to pharmacological therapy for menstrual distress. *Journal of Nurse-Midwifery* 23:34–44.

Melville, S.B. (1987). Relaxation techniques in acute myocardial infarction: the theoretic rationale. *Focus on Critical Care* 14(1):9–11.

Moreno, C.K. (1987). Concepts of stress management in cardiac rehabilitation. *Focus on Critical Care* 14(5):13–19.

Pollock, A., Weber, M., Case, D., & Laragh, J. (1977). Limitations of transcendental meditation in the treatment of essential hypertension. *Lancet* i:71–73.

Puente, A. (1981). Psychophysiological investigations on transcendental meditation. *Biofeedback and Self-Regulation* 6:327–342.

Shafii, M. (1973). Adaptive and therapeutic aspects of meditation. *International Journal of Psychoanalysis and Psychotherapy* 2:431–443.

Shafii, M., Lovely, R., & Jaffe, R. (1975). Meditation and the prevention of alcohol abuse. *American Journal of Psychiatry* 132:942–945.

Sugi, Y., & Akutsu, K. (1968). Studies on respiration and energy metabolism during sitting in Zazen. *Research Journal of Physical Education* 12:190–206.

Tart, C. (1971). A psychologist's experiences with transcendental meditation. *Journal of Transpersonal Psychology* 3:135–143.

Wallace, R. (1970). Physiological effects of transcendental meditation. *Science* 167:1751–1754.

Welwood, J. (1979). *The meeting of the ways: Explorations in east/west psychology.* New York: Schocken Books.

West, M. (1979). The psychosomatics of meditation. *Journal of Psychosomatic Medicine* 24:265–273.

_____. (1980). Meditation. *British Journal of Psychiatry* 135:457–467.

Woolfolk, R., Carr-Kaffashan, L., & McNulty, T. (1976). Meditation training as a treatment for insomnia. *Behavior Therapy* 7:350–365.

CHAPTER 19

SENSATION INFORMATION

(Note: Material in this chapter is based on content provided by A. Marilyn Sime for the first edition.)

BACKGROUND

The provision of sensation information as a strategy to prepare persons for upcoming stressful events has been investigated by a number of nurse researchers. The intervention is thought to enhance or stimulate cognitive processes that will reduce the emotional response experienced by patients encountering threatening stimuli and improve coping responses to the perceived stressful event. Because nurses frequently are responsible for the preparation of patients facing stressful diagnostic procedures and treatments, interventions that reduce patient distress and improve patient outcomes are important to include in nursing's armamentarium.

Definition

Sensation information (also termed sensory information) is the objective description of what a person will see, feel, hear, smell, and taste in a specific situation. The information concerns sense data, such as cold skin or sour taste, experienced by the individual as the result of direct stimulation of the sense organs. The information does not concern generalized reactions or affective states, such as comfort or fear. This is an important distinction. Unfortunately, the term sensation is often used to describe experiences ranging from sense organ stimulation to vague generalized states of being. Sensation information in this chapter will only be used to refer to objective descriptions of the experience of sense organs being stimulated.

Scientific Basis

An early investigation of the effects of sensation information on human responses to stressful situations was reported by Schachter and Singer (1962). They found that subjects who were told what bodily sensations they would experience from an injection of epinephrine responded with less emotion than subjects not told about these sensations.

Johnson (1973; Johnson & Rice, 1974) studied the threatening event of ischemic pain produced by the inflation of a blood pressure cuff. In a series of studies on the effects of sensation information Johnson learned:

1. Descriptions of typical sensations reduced the amount of distress experienced, but the intensity of pain was not decreased.
2. Attending to the sensations per se did not reduce distress.
3. Sensation information did not reduce the perceived danger of the threatening event or its expected intensity.
4. All typical sensations did not need to be described for distress reduction.
5. Atypical sensation descriptions resulted in elevated distress.

Johnson theorized that a cognitive process involving expectations about sensations to be experienced was the factor involved in distress reduction. Specifically, congruency between expected and experienced sensations reduced responses during threatening encounters.

In a series of studies involving endoscopy procedures (Johnson & Leventhal, 1974; Johnson et al., 1973), orthopedic cast removal (Johnson et al., 1975), pelvic examination (Fuller et al., 1978), and abdominal surgery (Johnson et al., 1978a, b), the following results were found:

1. Providing sensation information reduced negative emotional responses, heart rate, gagging, and restlessness and fewer tranquilizers were used.
2. Sensation information seemed to be most effective with persons who were relatively fearful before surgery. Sime (1976) found that increased amounts of preoperative information of an unspecified nature improved postoperative recovery only in patients with high anxiety.
3. Sensation information was not effective with all patients or with all populations.

Johnson concluded that knowing the sensations to be experienced provides reality-oriented cognitive images which in turn give the person a sense of control over the situation; this may bolster the person's ability to use available coping strategies. The conclusions from these clinical studies differ from those Johnson arrived at from her laboratory studies.

Leventhal et al. (1979) demonstrated that congruency or accuracy of the sensation information per se is not the critical factor in distress reduction. When a pain warning was added to sensation information, distress reduction was blocked. Leventhal interpreted this finding to mean that information on the potential strength of a stimulus elicits an emotional interpretation of the stimulus, rather than an objective encoding of the information. Arousal information, or descriptions of generalized states—such as apprehension, excitement, and tension—was demonstrated to have little impact on distress during the encounter with the stressor. According to Leventhal, such information does not seem to assist persons to construct a schema of the features of the stimulus. A schema provides a framework within which the person can interpret and understand the experience. If the schema is accurate, the person is assured that the experience is typical and will be more likely to cope effectively with the situation and not experience undue emotional distress.

INTERVENTION

Technique

First, sensation information that is common to a particular diagnostic procedure or treatment needs to be identified. Information that will allow the person to develop a schema of the upcoming event needs to be provided to the patient. The preparation contains information about the objective and subjective features of the event. The subjective features are the sensations the person would directly experience and are verifiable only by the person; the objective features are aspects of the situation verifiable by the experiencing person as well as anyone observing the event. Such objective features include the temporal ordering of activities and spacial features of the environment.

To develop sensation scripts for various procedures, patients who are undergoing the diagnostic test or treatment for which sensation information is being developed are interviewed. If the procedure is fairly lengthy, it may be best to break the procedure into specific segments and obtain information on each segment as the person's recall may not be accurate. Sime and Libera (1985) interviewed 10 patients who had periodontal surgery.

Clark and Gregar (1988) interviewed 30 patients to obtain sensations associated with femoral arteriography. Open-ended questions which elicited information on what patients saw, heard, tasted, smelled, or felt were used. Some patients may have difficulty describing their sensations. Others may use terms such as "had pain," which require follow-up questions on what is meant by pain. When patients describe behaviors such as "couldn't swallow" or "jumped," they are asked to describe any sensations that accompany these behaviors or responses. To obtain a complete description of the sensations experienced throughout the procedure, patients sometimes have to be asked about aspects of the procedure not initially described. It is important to ascertain the temporal order of the sensations the patient is reporting so that the sensations can be anchored with the specific objective features of the procedure.

Johnson suggests that sensations chosen for the script for a specific procedure be those that are reported by 50% of the respondents (Leventhal & Johnson, 1981). After the typical sensations are identified, the list is then verified with another group who has undergone the same diagnostic test or treatment.

A script that includes the verified typical sensations is developed. Some, such as Sime and Libera (1985), advocate making an audiotape. Use of the audiotape helps prevent patients from misreading written materials or only partially reading them. A nurse giving a verbal presentation of the content may omit important information, inadvertently evaluate the experience, or unintentionally attach emotion to particular passages. A portion of the script developed by Sime and Libera (1978) for patients having periodontal surgery follows:

> After the sheets have been placed on you, your student will use a cotton tipped swab and will apply a type of ointment to the gums surrounding the area where the surgery is to be done. This is a surface anesthetic to help numb the area. You'll probably notice a bitter taste as a result of this application. This student will then inject an anesthetic in the gum area that is to be treated. The injection usually feels like a sharp prickling sensation. A few minutes after the injection, your lips and cheek will feel numb.

Notice that no evaluative statements are included.

Photographs may be used to help depict a procedure. Care should be taken to eliminate irrelevant aspects from the photographs.

Sensation information is provided to the patient prior to the event. In fairly short-duration procedures, such as dental procedures, nasogastric intubation, pelvic examinations, and cast removal, the preparatory information has been given just before the procedure. For surgical procedures, the preparation has been given the evening before surgery (Johnson et al., 1978b). However, the advent of same-day surgery may alter this approach.

Measurement of Effectiveness

As the intervention is thought to stimulate cognitive processes that will reduce emotional responses to stressors and improve coping responses, measuring the patient's emotional state and coping processes during and after the procedure is indicated. Self-reported moods such as anxiety, depression, distress, anger, and tension have been measured. Observations of the patient's behaviors during and following the procedure have been made. These would reveal information on emotional states. Interviews may be conducted following the procedure to determine specific coping strategies that the patient used. Hill (1982) examined how soon the patient ventured from home to assume normal, everyday activities after cataract surgery. This was viewed as being indicative of successful coping.

The nurse using sensation information will need to identify the specific outcomes desired with specific diagnostic tests or procedures. The desired outcomes may vary according to the age of the patient, the patient's typical responses to the event, and the required or desired cooperative activities of the patient during the event.

Table 19.1
Procedures/tests for Which Sensation Information Has Been Used

Amniocentesis (Ruiz-Bueno, 1987)
Barium enema (Hartfield, Cason, & Cason, 1981)
Cardiac catheterization (Anderson & Masur, 1989; Kendall et al., 1979)
Cast removal (Johnson et al., 1975)
Dental surgery (Sime & Libera, 1985)
Endoscopy (Johnson et al., 1973)
Femoral arteriography (Clark & Gregor, 1988)
Surgery (Hill, 1982; Johnson et al., 1978a)

USES

The judgment of whether or not to use sensation information as an intervention is based on the nature of the diagnostic test or procedure, characteristics of the patient, and desired outcomes. The procedure would be one that constitutes a potential threat to the individual.

A number of procedures that have been deemed to be threatening to patients have been identified by health care workers. Ones for which sensation information have been used are listed in Table 19.1. Few studies have included the script that was developed. Thus, nurses wishing to use developed scripts need to contact individual investigators.

Individual patient characteristics is another factor to consider in selecting sensation information as an intervention. This factor has received limited attention in research studies. Although most of the research has involved adults, it has been shown to be effective with children (Johnson et al., 1975; Kendall et al., 1979). When the level of anxiety before the threatening situation is considered, patients with high anxiety have benefited more from the intervention than have patients with low anxiety (Johnson et al., 1978a). Sime and Libera (1985) found that persons with low anxiety may be disadvantaged by the use of sensation information. More research on the effectiveness of the intervention with patients with particular characteristics is needed.

Precautions

Some findings suggest that sensation information may have negative effects on some people. In a study of nasogastric insertion, Padilla et al. (1981) found the intervention of sensation information to be detrimental to patients who desired no control over their experience. However, Padilla and colleagues caution that their preparatory script probably contained some emotionally arousing evaluative content.

Use of the intervention with persons who have low anxiety prior to the procedure may produce negative effects. Although sensation information reduced tension and distress in patients with high anxiety, Sime and Libera (1985) found that it reduced the number of reported positive self-statement in persons with low anxiety. They did not measure behavioral coping during surgery or any measures of long-term effects; it is unknown whether or not negative findings occurred with respect to these variables. Sime and Libera (1985) suggest that sensation information may interfere with established coping responses in patients with low anxiety.

RESEARCH

Although the effectiveness of sensation information has been investigated in a number of studies, a number of theoretical and research questions remain. The following are some of the areas in which studies are needed.

1. Suls and Wan (1989) did a meta-analysis of the effects of sensory and procedural information on coping with stressful medical procedures. Their analysis included a number of nursing studies, but the number was limited. Such an analysis of nursing studies on sensation information would be beneficial.
2. A number of studies have combined sensation and procedural information. The designs have often precluded determining the effects of each type of information. Thus, studies need to be designed that will allow the determination of effects from each type of intervention. Likewise, the content of scripts needs to be evaluated to ascertain if only sensation information is included.
3. Further systematic investigation of the characteristics such as level of fear arousal and coping dispositions and preference is required in order to select the optimum intervention for an individual.

REFERENCES

Anderson, K.O., & Masur, F.T. (1989). Psychologic preparation for cardiac catheterization. *Heart & Lung* 18:154–163.

Clark, C.R., & Gregor, F.M. (1988). Developing a sensation information message for femoral arteriography. *Journal of Advanced Nursing* 13:237–244.

Hartfield, M.T., Cason, C.L., & Cason, G.J. (1981). Effects of information about a threatening procedure on patient's expectations and emotional distress. *Nursing Research* 31:202–206.

Hill, B.J. (1982). Sensory information, behavioral instructions and coping with sensory alternation surgery. *Nursing Research* 31:17–21.

Johnson, J.E. (1973). Effects of accurate expectations about sensations on the sensory and distress components of pain. *Journal of Personality and Social Psychology* 27:261–275.

Johnson, J.E., Fuller, S.S., Endress, M.P., & Rice, V.H. (1978a). Altering patients' responses to surgery: An extension and replication. *Research in Nursing and Health* 1:111–121.

Johnson, J.E., Kirchhoff, K., & Endress, M.P. (1975). Altering children's distress behavior during orthopedic cast removal. *Nursing Research* 24:404–410.

Johnson, J.E., & Leventhal, H. (1974). The effects of accurate expectations and behavioral instruction on reactions during a noxious medical examination. *Journal of Personality and Social Psychology* 29:710–718.

Johnson, J.E., Morrissey, J.F., & Leventhal, H. (1973). Psychological preparation for an endoscopic examination. *Gastrointestinal Endoscopy* 19:180–182.

Johnson, J.E., & Rice, V.H. (1974). Sensory and distress components of pain: Implications for the study of clinical pain. *Nursing Research* 23:203–209.

Johnson, J.E., Rice, V.H., & Endress, M.P. (1978b). Sensory information, instruction in a coping strategy, and recovery from surgery. *Research in Nursing and Health* 1:4–17.

Kendall, P.C., Williams, L., Pechacek, T.F., Graham, L.E., Shisslack, C., & Herzoff, N. (1979). Cognitive-behavioral and patient education interventions in cardiac catheterization procedures: The Palo Alto Psychology Project. *Journal of Consulting and Clinical Psychology* 47:49–58.

Leventhal, H., Brown, D., Schacham, S., & Engquist, G. (1979). Effects of preparatory information about sensation, threat of pain, and attention on cold pressor distress. *Journal of Personality and Social Psychology* 37:688–714.

Leventhal, H., & Johnson, J.E. (1981). Laboratory and field experimentation: Development of a theory of self-regulation. Pp. 189–262 in P. Woolridge, R. Leonard, & M. Schmitt eds., *Behavioral science and nursing theory*. St. Louis: C. V. Mosby.

Padilla, G.V., Grant, M.M., Rains, B.L., Hansen, G.C., Bergstrom, N., Wong, H.L., Hanson, R., & Kubo, W. (1981). Distress reduction and the effects of preparatory teaching films on patient control. *Research in Nursing and Health* 4:375–387.

Ruiz-Bueno, J. (1987). *Preferences for health care, pre-event anxiety, informational interventions and coping during genetic amniocentesis.* Unpublished doctoral dissertation, University of Minnesota, Minneapolis, MN.

Schachter, S., & Singer, J.E. (1962). Cognitive, social, and physiological determinants of emotional state. *Journal of Consulting and Clinical Psychology* 48:785–787.

Sime, A.M. (1976). Relationship of preoperative fear, type of coping and information received about surgery to recovery from surgery. *Journal of Personality and Social Psychology* 48:716–724.

Sime, A.M., & Libera, M.B. (1978). Sensation information for periodontal surgery. Unpublished script.

_____. (1985). Sensation information, self-instruction and responses to dental surgery. *Research in Nursing and Health* 8:41–47.

Suls, J., & Wan, C.K. (1989). Effects of sensory and procedural information on coping with stressful medical procedures and pain: A meta-analysis. *Journal of Consulting and Clinical Psychology* 57:372–379.

SECTION 4

SENSORY INTERVENTIONS

CHAPTER 20

THERAPEUTIC TOUCH

Ellen C. Egan

BACKGROUND

Touching, as a part of nursing care, has been used throughout the history of nursing to convey compassion, provide comfort, and ease pain. Touch is associated with so many basic nursing skills that Krieger et al. (1979) call touch the imprimatur of nursing.

In nursing literature, touch is commonly described as a form of nonverbal communication (Barnett, 1972; Goodykoontz, 1979; McCorkle, 1974) or interaction (Weiss, 1979). Barnett (1972) organized concepts of touch into five broad categories, all of which involve communication. They are: (a) mechanisms of communication, (b) a means of communication, (c) a basis for establishing communication, (d) a means of communicating emotions, and (e) a means of communicating ideas.

For a more encompassing view, Ujhely (1979) provided eight different meanings for the word "touch": (a) active striving to connect with another, (b) a means of expressing something or conveying something to the other, (c) a quality, (d) a mode of perception, (e) an experience, (f) a means of defining oneself to and differentiating oneself from the other, (g) taking from or being taken by, and (h) the relation between subject and object via touch. Each of these meanings implies some kind of meeting or encounter between people or nurse and client, but they do not all include physical contact. From an analysis of the research on touch from 1960 to 1985, Weiss (1988) concluded that touch does not have a universal meaning, rather the meaning of touch gestures may be context-dependent and person-specific.

From these concepts and interpretations of touch, it can be seen that there are many uses of touch as a nursing intervention or an assessment technique. However, therapeutic touch, the use of touch with the intention to transfer energy to another, is a relatively recent nursing intervention. It can be differentiated from other types of touch by the intention of the action or purpose for which each specific action is used. (See more about the intervention of purposeful touch in Chapter 25.)

Weber (1984) identifies models of touch that roughly correspond to cultural and philosophical contexts as well as three definitions of touch. The physical-sensory model, the psychological-humanistic model, and the field model are related respectively to "being in contact with," "reach and communicate" and "lay the hand or hands on (therapeutic touch)" definitions of touch. Weber indicates that the physical-sensory model fits the aims and assumptions of Anglo-American philosophy, the psychological-humanistic model expresses the concerns of contemporary continental philosophy (especially phenomenology and existentialism), and the field model as well as therapeutic touch harmonize with Eastern philosophy and its holistic world view. Eastern philosophy depicts human beings and nature as inherently linked as one and postulates the existence of energies which seem to play a distinct role in human well-being. Such an energy is prana which is thought in Eastern philosophies to be a key factor in human health and well-being.

Definition

Therapeutic touch is a process by which energy is transmitted from one person to another for the purpose of potentiating the healing process of one who is ill or injured. Krieger (1979) calls therapeutic touch a healing meditation in that the primary act of the intervener is to "center" herself and to maintain that center throughout the process. Therapeutic touch consists of four phases: (a) centering oneself, (b) assessing the client's energy field for differences in the quality of the energy flow, (c) mobilizing areas in the client's energy field that are perceived as nonflowing, and (d) directing energy through the hands to the client (Krieger, 1979).

Dolores Krieger (1979), who coined the term "therapeutic touch," learned the process from Dora Kunz and then began teaching other nurses the process in the early 1970s. This intervention, like many other nursing interventions, was practiced for some years before research studies were conducted to measure its effects. Unlike many other nursing interventions, therapeutic touch has attracted skepticism because the action of energy transfer is intangible and uses "laying-on of hands," which is associated with faith healing. It is to be noted, however, that the use of touch or the therapeutic use of hands has a long history. There are repeated references to it in Eastern, European, and religious literature (Krieger, 1979; Zefron, 1975). In these references, the laying-on of hands is thought to be used for healing or actually curing disease. Therapeutic touch, however, is considered to be different in that it is not done within a religious context nor does it bring about cures. Furthermore, unlike faith healing the client does not need to have faith in therapeutic touch for it to be effective.

Scientific Basis

Assumptions that are cited as basic to therapeutic touch include that a human being is an energy field in mutual simultaneous interaction with the environmental field that surrounds the human field (Boguslawski, 1979, 1980; Miller, 1979). Another important assumption is that energy can be intentionally channeled from one person to another.

It is thought that in health the human energy field is in harmonious integration as well as in harmony with the environmental field. In illness, however, the energy field is in disharmony so that there are disorderly, imbalanced, and unsynchronous energy patterns (Boguslawski, 1979). It is the energy pattern imbalances that are noted during assessment and are characterized as blocks, congestion, or asymmetrical densities. In nursing, the purpose of therapeutic touch is to restore order and harmony of the energy pattern by intentional and specific interaction between the nurse's energy field and the energy field of the client. This has been referred to as stimulating or calming the client's energy patterns.

Fanslow (1983) identified two principles that accompany the process of therapeutic touch, compassion and intentionality. Fanslow describes compassion as pure caring such that the person wants to help but without expectations for the outcome. Intentionality is the intent to help or heal and is the conscious direction of energy to the patient experiencing a deficit of energy. Compassion serves as the catalyst for the energy exchange process and intentionality the means of transmitting energy.

Krieger (1975), in explaining the healing process, believed prana, roughly translated to mean vitality or vigor, to be the basis of the transfer of energy. Eastern literature describes the healthy person as having an abundance of prana and the ill person a deficit. Prana can be activated by will and transferred to another. Because of the relationship between prana and the oxygen molecule, Krieger selected hemoglobin as a variable to be used to measure the effects of therapeutic touch.

How therapeutic touch works is not clear. It is assumed that energy is transmitted through the hands during the process, but it is not clear how the transmitted energy compensates for an energy deficit or serves to balance the energy patterns of the recipient. Also, how recipients use the energy to enhance their self-healing processes is not understood.

Boguslawski (1980) has set forth several possible explanations of the mechanisms of therapeutic touch in pain relief. These explanations include: (a) interruption of the transmission of pain impulses, (b) reduction of local edema, and (c) the production of endorphins and enkephalins. Boguslawski suggests that the mechanisms of acupuncture and therapeutic touch may be similar.

Research

Krieger (1975) began the systematic study of the effects of therapeutic touch on human subjects in the early 1970s. She selected changes in hemoglobin level as a measurement of the effect of therapeutic touch based on an assumed relationship between prana and hemoglobin. In each of three studies, Krieger was able to demonstrate that the level of hemoglobin increased significantly in groups who were treated with therapeutic touch, whereas there were no significant increases in control groups. Each of the studies used different subjects and therapists. These studies have been questioned in regard to the use of hemoglobin as a dependent variable and the methods used in the studies (Clark & Clark, 1984).

Krieger et al. (1979) measured physiological changes that occurred in the therapist and the client during therapeutic touch. The main finding measured by electroencephalogram (EEG) was a preponderance of fast beta activity present in the healer. This was interpreted as a type of meditative process. Although no significant changes were seen in the patients' EEG, electrocardiogram, electromyogram (EMG), galvanic skin response, or temperature, all patients showed a relaxed state. The abundance of large amplitude alpha activity with eyes opened and closed was interpreted as relaxation. Subjects also reported that therapeutic touch was relaxing. In a similar study of therapeutic touch practitioners Brown and associates (1977) also found that beta frequencies dominated and suggested that the beta frequencies might possibly serve to define the state of therapeutic touch healing in their group of subjects. They indicated that such beta activity has been associated with feeling states such as focused attention, visual scanning, and concentration.

Several studies have been conducted to ascertain the effect of therapeutic touch on state anxiety. Heidt (1981) demonstrated that subjects who received therapeutic touch with physical contact experienced significantly greater decrease in state anxiety than subjects who received casual (pulse taking) or no touch (conversation).

In a later study, Quinn (1984) demonstrated that subjects who experienced noncontact therapeutic touch had a significantly greater decrease in post-test state anxiety scores than the subjects treated with the noncontact mimic intervention. The results of Heidt's and Quinn's studies are similar. Both indicated an average of 17% decrease in anxiety after contact and noncontact therapeutic touch in hospitalized cardiovascular patients. In addition, both studies support that the placebo effect is small, accounting for an average of 4.5% decrease in state anxiety.

In later studies of the effects of therapeutic touch on anxiety levels among hospitalized adults, significant results were not found. Hale (1986) utilized three treatment groups: therapeutic touch, simulated therapeutic touch, and routine care. No significant differences between treatment groups were found for any of the dependent variables—state anxiety measured two hours after the treatment, systolic and diastolic blood pressure and pulse rate measured immediately and two hours after the treatment. In a study of elderly patients, Parkes (1985) designated groups that received either therapeutic touch or one of two kinds of mimicked therapeutic touch. No significant differences were found between groups; however, all three groups had a slight increase in anxiety at the post-test measurement time. Quinn (1989) studied the effect of therapeutic touch on state anxiety, blood pressure, and heart rate. No significant differences were found between groups—therapeutic touch without eye or facial contact, mimicked therapeutic touch, and no treatment—on any of the anxiety measures.

Randolph (1984) studied whether therapeutic touch produces a relaxation response such that subjects would be less responsive to stressful stimuli. Experimental and control groups observed a film that served as a stressful stimulus. The experimental group received therapeutic touch during the film and the control group were touched in a similar manner without therapeutic touch. No differences in the skin conductance level, electromyogram, or skin temperature were found between the two groups. Consequently, therapeutic touch was not demonstrated to be useful in decreasing the response to stressful stimuli using the methodology of this study.

Fedoruk (1984) studied the effect of therapeutic touch on stress associated with measuring infants' vital signs. Stress behavior and transcutaneous oxygen pressure were used to measure stress. Infants served as their own controls so all infants received therapeutic touch, mock therapeutic touch, and no treatment. Therapeutic touch was effective in reducing the behavioral stress of infants, but not physiological stress. An increase in stress with mock therapeutic touch was an unexpected finding.

The effect of therapeutic touch in the alleviation of pain has also been investigated. Meehan (1985) investigated the effect of therapeutic touch on acute pain in postoperative patients using three treatment groups: therapeutic touch, a mimicked therapeutic touch treatment, and the standard treatment (analgesics such as demerol or morphine injections). Results indicated that there was a difference between the therapeutic touch and mimicked therapeutic touch groups, but not enough to be significant. The standard treatment was significantly more effective than therapeutic touch. In another pain study, Keller and Bzdek (1986) studied the effect of therapeutic touch on tension headaches. The two treatment groups received either therapeutic touch or a simulation of therapeutic touch. Results indicated a significantly greater reduction of pain in the therapeutic touch group immediately following the treatment and four hours later. However, there was a 37% average pain reduction in the placebo group.

Quinn (1988) summarized eight research studies conducted to demonstrate the effects of therapeutic touch on such variables as hemoglobin, anxiety, physiologic response to stressful stimuli, response to stress, postoperative pain, and tension headache pain. Subjects included hospitalized adults, neonates, cardiovascular patients, college students, postoperative adult patients, gerontological hospitalized patients, and adults. The findings from these studies do not consistently support the effectiveness of therapeutic touch in alleviating anxiety and relieving pain. Quinn provided an analysis and possible explanations for the inconsistent findings. Quinn suggested that in the Randolph (1984) study the stress response would be considered a normal natural phenomenon and a protection from external threat. Therefore, it is questionable that therapeutic touch should be expected to cause the relaxation response in such a situation. In her analysis of the Fedoruk (1984) study, Quinn suggested reasons why the mimic therapeutic touch group may have experienced an increase in stress. Quinn indicated that the mimic therapeutic touch lasted 1 minute while the true therapeutic touch treatment lasted 5 minutes. The therapeutic touch treatment measurements were for 25 minutes while mimic therapeutic touch measurements were for only 23 minutes. Quinn suggested that the last two minutes of measurement may have made a difference in arousal in neonate subjects. In addition, the nurses counted aloud during the mimic therapeutic touch, which could have affected the arousal of the subjects. In discussing the Meehan (1985) study, Quinn stated that the investigator had indicated that a very conservative test of statistical significance had been used. As a consequence, even though the difference was very close to being significant, no significance was found. Of greater importance, Quinn pointed out that clinical practitioners typically administer therapeutic touch treatments of 15 minutes or longer to achieve pain relief. However, Meehan followed the established therapeutic touch research protocol and utilized only a five-minute therapeutic touch treatment. It is reasonable to assume that a longer treatment could have a greater effect.

From a review of the therapeutic touch research it can be concluded that the effectiveness of therapeutic touch has been demonstrated, but the results have not been consistent. Quinn's critique (1988), as well as the thoughtful analyses of other investigators, can be used to design studies that will facilitate the development of knowledge regarding the phenomenon of therapeutic touch.

INTERVENTION

Technique

The process of therapeutic touch consists of four steps: centering, assessment, unruffling, and transferring energy.

Centering

The first step of the process is centering. Centering is considered a meditative state in which one quiets oneself and directs attention inward. The centered person experiences integration and unity.

There are many ways of centering, but one of the simplest methods is to assume a comfortable sitting position, relax tension areas of the body, inhale deeply, exhale slowly, and mentally count "one" with each exhalation. Very quickly there is an experience of quiet, relaxation, and balance. Once centering has been achieved it can very easily be recreated again.

Centering is maintained throughout the therapeutic touch process and facilitates the remaining steps of the process. The centered person is in control and can direct energies and attention. There is a sense of detachment that enhances sensitivity and the person has less personal involvement in the outcomes of therapy.

Assessment

After the therapist is centered, the assessment process begins. The purpose of the assessment process is to find differences in the quality of the energy flow of the client. Differences in the energy flow are detected by sensing heat, cold, tingling, congestion, pressure, emptiness, or other sensations. These sensations usually are asymmetrical, present on one side of the body but not on the other.

Before assessment, the patient is encouraged to assume a comfortable position. Depending on the condition of the client, this may be standing, sitting sideways on a chair, or lying down.

The process of assessment is a scanning process. Both hands are used to establish a field and the palms are held two to three inches from the skin surface of the client. Usually the scanning is started with assessment of the head and slowly progresses down the entire front of the client. This is followed by the scanning from head to toe down the back of the client. The practitioner makes mental notes of the sensations that are perceived during the scanning. When there are doubts about areas, scanning can be repeated in those areas.

From the information obtained during assessment, the practitioner identifies areas of the body where the quality of the energy flow is different. The information is synthesized and used to determine where, how, and what kind of energy will be directed to the client. Thus, the intervention plan is developed.

The assessment process can be done by one practitioner or two. If two practitioners work together, one practitioner scans the front of the patient and the other practitioner simultaneously scans the back. By simultaneously scanning the front and back, a field is maintained between the hands of the two practitioners.

Unruffling the Field

Krieger (1979) equates the sensation of a congested energy field with the word "ruffled." The sensation is one of pressure and overlapping layers of densities, like ruffles. When this is encountered, "unruffling" can be used to mobilize the flow of energy in these areas of the energy field.

The "unruffling process" is accomplished by moving the hands (palms facing the client) from the area where pressure was perceived in a sweeping-away motion. This sweeping motion of the hands is continued down the body following the long bones. The unruffled field or mobile field seems to enhance the transfer of energy from the practitioner. The client's field seems to be more receptive of energy.

Transferring Energy

The actual transferring of energy is brought about by the intention of doing so. In other words, by intending to transfer energy, energy will be transferred from the practitioner through the hands to the client. This seems the simplest part of the intervention and can be accomplished by most people who engage in the process. It does, however, necessitate having the intention to help another.

The complex parts of the process are to know the form of energy to use, how to modulate energy, and where to apply the energy. The form of energy is related to colors. Blue energy is a sedating kind of energy, yellow energy is stimulating and energizing, and green is harmonizing. Because of the different effects of the forms of energy, different forms are used for different conditions of the client. Blue energy is used to calm, relieve pain, and to reduce edema. Yellow energy is used to restore energy for someone fatigued or depleted of energy. Green energy is used to restore the harmony of the person.

The way energy forms are modulated is through visualization of the color of the particular energy. For example, the practitioner would visualize light streaming through a blue stained-glass window when wishing to transfer blue energy. Similarly, visualizing yellow or green light streams would be used to modulate these energy forms. This part of the process then requires that the practitioner can mentally visualize colors.

Where to apply energy is dependent on the assessment. In some instances the energy is applied directly to a particular area, as when the client has pain in a particular place. In some instances, such as when the client is fatigued, the energy is applied to one of the chakras located in the thoracic or solar plexus areas. (Chakras are special channels or centers within the energy field that serve as entry areas for energy from the environment. See Chapter 4 for a discussion of the chakras.) Energy also may be applied in minimal amounts by keeping the hands in motion over particular areas of the entire body using a motion similar to the sweeping motion of unruffling. This might be used in the area of the head or with infants where only minimal amounts of energy are used.

Usually it is desirable for the flow of energy through the extremities to be enhanced and for energy to be distributed. This has been called "grounding," in that the energy flows through the extremities and the hands or feet while the practitioner serves as a grounding rod. The flow of energy through an arm can be accomplished by placing one hand between the shoulder blades and the other hand palm to palm with the client. Energy is transferred through the thoracic chakra and out the secondary chakra of the palm. When the flow of energy is established, the energy can be felt in the receiving palm. To facilitate the flow of energy, the hand that was placed on the palm of the client can be cupped and moved down the arm in the manner of pushing a pressure ridge down the arm and out of the hand. A similar process is used with the legs. Energy can be distributed by using a sweeping motion of the hands from a particular area to surrounding areas. The unruffling motion can be used to distribute energy over the entire body. In some instances it is desirable to keep the hands in constant motion when directing energy. This motion serves to control the amount of energy given, such that small amounts of energy are given to sensitive areas or individuals.

As stated earlier the decision for treatment begins with the assessment process. Usually what is sensed during assessment indicates an underlying problem. If an area is sensed to be hot, there can be an inflammatory process, pain, injury, or other pathological problem present in the underlying area. An area of coldness indicates a block in the flow of energy to the area. If the sensations are of emptiness, this usually indicates a general lack of energy. Congestion or heavy areas indicate a situation of uneven or poor energy flow. Most clients will tell the practitioner their medical diagnosis or what is troubling them. This information also can be used in determining the nature of the treatment.

Generally, if an area is hot, blue energy is given directly to the area. If the blocking of energy was assessed, blue energy is given through the thorax or solar plexus and directed through the arms or legs. When a condition of low energy is detected, yellow energy is given through the solar plexus or kidney areas. If areas are determined to be congested, the field is smoothed by using sweeping motions. See Table 20.1 for examples of the energy forms and the application locations for various conditions.

Experienced practitioners seem to develop a tacit knowledge of the kind and direction of energy to use in different situations. The knowledge seems to be derived from the assessment and response to treatment, and it is as if the practitioner's hands are drawn to certain areas.

Procedure

The general procedure for engaging in transferring energy begins by having the client seated comfortably sideways on an armless chair or lying on his or her back, side, or abdomen. The client's arms and legs should be uncrossed with shoes removed, if treatment will involve the feet. If the client is relaxed there is greater reception of energy. Relaxation can be facilitated by briefly massaging the client's shoulders and/or having the client take a few deep breaths.

Table 20.1
Examples of Forms of Energy and Application Locations for Various Conditions

Assessment	Conditions	Form of Energy	Application Location
Hot	Inflammatory process, pain or injury	Blue	Affected area
Cold	Block of energy flow	Blue	Thorax or solar plexus
Empty	Lack of energy	Yellow	Solar plexus
Heavy	Uneven energy flow	_____	Sweeping motion, unruffling
_____	Arthritic pain	Blue	Solar plexus affected area, gently
_____	Lung congestion, asthma	Blue	Thorax with grounding
_____	Abdominal ulcers	Blue, calm thoughts	Solar plexus
_____	Tension, anxiety	Blue	Thorax or solar plexus
_____	Disharmony, imbalance or depression	Green	Solar plexus with grounding

The practitioner's hands are placed on a predetermined area or can be held two to three inches from the skin surface as during assessment. Both hands are always used to maintain a field for balance and distribution of energy. The hands are held over a particular area only for a few moments at a time so that too much energy is not given in one area. The energy can be distributed from the area by sweeping motions of the hands. Depending on the assessment, energy may be given generally through the chakras, to one or more particular area, to an area with sweeping motions, or a combination of the above. When energy is given through the thoracic of solar plexus area, the flow of energy through the arms or legs is usually established by the practitioner.

Clients tend to draw energy. They will usually experience heat or warmth in the area where the energy is directed. A relaxation response exhibited by deeper breathing and a flushed appearance usually results. Krieger (1981) describes the relaxation following therapeutic touch as follows:

> These changes essentially constitute a relaxation response and occur as follows: (1) the first observable change noted is that the voice level of the healee drops several decibels; (2) there is then a noted change in respirations in which the respirations become slower and deeper; (3) following this, an audible sign of relaxation occurs and is usually signaled by a deep inhalation, a sigh, or an actual statement such as "I feel so relaxed"; (4) another interesting sign is that a peripheral flush will be noted in the healee; this is a generalized slight pinking-up of the skin that occurs throughout the body but is most readily perceived on the healee's face. [p. 145]

The treatment is stopped when the practitioner senses a cessation or decrease of sensations in her hands, a feeling of rebound of energy from the client, or cessation of reception by the client. The practitioner also will stop the treatment when it is thought enough energy has been given for a treatment. At the conclusion some practitioners distribute the energy by using the unruffling motion. Wyatt and Dimmer (1988) describe "balancing" (shifting energy from areas of congestion to areas of deficit) in order to smooth out the entire energy field after depleted areas of the field have been energized. The energy field can be reassessed to determine whether the field is symmetrical as a means of validating that the treatment is completed. After the treatment is completed clients are encouraged to rest.

General Comments About the Process

Although the process of therapeutic touch has been presented as sequential steps, only step one is sequential in that the process is always started by centering oneself and maintaining centering throughout the process. The other steps of the process might be engaged in more than once or in different orders, depending on the experience of the practitioner and the condition of the client.

As the practitioner gains skill and experience, she/he may develop a more individual type of practice (Bulbrook, 1984; Wyatt & Dimmer, 1988). For example, some practitioners use unruffling as part of the assessment process to obtain a deeper assessment. Other practitioners use unruffling to mobilize energy during the process of transferring energy. Some practitioners do a modified assessment when the client is expressing acute pain or the condition of the client is well known.

Macrae (1979) described using therapeutic touch with children in a holistic manner. She found that by not actually touching the patient she was able to more easily perceive dysrhythmia and the healing process proceeded more rapidly. She described moving the areas of congestion or pain out of the energy field.

In addition to directing energy and modulating energy through visualizing colors, practitioners use mental images or thoughts to convey complementary messages. These thought messages may be of wholeness, wellness, peace, calmness, harmony, etc., and are selected as appropriate for the client's condition.

While the practitioner is engaging in therapeutic touch or transmitting orderly healing energies, several conditions are necessary for successful and effective treatment: the practitioner is centered, has the intent to help the client to be well and whole, has compassion for the client as well as detachment, can concentrate on the therapy, has the ability to mentally visualize colors and thought messages, and is in a rested and well condition.

Boguslawski (1979, 1980) suggests that other therapies can be used in conjunction with therapeutic touch to repattern energy. Meditation can be used by the client to relax, gain insight regarding behavior patterns, and to acquire a sense of wholeness. Visualization can be used by the client to channel, direct, and repattern energy. Other practitioners use other therapies depending on the needs and receptivity of their clients.

USES

When humans are viewed as energy fields in constant interaction with the environmental energy field, changes in the energy field are expected. Energy is channeled to maintain the integrity of the field, in response to the environmental field and as directed by the individual. Prolonged or extreme changes in the energy field are manifested as a disharmony of the energy field. Illness, whether physical or mental, could be viewed as the manifestation of disharmony or an unbalanced energy field.

Therapeutic touch is used to help restore the balance of the energy field and to provide additional energy to be used in the recuperative and self-healing process of the client. Therapeutic touch does not bring about miraculous cures or restore structural damage. Therapeutic touch is not an alternative for medical care, but is regarded as complementary to medical treatment. Two notable consequences of therapeutic touch are a generalized relaxation response and relief of pain. (Research studies that measured the effectiveness of therapeutic touch in reducing anxiety and relieving pain were described earlier.) The relaxation produced by therapeutic touch has been capitalized on for persons experiencing tension or anxiety. There can be an immediate response and the duration of the effect may vary. However, the sense of relaxation can be very beneficial to promoting rest and sleep, to facilitating a successful encounter with stressful situations, or to complementing therapy for hypertension.

The most dramatic response to therapeutic touch is the relief of pain. Pain can begin to ease in a few minutes and the effects can last for a few hours to several days. The amount and duration of pain relief depends on the cause and nature of the pain. Therapeutic touch has been effective in the treatment of both acute and chronic pain (Boguslawski, 1980). Tense muscles, often present during pain, can contribute to the amount of pain experienced. Relaxation of these tense muscles, as part of the relaxation response to therapeutic touch, enhances pain relief.

Providing energy to clients with acute or chronic illness has been useful in diminishing fatigue, promoting sleep and rest, and promoting a sense of well-being.

Examples of the usefulness of therapeutic touch for selected conditions and populations follow. Therapeutic touch has been used with mothers and babies for a number of different conditions. Wolfson (1984) described the use of therapeutic touch in the practice of midwifery. Therapeutic touch was used as a therapy for the treatment of anxieties, discomforts, and complications related to pregnancy and birth, including alleviating the painful sensations of labor contractions, enhancing relaxation, stimulating the baby immediately following birth, and helping stimulate contractions to facilitate delivery of the placenta. Leduc (1987) described the use of therapeutic touch with ill babies. Therapeutic touch was used to calm fussy babies, improve respiratory distress in babies with transient tachypnea and moderate meconium aspiration, and provide energy to babies with chronic lung disease or bronchopulmonary dysplasia. Leduc also described treating the babies' mothers and teaching the mothers to do therapeutic touch so that they could treat their babies at home.

Other populations that have benefited from therapeutic touch are the elderly, dying patients, and rehabilitation patients. Fanslow (1984) described the use of therapeutic touch with the elderly who had arteriosclerotic heart disease to improve ambulation and mobility; with arthritic patients to decrease the symptoms of pain, inflammation, and joint swelling; and with hemiplegic stroke patients to decrease pain and spasticity of the involved upper extremity. Fanslow also used therapeutic touch with dying patients. These patients reported a deep warmth and a sense of peace and deep calm. Payne (1989) described the use of therapeutic touch with rehabilitation patients and achieved responses such as: clearer speech in expressive aphasic clients, falling asleep when requesting therapeutic touch treatments at bedtime, being able to void after difficulty initiating a stream of urine following Foley catheter removal, and verbalization of upsetting feelings regarding their disability.

Newshan (1989) described the use of therapeutic touch to alleviate symptoms associated with AIDS. She described using therapeutic touch to ease the dyspnea and cough associated with respiratory complications, hiccups, diarrhea, cramping abdominal pain, constipation, fever, pain, and anxiety.

Precautions

As a general rule, the client will absorb the amount of energy that is needed and then will stop drawing from the energy source; however, in some instances precautions must be taken. Infants and children are very sensitive to treatments. Energy should be given slowly and gently in small amounts by an experienced practitioner (Boguslawski, 1979). Aged, extremely ill, or dying individuals may require modifications in treatment or gentle energy input. The head is also very sensitive, so only cooling sweeping motions are used in the head area. Patients with cancer are treated in such a way that energy is not concentrated in a particular area.

A final precaution is directed to the learner of therapeutic touch. Although it is possible to learn to transfer energy in a short time, knowing when and how to use therapeutic touch requires greater practice and experience. Therapeutic touch is learned through an apprenticeship experience. This learning process with a mentor may take one to two years to perfect a knowledgeable practice.

RESEARCH QUESTIONS

Documentation of the process and effects of therapeutic touch is minimal and has been inconsistent. A few suggestions for research endeavors would include:

1. Empirical validation of the energy exchange process.
2. Determination of appropriate protocols for the administration of therapeutic touch with varying conditions amenable to therapeutic touch.
3. Differentiation of the placebo effect and therapeutic effect of therapeutic touch.
4. Examination of the longitudinal effects of therapeutic touch.
5. Examination of the characteristics of subjects who benefit from therapeutic touch.
6. Correlation of changes in physiological variables with changes in subjective measures of anxiety.
7. Continued validation of the pain relief effects of therapeutic touch.

REFERENCES

Barnett, K. (1972). A theoretical construct of the concepts of touch as they relate to nursing. *Nursing Research* 21: 102–103.

Boguslawski, M. (1979). The use of therapeutic touch in nursing. *The Journal of Continuing Education in Nursing* 10(4): 9–15.

_____. (1980). Therapeutic touch: A facilitator of pain relief. *Topics in Clinical Nursing* 2(1):27–37.

Brown, C.C., Fischer, R., Wagman, A.M.I., Horrom, N., & Marks, P. (1977). The EEG in meditation and therapeutic touch healing. *Journal of Altered States of Consciousness* 3:169–180.

Bulbrook, M.J. (1984). Bulbrook's model of therapeutic touch: one form of health and healing in the future. *The Canadian Nurse* 80(11):30–34.

Clark, P.E., & Clark, M.J. (1984). Therapeutic touch: Is there a scientific basis for the practice? *Nursing Research* 33:37–41.

Fanslow, C. A. (1983). Therapeutic touch: A healing modality throughout life. *Topics in Clinical Nursing* 5(2):72–79.

_____. (1984). Touch and the elderly. Pp. 183–189 in C.C. Brown ed., *The many facets of touch*. Skillman, NJ: Johnson & Johnson Baby Products Co.

Fedoruk, R.B. (1984). Transfer of the relaxation response: Therapeutic touch as a method for reduction of stress in premature neonates. *Dissertation Abstracts International* 46:978B. (University Microfilms No. ADG85-09162)

Goodykoontz, L. (1979). Touch: Attitude and practice. *Nursing Forum* 18:4–17.

Hale, E.H. (1986). A study of the relationship between therapeutic touch and the anxiety levels of hospitalized adults. *Dissertation Abstracts International* 47:1928B. (University Microfilms No. ADG86-18897)

Heidt, P. (1981). Effect of therapeutic touch on anxiety level of hospitalized patients. *Nursing Research* 30:32–37.

Keller, E., & Bzdek, V. (1986). Effects of therapeutic touch on tension headache pain. *Nursing Research* 35:101–106.

Krieger, D. (1975). Therapeutic touch: The imprimatur of nursing. *American Journal of Nursing* 75:784–787.

_____. (1979). *The therapeutic touch: How to use your hands to help or heal.* Englewood Cliffs, NJ: Prentice-Hall.

_____. (1981). *Foundations for holistic health nursing practices.* Philadelphia: J.B. Lippincott Co.

Krieger, D., Peper, E., & Ancoli, S. (1979). Therapeutic touch: Searching for evidence of physiological change. *American Journal of Nursing* 79:660–662.

Leduc, E. (1987). Letter to the editor. *Neonatal Network* 5(6):46–47.

Macrae, J. (1979). Therapeutic touch in practice. *American Journal of Nursing* 79:664–665.

McCorkle, R. (1974). Effects of touch on seriously ill patients. *Nursing Research* 23:125–132.

Meehan, M.C. (1985). The effect of therapeutic touch on the experience of acute pain in postoperative patients. *Dissertation Abstracts International* 46:795B. (University Microfilms No. ADG85–10765)

Miller, L.A. (1979). An explanation of therapeutic touch: Using the science of unitary man. *Nursing Forum* 18:278–287.

Newshan, M.A. (1989). Therapeutic touch for symptom control in persons with AIDS. *Holistic Nursing Practice* 3(4): 45–51.

Parkes, B.S. (1985). Therapeutic touch as an intervention to reduce anxiety in elderly hospitalized patients. *Dissertation Abstracts International* 47:573B.

Payne, M.B. (1989). The use of therapeutic touch with rehabilitation clients. *Rehabilitation Nursing* 14:69–72.

Quinn, J.F. (1984). Therapeutic touch as energy exchange: Testing the theory. *Advances in Nursing Science* 6(2):42–49.

____. (1988). Building a body of knowledge: Research on therapeutic touch 1974–1986. *Journal of Holistic Nursing* 6(1):37–45.

____. (1989). Therapeutic touch as energy exchange: Replication and extension. *Nursing Science Quarterly* 2(2):79–87.

Randolph, G.L. (1984). Therapeutic and physical touch: Physiological response to stressful stimuli. *Nursing Research* 33:33–36.

Ujhely, G.B. (1979). Touch: Reflections and perceptions. *Nursing Forum* 18:18–33.

Weber, R. (1984). Philosophers on touch. Pp. 3–12 in C. C. Brown ed., *The many facets of touch*. Skillman, NJ: Johnson & Johnson Baby Products Co.

Weiss, S.J. (1979). The language of touch. *Nursing Research* 28:76–80.

____. (1988). Touch. Pp. 3–27 in J.J. Fitzpatrick, R.L. Taunton, & J.Q. Benoliel eds., *Annual Review of Nursing Research,* vol. 6. New York: Springer Publishing Co.

Wolfson, I.S. (1984). Therapeutic touch and midwifery. Pp. 166–172 in C.C. Brown ed., *The many facets of touch*. Skillman, NJ: Johnson & Johnson Baby Products Co.

Wyatt, G., & Dimmer, S. (1988). The balancing touch. *Nursing Times* 84(21):40–42.

Zefron, L.J. (1975). The history of the laying-on of hands in nursing. *Nursing Forum* 14:350–363.

CHAPTER 21

MUSIC

BACKGROUND

Music has been used since ancient times as a treatment modality. Over 4000 years ago the Egyptians noted that incantations affected the fertility of women. The *Bible* details how David used the harp to cure King Saul's depression. Plato and Aristotle have been designated by Alvin (1975) as the fathers of music therapy; they prescribed music for treating numerous diseases. According to Plato, health of mind and body could be obtained through music. Aristotle provided hyperactive children with musical rattles for the purpose of calming the youngsters. Since the time of Aeschulapius, music has been used to treat the mentally ill. Cicero and Seneca studied the effects that music had on behavior. Therapeutic use of music has not been confined to Western cultures. Shamans, priests, and healers in all cultures have used music as a healing force (Moreno, 1988).

Music therapy evolved as a distinct profession in the late 1940s. Although music therapists are found in many larger health care facilities and would be chiefly responsible for planning and instituting the therapeutic use of music, many occasions and situations exist in which nurses are in a prime position to implement music as an intervention. Herth (1978) stated that the nurse can judiciously integrate music into the patient's care plan. Music has been used with many patient populations, but it has been used most extensively with patients with psychiatric disorders. Although the majority of literature on the use of music in nursing is anecdotal, the number of experimental design studies on the use of music as an intervention is increasing.

Definition

Webster's dictionary (Woolf, 1979) defined music as:

> The science or art of ordering tones or sounds in succession, in combination, and in temporal relationships to produce a composition having unity and continuity. [p. 752]

Music used for therapeutic purposes has been termed music therapy. Munro and Mount (1978) defined music therapy as:

> the controlled use of music and its influence on the human being to aid in physiologic, psychologic, and emotional integration of the individual during treatment of an illness or disability. [p. 1029]

One element missing from this definition that is critical to nursing is the use of music to promote health and well-being.

Alvin (1975) delineated five elements of music. These, particularly the rhythm, greatly influence the responses effected. The five elements are:

1. Frequency (pitch)
2. Intensity
3. Tone color
4. Interval (creates melody and harmony)
5. Duration (creates rhythm and tempo)

The character of the music and its effects depend on the qualities of these elements and their relationships to each other.

Pitch is produced by the number of vibrations of a sound. Rapid vibrations tend to act as a stimulant, whereas slow vibrations bring about relaxation.

Intensity creates the volume of the sound. It is related to the amplitude of the vibrations. A person's like or dislike of a musical piece often depends on the intensity of the music. Intensity can be used to produce effects such as intimacy (soft music), protection (loud music), and power (alternating volumes). Emotions are affected by the intensity of the music. Results from Riegler's (1980a) study revealed that elderly persons preferred softer music.

Tone color is a nonrhythmical, purely sensuous property and results from the harmony present. Psychological significance results from the tone color of a piece, because the person associates it with past events or feelings. A musical piece sung by two different artists can produce very different effects on an individual because of the tone color (Alvin, 1975).

The interval is the distance between two notes and is related to pitch. The sequence of intervals results in the melody and harmony of a piece. Cultural norms determine what is deemed enjoyable and pleasant. Musical compositions may contain dissonances, but the expectation in Western culture is that these will be resolved and that the ending of the piece will be a pleasant experience. The harmonic progression in a musical piece holds the person's attention until the conclusion. Modern music often deviates from these forms.

Duration and the rhythm are similar. Duration refers to the length of sounds, and rhythm is a time pattern fitted into a certain speed. Rhythm is the most dynamic aspect of music and is a key factor for selecting particular pieces to use in specific situations. Rhythms (respiration, heartbeat, speech, gait) are an integral part of human life, and music can play an instrumental role in harmonizing these internal rhythms. In some pieces, the rhythm conveys peace and security. Repetitive rhythms can elicit feelings of depression. Continuous sounds that are repeated at a slow pace and become gradually slower produce decreased levels of responsiveness. Strong rhythms can awaken feelings of power and control. Primitive rhythms evoke a myriad of feelings. Although all of the five elements are important to consider in selecting music for a patient population or individual, rhythm requires the closest scrutiny.

Scientific Basis

Music affects all aspects (physiological, psychological, spiritual) of human beings, and it is difficult to differentiate the precise effects because of the constant interplay between and among them. Over the centuries philosophers, musicians, and psychologists have debated whether the physiological or psychological system is affected first. Alvin (1975) stated:

> Throughout history man's responses to music have been basically similar and influenced by the same factors, namely man's physical receptivity to sound, his innate or acquired sensitiveness to music, and his state of mind at the time. Conditioning due to prejudices, environment, education and other non-musical factors play an important part in these responses. We cannot ignore them. [p. 74]

Music affects the limbic system, which is integrally involved in emotions and feelings. In particular, the pitch and rhythm of the music affect the limbic system (Guzzetta, 1988). Psychophysiologic responses occur because of the impact the musical selection has on the limbic system. Guzzetta (1988) notes that musical vibrations that are in harmony with a person's fundamental vibratory pattern may produce healing throughout the body and restore regulatory functions. Body–mind–spirit are brought into harmony.

INTERVENTION

Adequate assessment is needed before using music as an intervention. Determination of a patient's likes and dislikes regarding musical selections is essential. This assessment will provide information on how frequently the patient listens to music, the type of musical selections that are liked and disliked, and the purpose for which the person listens to music. The purpose for listening to music for some persons may have been for relaxation and restfulness while others may have listened to music to stimulate and invigorate them. It is only after sufficient data have been gathered that decisions can be made regarding the type of selections and the technique that would be most feasible to use.

Technique

Use of music can take many forms ranging from listening to a recording to singing or to playing an instrument. The nurse must keep a number of factors in mind when considering the use of music as an intervention: type of music, active vs. passive involvement, use in a group or on an individual basis, length of time to use music, and the desired outcomes.

Listening

Providing means for patients to listen to musical selections is the technique most frequently employed. Modern-day tapes and compact discs make it easy to provide music for patients in all types of settings. Tapes have many advantages. The machines are relatively inexpensive; they are small and can be used in even the most crowded confines such as critical care units. For a very modest outlay of money, a nursing unit can establish a tape library containing a wide variety of selections. It is also easy to individualize tapes to meet the likes of each patient. In her study on the effects of music on patients participating in group play therapy, Hinds (1980) used 120-minute tapes that included 15 minutes of silence interspersed with the music. Tapes of this length with built-in periods of quiet reduce demands on the nursing staff. Attention to copyright laws, however, is needed in producing such tapes. Permission from the production company is needed. A number of commercial companies, such as Halpern Sounds, produce long-playing tapes that are appropriate for hospital use. The availability of headphones allow patients to listen to music and not disturb others.

A variety of types of music is readily available on the radio. Commercial messages and talk are deterrents to its use in music therapy. The quality of reception also is uncertain.

Active Involvement

The purpose for which music is being used dictates the type of patient involvement. Active involvement is often used to elicit responses from withdrawn patients. Hoskyns (1982) had a group of patients with Huntington's Chorea play instruments as a means of stimulation and to increase involvement with others. Mason (1978) used tambourines, triangles, castanets, sleigh bells, chime bars, cymbals, and drums with an elderly population as a means for increasing social interaction. Playing instruments was used to improve joint movement and coordination. Active participation requires more planning and time involvement on the part of the nurse than does the use of tapes for listening.

Type of Music

Careful attention to the selection of the music contributes to the therapeutic effects obtained. Because past experiences influence a person's response to music, careful assessment of the patient precedes initiation of the therapy. Specific songs may be associated with happy or sad past experiences. Desired responses, sedative or stimulative effect, dictates the type of musical selections used. A number of sources suggest music to use specific types of situations (Long & Johnson, 1978; Mason, 1978). Mason recommended having available recordings of old-time songs and dances; theme music from plays, television and radio programs, and movies; national and folk songs; Vienese waltzes, polkas, and marches; and popular classics. Findings in a study by Gibbons (1977) revealed that elderly preferred music that was popular when they were young; no differences in preference were found between stimulation and sedative music.

Religious music may be welcomed by many. Hymns are not readily available on the radio, and providing tapes will fill a void for many who are unable to attend church or synagogue services. Playing these at the time of the scheduled service may help to make the person feel less isolated.

New-age or nontraditional music has become very popular. This type of music differs from traditional music that is characterized by tension and release (Guzzetta, 1988). New-age music allows the individual to choose his or her response mode. According to Guzzetta (1988), new-age music "is a vibrational language that helps the bodymind attune itself with its own pattern or resonance" (p. 273). New-age music is frequently used in promoting a relaxed state.

Individual Versus Group

Music has been used widely for groups of patients. It is the most social of all the arts (Alvin, 1975). Alvin viewed music as a powerful integrating force in a group of people. Music creates interrelationships among the members, and between the listener and the music. Music has been used as a modality for fostering group social interaction with the elderly and with persons who have psychiatric disorders. Unless an appropriate research design is used, it is difficult to determine if the effects obtained from the use of music are due to the music or to the interaction and support provided from being part of a group.

Diversity in the preferences of individuals in a group or the lack of an appropriate site for a group session may necessitate implementing music on an individual basis. Assessment findings provide data from which the nurse makes the decision about which method is the preferred one for a specific patient.

Measurement of Effectiveness

The outcome indices selected for evaluating the effectiveness of music vary depending on the purpose for which music was implemented. Outcomes may be a decrease in anxiety, an increase in arousal, an increase in social interaction, and an increase in overall well-being. Improvement in various physiological parameters may also be measured. References provided in Table 21.1 provide the reader with measurement indices that have been used with specific populations.

USES

Music has been prescribed as a therapeutic intervention for many different patient populations. Table 21.1 lists populations for whom music has been used as an intervention. General purposes for the use of music are orienting persons, decreasing anxiety, increasing movement, stimulating persons, and improving well-being.

Table 21.1
Uses of Music

___

Orientation
    Elderly (Riegler, 1980b)
    Psychiatric patients (Cassity, 1976; Hinds, 1980)

Decreased Anxiety
    Relief of Pain
        Burn patients (Christenberry, 1979)
        Postoperative patients (Locsin, 1981; Herth, 1978)
        Chronic pain (Wolfe, 1978)
        Childbirth (Livingston, 1979; Hanser et al., 1983)
        Oncology (Cook, 1981)
    Tests
        (Blanchard, 1979)
    Operating Room
        (McClelland, 1979)

Chemotherapy
    (Frank, 1985)

Increased Intracranial Pressure
    (Wincek, 1989)

Coronary Care Units
    (Zimmerman et al., 1988)

Stimulation
    Comatose (Sisson, 1979)
    Elderly (Needler & Baer, 1982)
    Blind (Maas, 1982)
    Advanced stages of dementia (Norberg et al., 1986)

Increased/improving Movement
    Cerebral palsy (Scartelli, 1982)
    Huntington's Chorea (Hoskyns, 1982)
    Elderly (Mason, 1978)
    Parkinson's (Mason, 1978)
    Postoperative (Herth, 1978)
    Speech therapy (Mason, 1978)

___

Orienting

Music is viewed as an integrating force of body–mind–spirit. As a person listens to music or engages in singing or playing an instrument, the individual becomes more aware of his/her entire being. Kinesthetic sense is awakened as the body responds to the music. Music with a strong beat helps persons gain this awareness. Music compositions that awaken sensitivity are also appropriate.

Music has been used extensively with patients who have psychiatric problems (Cassity, 1976; Hinds, 1980) to promote wholeness (schizophrenia), to reduce hyperactivity (mania), and to improve affect (depression).

Elderly who are confused are another group with whom music has been used to achieve therapeutic outcomes (Phillips, 1980; Needler & Baer, 1982). Phillips noted that music assists the elderly to repattern mental behaviors. Music stimulates free association of ideas, helping the person recall past experiences, events, and feelings and integrating these past experiences into the present. Playing familiar songs prompts reminiscing capabilities and stimulates the memory to recall past events associated with the music (Phillips, 1980). Use of music in a group both facilitates orientation and improves social interaction. Needler and Baer (1982) used music to improve movement and remotivation in addition to orientation. Their anecdotal accounts addressed the effectiveness of these methods. The exact role that music played in the success is not demonstrable, but it appeared to have been a vital element. Riegler (1980b), comparing the effects of music-based reality therapy and traditional reality therapy, found that the groups receiving music-based reality orientation showed marked improvement while the traditional reality orientation method group remained the same.

Decreasing Anxiety

Music has been used for reducing anxiety in a variety of populations (Standley, 1986). Blanchard (1979) and Stoudenmire (1975) explored the effects music had on anxiety in college students who were taking an examination. Pulse rate and blood pressure were lower in subjects who listened to music as compared to subjects in the control group. Stoudenmire compared the effects of music and progressive relaxation on anxiety reduction in college students. Both interventions were effective in reducing state anxiety.

Cook (1981) used soothing music with oncology patients who were receiving betatron radiation therapy. Subjects in the experimental group had significantly lower anxiety scores 10 days into the treatment than did subjects in the control group. Subjects stated that the music made the treatment go faster, the noise level of the environment was reduced, and it made the treatment less stressful. Frank (1985) reported that oncology patients who had listened to music and imagery tapes had lower anxiety scores after listening to these tapes. Likewise, patients perceived that their vomiting had been reduced.

Music has been used extensively with patients experiencing acute and chronic pain. Music may serve as a distractor from the pain stimuli or produce relaxation. Wolfe (1978) used music with a group of patients in a treatment center for chronic pain; findings showed an increase in verbalizations and interactions, indicating that the patients were experiencing less discomfort after they had listened to music. Locsin (1981), investigating the effects of preferred music on postoperative pain, found that patients in the experimental group had lower musculoskeletal and verbal pain scores and lower blood pressure and pulse rates than those in the control group. He played music selections preferred by the patient for 15 minutes every 2 hours for the first 48 hours post surgery with the experimental group and non-preferred music with the control group. Findings from a study of mothers in labor revealed decreased responses to pain when music was employed (Hanser et al., 1983). Curtis (1986) used music with patients who were terminally ill; her findings suggest that music was effective in promoting comfort. In a laboratory study conducted by Geden and colleagues (1989), subjects who used imagery and music reported less subjective pain than subjects in other groups.

Morosko and Simmons (1966) applied the term "audio-analgesia" in discussing the use of white noise to suppress pain during dental procedures. They found audio-analgesia to be effective in reducing both pain threshold and pain tolerance. However, this intervention is no longer used.

According to Mason (1978), music decreased tension in elderly persons with neurological disease, resulting in a decrease in symptoms associated with Parkinson's disease and disseminated sclerosis. By promoting relaxation in persons with Huntington's Chorea, music subsequently resulted in a reduction in choreic movements (Hoskyns, 1982).

Soothing music is the most appropriate type of music to use to reduce anxiety, but the personal preference of the patient is very important. Pieces with repetitive rhythms are believed to inhibit functioning of the central nervous system (Farber, 1982). Blanchard (1979) found that both rock n' roll and classical music were effective in reducing anxiety. New-age music is aimed at promoting relaxation.

Increasing Movement

Both listening to music and playing musical instruments have been used to improve movement and coordination. Livingston (1979) used music during exercise sessions to help pregnant women condition their bodies; these exercises helped in controlling breathing and concentration during pregnancy, childbirth, and postpartum periods.

Herth's (1978) anecdotal reports revealed that music enticed an elderly patient who was hemiplegic to do range of motion exercises. She noted that muscular energy increased with the intensity and pitch of sound stimuli. Herth reported use of music to decrease the discomfort associated with dangling and ambulation in postsurgical patients; playing music for five minutes before ambulating patients decreased the lightheadedness and pain associated with dangling and ambulation. These patients ambulated more readily than patients who had not listened to music.

In working with patients who had Huntington's Chorea, Hoskyns (1982) found that the patient's ability to speak improved after listening to music. Music tended to decrease choreic movements, but these increased if the person was asked to play an instrument. The thought of playing may have increased the patient's anxiety which would, in turn, increase choreic movements. Thaut (1988) documented the effectiveness of music in gait rehabilitation. Mason (1978) reported that certain songs convey movement and assist persons to do their exercises. Marches lend to foot tapping while waltzes suggest gentle swinging. She advocated using slower tempos with the elderly. In addition to improving musculoskeletal function, movement improves circulation and muscle tone (Phillips, 1980).

Stimulation

Music can be used to both calm patients (inhibitory) and as a means of stimulation (facilitory). The type of music selected for each will vary. Sisson (1979) played cassette recordings of *A Fifth of Beethoven* and *Theme from Grease* for patients who were unresponsive after head trauma. Observations of behavior, Glasgow Coma Scale scores, and electroencephalogram recordings indicated varying responses to the musical stimulation, with some of the patients manifesting increased arousal.

Several authors reported positive effects of music on improving social interaction of elderly persons who had been withdrawn. Mason (1978) used music to arouse the interest of apathetic patients and to intellectually stimulate withdrawn persons. Social awareness and communication between patients were increased. Music has been used to stimulate associations between items mentioned in the songs and everyday life; this resulted in improved social interactions and increased awareness of the outside world (Needler & Baer, 1982).

Precautions

Adaptation occurs if the auditory system is continually exposed to the same type of stimulus (Farber, 1982). Neural adaptation occurs after three minutes of continuous exposure. Music no longer is the stimulant or calming influence that it was intended to be. Use of stimulation, such as music, in Phase I following head injury may increase intracranial pressure. Music of a stimulating quality should be delayed until the autonomic nervous system has stabilized. Quiet music may be used to induce relaxation and block the irritating sounds from the environment.

Careful control of volume is essential. Permanent ear damage results from exposure to high frequencies. Decibels higher than 90 dBSL cause discomfort (Idzoriek, 1982). Fatigue occurs more frequently when stimulation is at higher frequencies (Farber, 1982).

Initiating music as an intervention without first assessing the patient's likes and dislikes may produce deleterious effects. A patient may have emotional links to a particular musical piece that may produce an unintended response. Long and Johnson (1978) stated that this was more likely to occur with vocal music rather than with instrumental music.

Before using music for therapeutic purposes, nurses need to have some knowledge of music and the effects that particular types of music can produce. Thought needs to be given to the type of music to use, when to use it, and for how long a period. Just placing a radio at a patient's bedside does not constitute music therapy.

RESEARCH QUESTIONS

The majority of articles on the use of music in nursing contain anecdotal accounts about its use and effectiveness. Although studies from other disciplines, especially music therapy, are helpful to nurses, research is needed to establish parameters for its use as a nursing intervention. Findings from the studies that have been conducted have produced inconsistent results. Some of the statistically nonsignificant results may be due to the small sample sizes that were used. Standley (1986) did a meta-analysis on studies in which music had been used in the health care sciences. This article provides an excellent overview of the measurements used and the results obtained.

1. Is music more effective when used in conjunction with other therapies, such as imagery, than when used alone? If multiple modalities are used, studies need to be designed to ascertain the effect that each contributes to the end result. This is particularly true in the studies on the elderly in which multiple modalities are being used.
2. What is the most advantageous time period for which to play music? Few studies have addressed this issue. When does music shift from being a calming influence to being an irritant?
3. Does playing sedative music during painful procedures for patients who are prone to increases in intracranial pressure prevent significant pressure increases? The efficacy of music in decreasing discomfort resulting from painful procedures could also be determined.
4. New-age music has been widely promoted as producing relaxation. However, the findings of Bruya and Severtsen (1984) and the review article by Hanser (1988) question this contention. Bruya and Severtsen's findings suggest that a number of persons may find classical music to be more relaxing than new-age music. Research is needed to evaluate the effects of new-age music.

REFERENCES

Alvin, J. (1975). *Music Therapy.* New York: Basic Books.

Blanchard, B. (1979). The effect of music on pulse rate, blood pressure and final exam scores of university students. *The Journal of School Health* 49:470-471.

Bruya, M.A., & Severtsen, B. (1984). Evaluating the effects of music on electroencephalogram patterns of normal subjects. *Journal of Neuroscience Nursing* 16:96-100.

Cassity, D. (1976). The influence of a music therapy activity upon peer acceptance, group cohesiveness, and interpersonal relationships of adult psychiatric patients. *Journal of Music Therapy* 13:66-76.

Christenberry, E. (1979). The use of music therapy with burn patients. *Journal of Music Therapy* 16:138-148.

Cook, J. (1981). The therapeutic use of music: A literature review. *Nursing Forum* 20:252-266.

Curtis, S.L. (1986). The effect of music on pain relief and relaxation of the terminally ill. *Journal of Music Therapy* 23:10-24.

Farber, S. (1982). *Neurorehabilitation.* Philadelphia: W.B. Saunders.

Frank, J.M. (1985). The effects of music therapy and guided visual imagery on chemotherapy induced nausea and vomiting. *Oncology Nursing Forum* 12(5):47-52.

Geden, E.A., Lower, M., Beattie, S., & Beck, N. (1989). Effects of music and imagery on physiologic and self-report of analogued labor pain. *Nursing Research* 38:37-41.

Gibbons, A. (1977). Popular music preferences of elderly people. *Journal of Music Therapy* 14:180-189.

Guzzetta, C.E. (1988). Music therapy: Hearing the melody of the soul. Pp. 263-288 in B. Dossey, L. Keegan, C. Guzzetta, & L. Kalkmeier eds., *Holistic nursing—a handbook for practice.* Rockville, MD: Aspen.

Hanser, S.B. (1988). Controversy in music listening/stress reduction research. *The Arts in Psychotherapy* 15:211-217.

Hanser, S.B., Larson, S., & O'Connell, A. (1983). The effect of music on relaxation of expectant mothers during labor. *Journal of Music Therapy* 20:50–58.

Herth, K. (1978). The therapeutic use of music. *Supervisor Nurse* 9(10):22–23.

Hinds, P. (1980). Music: A milieu factor with implications for the nurse-therapist. *Journal of Psychiatric Nursing and Mental Health Services* 18(6):28–33.

Hoskyns, S. (1982). Striking the right chord. *Nursing Mirror* 154(June 2):14–17.

Idzoriek, P. (1982). *Comparison of auditory and strong tactile stimuli on responsiveness.* Unpublished Plan B Project. University of Minnesota, School of Nursing, Minneapolis.

Livingston, J. (1979). Music for the childbearing family. *JOGN Nursing* 8:363–367.

Locsin, R. (1981). The effect of music on the pain of selected post-operative patients. *Journal of Advanced Nursing* 6: 19–25.

Long, L., & Johnson, J. (1978). Using music to aid relaxation and relieve pain. *Dental Survey* 54(8):35–38.

Maas, J. (1982). An introductory to music therapy. Pp. 87–100 in E. Nickerson & K. O'Laughlin eds., *Helping through action: Action oriented therapies.* Amherst, MA: Human Resources Development Press.

Mason, C. (1978). Musical activities with elderly patients. *Physiotherapy* 64(3):80–82.

McClelland, D. (1979). Music in the operating room. *AORN* 29:252–260.

Moreno, J.J. (1988). The music therapist: Creative arts therapist and contemporary shaman. *The Arts in Psychotherapy* 15:271–280.

Morosko, T., & Simmons, F. (1966). The effect of audio-analgesia on pain threshold and pain tolerance. *Journal of Dental Research* 45:1608–1617.

Munro, S., & Mount, B. (1978). Music therapy in palliative care. *Canadian Medical Association Journal* 119:1029–1034.

Needler, W., & Baer, M. (1982). Movement, music, and remotivation with the regressed elderly. *Journal of Gerontological Nursing* 8:497–503.

Norberg, A., Melin, E., & Asplund, K. (1986). Reactions to music, touch and object presentation in the final stage of dementia. An exploratory study. *International Journal of Nursing Studies* 23:315–323.

Phillips, J. (1980). Music in the nursing of elderly persons in nursing homes. *Journal of Gerontological Nursing* 6:37–39.

Riegler, J. (1980a). Most comfortable loudness level of geriatric patients as a function of seashore loudness discrimination scores, detection threshold, age, sex, and musical background. *Journal of Music Therapy* 17:214–222.

____. (1980b). Comparison of a reality orientation program for geriatric patients with and without music. *Journal of Music Therapy* 17:26–33.

Scartelli, J. (1982). The effect of sedative music on electromyogram biofeedback assisted relaxation training of spastic cerebral palsied adults. *Journal of Music Therapy* 19:210–218.

Sisson, R. (1979). *The effect of stimuli on patients with closed head injuries.* Unpublished doctoral dissertation, University of Texas, Austin.

Standley, J.M. (1986). Music research in medical/dental treatment: Meta-analysis and clinical application. *Journal of Music Therapy* 23:56–122.

Stoudenmire, J. (1975). A comparison of muscle relaxation training and music in the reduction of state and trait anxiety. *Journal of Clinical Psychology* 31:490–492.

Thaut, M.H. (1988). Rhythmic intervention techniques in music therapy with gross motor dysfunction. *The Arts in Psychotherapy* 15:127–137.

Wincek, J. (1989). Effects of auditory control measures on children with cerebral edema. *Research Review* 5(4):3.

Wolfe, D. (1978). Pain rehabilitation and music therapy. *Journal of Music Therapy* 15:162–178.

Woolf, H. (ed.) (1979). *New collegiate dictionary.* Springfield, MA: G & C Merriman Company.

Zimmerman, L.M., Pierson, M.A., & Marker, J. (1988). Effects of music on patient anxiety in coronary care unit. *Heart & Lung* 17:560–566.

CHAPTER 22

HEAT AND COLD

BACKGROUND

The sight of a nurse applying a cool washcloth to the forehead of a person in pain is a commonly portrayed image of nurses. Heat and cold have been used in the practice of nursing for years. Heat has been used to relieve pain since humans first experienced the therapeutic effects of the sun (Licht, 1982). Cold also has been used throughout time as a mode of treatment. Hippocrates prescribed cold drinks to alleviate fever (Lehmann & DeLateur, 1982a). Savonarola treated constipation by having persons walk on cold, wet marble floors. New uses for heat and cold are continually being explored.

Using heat and cold as treatment modalities is not unique to nursing; many professions use these therapies. Physical therapy and sports medicine make extensive use of these modalities. Research findings from these disciplines provide guidance for the use of heat and/or cold in nursing. This chapter will provide an overview of the use of the two modalities in nursing and suggest areas in which further research is needed.

Scientific Basis

Heat

Heat produces the following therapeutic effects:

1. Increases extensibility of collagen tissue.
2. Decreases joint stiffness.
3. Lessens pain.
4. Relieves muscle spasms.
5. Helps resolve inflammatory infiltration, edema, and exudates.
6. Increases blood flow.

The physiological effects of heat in relief of pain and in the resolution of edema will be presented. Various mechanisms may be operant in heat applications for reducing pain. Heat reduces muscle spasms which may contribute to pain. Ischemia frequently is found in pain associated with tension; heat increases blood flow to the region and thus reduces pain. Heat enhances the absorption of exudate and fluid, thus decreasing pressure on nerves. However, Michlovitz (1990a) noted that the mild inflammatory reaction created by heat application to the skin may increase capillary hydrostatic pressure and permeability resulting in mild edema. Heat applied over a peripheral nerve increases the pain threshold (Michlovitz, 1990a).

Local application of heat causes vasodilatation and an increase in blood flow to the region. Several hypotheses for vasodilatation have been proposed. Crockford et al. (1962) believed that the dilatation results from direct action of heat on the smooth musculature of the vessels and is not a result of an autonomic response. Fox and Hilton (1958) concluded that vasodilatation of the skin following exposure to heat was caused by the release of bradykinin from sweat glands. A spinal cord reflex is elicited from the application of heat to the skin (Michlovitz, 1990a); a decrease in postganglionic sympathetic nerve activity occurs. A consensual response also occurs; if heat is applied to one extremity, there will be a slight elevation in temperature of the other extremity.

Cold

Cryotherapy (cold) produces the following therapeutic effects:

1. Vasoconstriction with subsequent reduction of bleeding and edema.
2. Reduction of spasticity and muscle tone.
3. Elevation of pain threshold.
4. Facilitation of muscle contractions in re-education of muscles.

Cold causes vasoconstriction with a subsequent decrease in the blood flow to the areas (Michlovitz, 1990b). This effect occurs from the stimulation of the cold thermal sensors in the skin; in turn, a reflex excitation of sympathetic adrenergic fibers is initiated resulting in vasoconstriction. Lehmann and DeLateur (1982b) viewed this action as the principal therapeutic mechanism for the use of cold. Decreasing blood flow to a traumatized area lessens formation of edema. Less histamine is released with less capillary breakdown occurring. Lowering of the temperature of tissue decreases cell metabolism and diminishes the oxygen and nutrient needs of the affected tissue cells.

Cold reduces pain by altering the conduction velocity and synaptic activity of peripheral nerves (Michlovitz, 1990b). Synaptic transmission is slowed or blocked; the effect depends on the temperature of the application and the amount of time it is in place. The nerves most sensitive to cold applications are the small-diameter myelinated fibers.

INTERVENTION

Technique

Heat

Many modalities can be used to increase the temperature of an area. Heat is transmitted via three modes: convection, conduction, and radiation. Of these, conduction, the direct contact of the body area with a heated substance, is the most commonly used mode in nursing.

Hot packs are frequently used by nurses to achieve various outcomes. The chief means of heat transfer from the hot pack to the patient is by conduction, with minimal heat transfer by radiation and convection. According to Lehmann and DeLateur (1982a):

> The amount of heat [H] which flows through a body by conduction is directly proportional to the time of flow [t], the area through which it flows [A], the temperature gradient [xT], and the thermal conductivity [k] and is inversely proportional to the thickness of the layer [xL] across which the temperature gradient is measured. The formula for this is: $H = kAt[xT/xL]$. [p. 429]

Increased thicknesses of toweling reduce the amount of heat the body receives. Heat is conducted more rapidly through wet towels than through dry cloths. Transfer of heat from hot packs to deep muscles is usually not significant because the thermal fat acts as an insulator. The increased blood flow to the skin carries away the heat that has been applied externally. The temperature of the Kenny pack (woolen cloth that has been steam heated) drops to 100°F within five minutes after application (Lehmann & DeLateur, 1982a). Commercial hot packs, usually filled with bentonite, are frequently used instead of the traditional Kenny pack. Care is taken to reduce the space between the hot pack and the skin as air is a poor conductor of heat (Lehmann & DeLateur, 1982b). Packs are frequently left in place for 30 minutes.

In addition to hot packs, a number of other modalities are used for applying heat to a localized area. These include hot water bottles, commercial pads (K-matic®) that have water flowing through them, electric heating pads, and electrically controlled moist heating packs such as Thermophore. The nurse needs to take into account the desired effects and which modality would be most appropriate for the specific patient.

Cold

Many modalities are used to apply cold: chipped ice in a bag, frozen gel, chemical ice envelope, ice baths, refrigerant-inflated bladders, ice water, vapocollants, ice massage, and cold packs (Halkovich et al., 1981; Lehmann & DeLateur, 1982b). Research findings have been inconclusive on the most effective cold modality. In comparing the effectiveness of chipped ice, frozen gel, chemical ice envelopes, and refrigerant-inflated bladders, McMaster et al. (1978) found that chipped ice was the most efficient means with frozen gel a close second. Local freezing sprays produce only superficial cooling and therefore are not effective in the treatment of tissue trauma. Ice massage (rubbing the skin with ice) is advocated by Bugaj (1975) as it more quickly produces greater temperature reduction. Ice massage causes less patient discomfort than other forms of cryotherapy.

The manner in which ice is applied affects the degree of tissue cooling. LaVelle & Snyder (1985) tested the amount of cold that penetrated various barriers (ace bandage, dry washcloth, no barrier, damp washcloth, and padded ace bandage) placed over an ankle. They found that cold did not penetrate through a padded ace bandage. The greatest reduction in skin temperature occurred with the use of chipped ice in a baggie that was placed over a damp washcloth; skin temperature after 30 minutes was 9.9°C. A greater reduction was found with this method than when the ice bag was placed directly on the skin; the mean skin temperature after 30 minutes was 10.8°C when ice was placed directly on the skin. The mean temperature for the padded ace bandage group was 30.5°C, 20.5°C for the ace group, and 17.8°C for the dry washcloth group. The most drastic cooling occurred during the first two minutes of application. Although no subject in the study asked to have the ice removed during the study, several who had ice applied over the wet washcloth commented that they would not use this method at home if it were prescribed because of the discomfort experienced.

The amount of subcutaneous fat is a determinant in the time it takes to achieve a specific tissue temperature. Lehmann and DeLateur (1982b) reported that in subjects with less than 1 cm of subcutaneous fat there is a significant reduction in muscle temperature after 10 minutes of application of cold. However, if the person has more than 2 cm of subcutaneous fat, only a minimal change in temperature occurs after 10 minutes.

The length of time ice should be applied is debated. LaVelle and Snyder (1985) applied ice for 30–45 minutes, noting that the greatest decrease occurred during the first two minutes. Lehmann et al. (1974) recommended applying the cold for 30 minutes; a longer period may be needed if the effect is to be on deep tissue. If cold packs are left in place longer than 30 minutes, blood flow to the area is alternately increased and decreased (Lehmann et al., 1974). Hocutt et al. (1982) established 15 minutes as the minimum time for applying ice to obtain therapeutic effects. Table 22.1 presents the stages of sensation experienced by persons at various times after ice has been applied.

Table 22.1
Four Stages of Sensation Experienced by Persons Receiving Cryotherapy

Sensation	Length of Time
Cold feeling	1–3 minutes after application
Burning and aching	2–7 minutes after application
Local numbness	5–12 minutes after application
Reflex deep tissue vasodilatation and increased metabolism	12–15 minutes after application

USES

Debate continues on when it is more advantageous to use heat rather than cold and vice versa. A generally accepted distinction is to use cold in acute situations while heat is more often used with chronic conditions. However, each situation needs to be carefully assessed. Hill (1989) found no significant differences in redness, ecchymosis, discharge, and skin approximation in women with episiotomies/lacerations when heat or cold were applied.

Heat

Hot packs are prescribed to decrease muscle spasms, to improve joint movements, decrease abdominal cramps, decrease menstrual cramps, resolve thrombophlebitis, and clear up localized infections (Lehmann & DeLateur, 1982a). Some investigators believe that heat increases the chances of embolism when it is applied during the acute stages of thrombophlebitis. Application of heat is frequently used to promote comfort. Michlovitz (1990b) noted that hot packs have been used to reduce cervical pain of varying origins: injury, arthritis, tension. Psychologically, heat may be better tolerated than cold.

Cold

Cryotherapy is indicated immediately following tissue trauma, particularly in ankle and other joint trauma. Hocutt et al. (1982) found that cold applied within 36 hours after trauma was the most effective modality in reducing tissue damage from sprains. Basur et al. (1976) reported that "Cryogel" applied hours after injury produced significantly better recovery than did only the use of compression dressings.

Cryotherapy also is used in the treatment of pain. Cold acts as a counterirritant. Spray cold is sometimes used in emergency departments for relief of pain during simple suturing procedures. This modality also is used to dull pain resulting from injuries received during athletic events. Caution needs to be taken so that further injury does not occur in the anesthetized area. Melzack et al. (1980) found ice massage to be effective in relieving low back pain.

Application of ice cubes was found to be effective in treating cold sores (Danziger, 1978). Applying ice for 90–120 minutes during the first 24 hours after symptoms appeared lessened the pain and the fluid in the vesicles was reabsorbed.

Precautions

Heat

Careful assessment is needed to detect photosensitivity to heat; a heat-induced urticaria develops in persons who are sensitive to heat (Willis & Epstein, 1974). Heat exacerbates symptoms in multiple sclerosis; extensive use of heat with this population is not recommended. Heat is contraindicated in persons with hemorrhagic diathesis and after trauma; application of heat increases blood flow to the area and may aggravate bleeding (Lehmann et al., 1974). Caution is needed in using heat with persons who have decreased levels of responsiveness or impaired sensation. They will be unable to communicate pain which may be an indicator of tissue damage. Heat is contraindicated in areas that have inadequate blood supply or decreased sensation.

Cold

Cryotherapy is contraindicated in persons with cold allergy and Raynaud's phenomenon (Hocutt et al., 1982). According to Lehmann et al. (1974), cold should not be used in persons with periarteritis nodosa and lupus erythematosus. It needs to be used with caution in persons with rheumatoid conditions (Michlovitz, 1990b). Wound healing may be impaired by the use of cryotherapy. Michlovitz (1990b) recommends not using cryotherapy during the first two weeks of healing.

Careful assessment of patients receiving cryotherapy is necessary. Nerve palsy may occur when ice is applied over joints (Drez et al., 1981). This complication can be avoided by not using ice for longer than 30 minutes at one time and protecting superficial nerves that are directly under the application. Frostbite is another untoward effect of cryotherapy, but tissue damage is a rare occurrence (Lehmann & DeLateur, 1982b).

RESEARCH QUESTIONS

Although nursing has used heat and cold as treatment modalities for years, a comparative dearth of published research reports in nursing was found. These two treatment modes appear to have many applications in nursing. Significantly more research is needed to provide a scientific basis for their use and to more clearly delineate the conditions for which each would be most appropriate. Some of the questions that need to be answered are:

1. For what conditions is heat more effective than cold, and vice versa? Is a combination of the two the best therapy for some conditions?
2. How long should heat or cold be applied to obtain maximum results? Does this differ for different applications and for different conditions?
3. How much cold from cryogel (and other modalities) is transferred through various barriers? How much heat is transferred through the various barriers used in treatment? Do persons with varying amounts of subcutaneous tissue require differing types of barriers for safe and effective therapy?
4. How can cold applications be made comfortable so that persons will continue to use them?
5. According to Kauffman (1987), little clinical research has been conducted to determine the response of elderly to heat applications even though heat is used extensively with this population. Therefore, research with this population is needed.

REFERENCES

Basur, R., Shepard, E., & Mouzas, G. (1976). A cooling method of ankle sprains. *Practitioner* 216:708–711.

Bujag, R. (1975). The cooling, analgesic, and rewarming effects of ice massage on localized skin. *Physical Therapy* 55: 11–19.

Crockford, G., Hellon, R., & Parkhouse, J. (1962). Thermal vasomotor responses in human skin mediated by local mechanisms. *Journal of Physiology* 161:10–20.

Danziger, S. (1978). *Lancet* i:103.

Drez, D., Faust, D., & Evans, J. (1981). Cryotherapy and nerve palsy. *The American Journal of Sports Medicine* 9:256–257.

Fox, R., & Hilton, S. (1958). Bradykinin formation in human skin as factor in vasodilatation. *Journal of Physiology* 142:219–232.

Halkovich, L., Personius, W., Clamann, M., & Newton, R. (1981). Effect of fluro-methane® spray on hip flexion. *Physical Medicine* 61:185–189.

Hill, P.D. (1989). Effects of heat and cold on the perineum after episiotomy/laceration. *Journal of Obstetric, Gynecologic, and Neonatal Nursing* 18:124–129.

Hocutt, J., Jaffe, R., Rylander, R., & Beebe, J. (1982). Cryotherapy in ankle sprains. *The Journal of Sports Medicine* 10:316–319.

Kauffman, T. (1987). Thermoregulation and use of heat and cold. Pp. 69–91 in O. Jackson ed., *Therapeutic considerations for the elderly*. New York: Churchill Livingstone.

LaVelle, B.E., & Snyder, M. (1985). Differential conduction of cold through barriers. *Journal of Advanced Nursing* 10: 55–61.

Lehmann, J., & DeLateur, B. (1982a). Therapeutic heat. Pp. 404–562 in J. Lehmann ed., *Therapeutic heat and cold.* Baltimore: Williams & Wilkins.

_____. (1982b). Cryotherapy. Pp. 563–602 in J. Lehmann ed., *Therapeutic heat and cold.* Baltimore: Williams & Wilkins.

Lehmann, J., Warren, C., & Scham, S. (1974). Therapeutic heat and cold. *Clinical Orthopedics and Related Research* 99:207–245.

Licht, S. (1982). History of therapeutic heat and cold. Pp. 1–34 in J. Lehmann ed., *Therapeutic heat and cold.* Baltimore: Williams & Wilkins.

McMaster, W., Liddle, S., & Waugh, T. (1978). Laboratory evaluation of various cold therapy and modalities. *The American Journal of Sports* 6:291–293.

Melzack, R., Jeans, M., Stratford, J., & Monks, R. (1980). Ice massage and transcutaneous electrical stimulation: Comparison of treatment for low-back pain. *Pain* 9:209–217.

Michlovitz, S.L. (1990a). Biophysical principles of heating and superficial heat agents. Pp. 63–87 in S. Michlovitz ed., *Thermal agents in rehabilitation.* Philadelphia: F.A. Davis.

_____. (1990b). Cryotherapy: The use of cold as a therapeutic agent. Pp. 88–108 in M. Michlovitz ed., *Thermal agents in rehabilitation.* Philadelphia: F.A. Davis.

Willis, I., & Epstein, J. (1974). Solar- vs heat-induced urticaria. *Archives of Dermatology* 110:389–392.

CHAPTER 23

MASSAGE

BACKGROUND

Massage has a long history of use as a nursing intervention. According to White (1988), the therapeutic effects of massage were described by Hippocrates in the fifth century B.C. Giving a back rub was one of the first "skills" the author learned as a nursing student. While little basis was given for its use three times a day, this author noted that patients most often looked forward to the back rub and seemed to be more comfortable and relaxed after the intervention. More recent nursing fundamental texts have devoted less attention to the back rub. Likewise, observation in the clinical areas points to the infrequent use of back rubs. Reasons for this decreased use are not clear, but it is ironic that nurses have decreased use of massage when the general public is seeking it as a means for decreasing stress and improving well-being. Most health spas and athletic clubs have masseurs or masseuses on their staffs. They are sought to "massage away" tension and relax the person. In addition to its use for reducing stress, the intervention of massage is beneficial for numerous other conditions. This chapter will provide a basis for nurses to prescribe and use massage for a variety of conditions.

Definition

Massage involves the manipulation of soft tissue for therapeutic purposes (Barr & Taslitz, 1970; Longworth, 1982). Maanum and Montgomery (1985) defined massage as, "a controlled form of touching meant to create a particular response" (p. 8). Wakim (1985) noted the holistic aspect of massage in that movement of tissue helps repair the human body. Two points pervade all definitions of massage: Therapeutic intent of the process and movement of soft tissue by the therapist's hands.

A number of strokes or movements are used in manipulating the soft tissue. Francon (1960) listed six: effleurage (stroking), friction, pressure, petrissage (kneading), vibration, and percussion. Combinations of these are used in giving a massage. The reader is referred to *The Book of Massage* (Lidell, 1984) or *The Complete Book of Swedish Massage* (Maanum & Montgomery, 1985) for diagrams of the movements described.

Effleurage is the slow, rhythmic stroking made by light contact with the skin. The palmar surface of the hands is used for larger surfaces, and the thumbs and fingers are used for smaller areas. On large surfaces, long, gliding strokes, 10–20 inches in length, are used. A pace of about 15 sweeps per minute has been found to be the most effective (Francon, 1960). Effleurage may be applied very superficially or more deeply. In most instances, a combination of the two intensities is used. Francon (1960) recommended using effleurage for at least 5 minutes but not for more than 20 minutes in any one area.

Friction movements involve the application of moderate, constant pressure to an area with the thumbs or fingers. They are held in place and moved in a circular fashion. The pressure stroke is similar, but it is done with the hand or hands on a circumscribed area. The pressure stroke is made slowly, 15 or less strokes per minute. Friction stroking of an area should not exceed 10 minutes.

Petrissage, or kneading, is another frequently used stroke. A large fold of skin along with the underlying muscle is raised and held between the thumb and fingers. The tissues are pushed against the bone, then squeezed and raised in circular movements (Francon, 1960). The therapist alternately tightens and loosens her grasp on the tissue held. The tissue is supported by one hand while the other kneads it. Variations of kneading include pinching, rolling, wringing, fist-kneading, and digital-kneading. Petrissage is used only in well-padded tissue areas. Strong kneading in an area should be limited to five minutes or less.

The vibration stroke can be given either with the entire hand or with the fingers. Very rapid, continuous strokes are used. Vibration demands much energy; therefore, mechanical vibrators are often used. Vibration should be limited to five minutes in a specific body location.

Percussion strokes are done with a quite rapid tempo over a large area. The wrist acts as the fulcrum for the hand; supple wrists are required. Tapping and clapping are variants of the percussion stroke. Francon (1960) cautioned that only experts knowledgeable about the technique should perform it. Percussion should not exceed five minutes in any one area.

Acupressure includes some of the strokes used in "ordinary" massage, but the emphasis is on the pressure strokes and the application to precise spots of the body. According to Lee and Whincup (1983), the use of massage techniques over acupoints has a reflexive effect on nerve functions, causing the excitatory and inhibitory processes of the nervous system to reach a relative equilibrium. Lee and Whincup present a good description of acupressure and its uses.

Scientific Basis

Massage produces therapeutic effects on multiple body systems: integumentary, musculoskeletal, cardiovascular, lymph, and nervous. Manipulating the skin causes it to become more supple and finer. Perspiration and sebaceous excretion are enhanced (Wakim, 1985). Massage has been used most extensively to produce therapeutic effects in the musculoskeletal system. It increases or enhances movement by reduction of swelling, loosening and stretching of contracted tendons, and aiding in the reduction of soft tissue adhesions. Muscle fatigue is lessened as the result of the more rapid removal of waste products. Friction on the skin and underlying tissue causes a release of histamines which, in turn, produce vasodilation (Wakim, 1985). Venous return is enhanced. Massage results in an overwhelming improvement in the flow of lymph; this may be as high of an increase as 25% (Wakim, 1985).

Barr and Taslitz (1970) examined the influence of back massage on the autonomic nervous system. They measured blood pressure, heart rate, galvanic skin response, axillary sweating, peripheral skin temperature, pupil diameter, and respiration rate. Ten normal females received three back massages from a female therapist. The subjects served as their own control. A control session was held on each evening preceding the massage session. Findings from their study indicated that sympathetic arousal rather than parasympathetic responses occurred during the back massage but not during the control period.

Longworth (1982) reported that after a six-minute slow back massage, the heart rate and electromyogram readings of her subjects (also females) had increased from the resting baseline period. The systolic and diastolic blood pressure, however, decreased. No appreciable changes were noted in the skin temperature. Scores on Spielberger's State Anxiety Questionnaire indicated that the subjects viewed the massage as relaxing. Self-reports verified these findings. A general increase in autonomic arousal was noted after three minutes of the back massage.

Variable results relating to the effect of massage on arousal also have been found in other studies (Rubin, 1978; Tyler et al., 1990). Rubin investigated the effect a back rub had on electrocardiogram (ECG) readings, blood pressure, pulse, temperature, and respiratory rates. Only slight changes were noted in ECG rhythms in 10% of the subjects. Tyler et al. (1990) found that a one-minute back rub increased heart rate and decreased Svo2 in a sample of critically ill patients. However, the investigators noted that although these changes were statistically significant, the changes were not clinically significant as the heart rate only increased four beats per minute.

Whereas the results of studies do not provide conclusive evidence to support the use of massage to provide relaxation, some basis for its use is given. Fakouri and Jones (1987) found that 10 minutes after the conclusion of the back rub, the skin temperature remained higher and the heart rate slower than were noted in the baseline rates. The majority of subjects in the studies reported being relaxed. Because the type of massage used was not clearly elaborated in a number of the studies, the nature of the massage technique may have had an impact on the findings. Longworth (1982) discerned that the underlying pathologies in subjects also may have contributed to the lack of congruity in the findings.

Slow-stroke back massage was used by Longworth (1982) with the express purpose of inducing relaxation. This technique may bring about relaxation by habituation to tactile stimuli and "inhibition of the muscle spindle by the passive stretch on the tendinous insertion of the muscles" (Longworth, 1982:50). Habituation occurs as the result of repetitive, monotonous stimuli. After a period of time, the frontal lobe no longer perceives these as threatening, and the arousal impact disappears. Stretching the tendon insertions temporarily relaxes the muscle, accounting for the relaxation experienced.

INTERVENTION

Massage may be used to achieve a number of different outcomes. The combination of strokes used varies depending on the desired outcome. Any one or combination of the six strokes described earlier in the chapter may be used. Two massage techniques, back massage and foot massage, will be presented. Although some may consider massage to be very elementary, evidence supports the fact that many nurses have never learned the basic elements for administering a therapeutic back massage or doing a foot massage. Michaelson (1978) noted that with the many advances in nursing, the back rub has been forgotten.

Technique

A number of persons recommend that the nurse center herself/himself before beginning the massage. Preparation for the back massage includes warming the lotion and one's hands. A cold stimulus startles the patient. Because a sizeable area of the patient's body will be exposed, the room also must be warm and comfortable. If the purpose of the back massage is relaxation, care is taken to eliminate any loud or distracting noises.

Michaelson's technique consists of eight steps:

1. Effleurage of the entire back.
2. Friction strokes next to spine.
3. Petrissage of shoulder area.
4. Hand pressure moving up back.
5. Effleurage and kneading of the upper back and shoulder.
6. Pressure stroke to spinal column.
7. Circular movements to the lower back.
8. Light effleurage movements to entire back.

Each of these movements will be described in the order of its listing.

Hands are placed next to the lower spine and moved upwards to the neck in effleurage. Moderate pressure is applied with a gradual diminishment as the hands are moved toward the neck. The hands are gradually lifted at the end of the stroke, almost lifted off the skin. The hands circle the shoulder blades and are moved lightly down the outside edge of the back. Francon (1960) recommended making 15 sweeps per minute. This number can be reduced if the purpose is to achieve relaxation. Also, one can initially use 15 strokes per minute and then reduce the number as the procedure continues.

After several minutes of effleurage, friction strokes are used next to the spine in the lower back. There is an alternation between the left and right sides until the waistline is reached. The hands are glided up to the neck.

Petrissage (kneading) is performed in the shoulder region. Points in the shoulder area are grasped and kneaded. Constant assessment is necessary to determine if the patient is experiencing any pain from the kneading. Pressure can be lessened or certain areas avoided if pain or discomfort are detected.

Hands are next placed at the outer edge of the back at the level of the hips. Moderate pressure is applied as the hands are simultaneously moved (walked) up and over the back to the opposite side. This crisscrossing of the hands is repeated until the top of the neck is reached.

Attention is given to the shoulder region as these muscles are often tense. Effleurage, with hand movements from the middle to the upper back and shoulder, is used. Gentle kneading of the upper arms with assessments of the patient's reaction is done.

A pressure stroke is used as the hands are moved from the lower spine to the top of the spine. One hand is placed on top of the other and pressure is applied to the palm of the hand on the spinal column. Light to moderate pressure is used.

Large circular movements are made on the lower back region by placing one hand on top of the other; moderate pressure is applied. The hands are moved on the outer side of the body from the waistline to the lower hip and then across the hip and up the spine.

Light effleurage is used to conclude the back massage. Pressure is lessened with each succeeding stroke. Strokes are made from the neck to the sacrum.

Francon (1960) cautioned against protracting the length of the massage. Massaging for too long can produce fatigue and negate the effects of the intervention. He advocated using effleurage for at least 5 minutes, but never more than 20 minutes. Effleurage in any one area should not exceed 10 minutes. More forceful movements should be of short duration and never exceed 5 minutes.

A number of variations of the back massage—such as the slow stroke massage, Swedish massage, holistic massage, and self-massage—exist. The slow-stroke back massage has been advocated by several persons as a method for inducing relaxation (Hofkash, 1980; Longworth, 1982). This technique consists primarily of stroking down both sides of the spine with the hands two inches from the spine. Sixty strokes per minute are administered for three minutes. Lee and Whincup (1983) described a method that a person can use to give a self-massage. The technique involves massaging or applying pressure on 20 points from head to foot. The authors stated that the technique can be used to strengthen the body, protect it from disease, and treat disease. The individual can use all 20 steps or selectively choose the ones for specific circumstances.

Technique for Foot Massage

According to Joachim (1983), foot massage is an important, but neglected, nursing intervention. It is easiest to massage the feet if the patient is recumbent. Rub the entire foot and ankle area with oil. Hold the patient's foot firmly and make circular strokes around the bones of the ankle. Cover the surface on the top of the foot with circular strokes. Use a finger to trace the space between the tendons, moving from the toes to the ankle. Next, massage the four sides of each toe, concluding with the squeezing of the tip of each toe. The bottom of the foot is massaged by using the fist in making circular motions. Massage the sides of the foot by moving the tissue between the index and third finger. Many patients enjoy having a pounding motion used on the sole of the foot. Firm, sweeping motions over the top and bottom of the foot are used to conclude the massage of each foot.

It is important to use firm strokes in massaging feet as light strokes may cause tickling. The nurse must also be alert to the facial expressions of the patient as some areas of the foot may be very sensitive.

Table 23.1
Uses of Massage

Decrease overall body tension and lessen fatigue (Fakouri & Jones, 1987; Longworth, 1982)
Chest physiotherapy (Chopra et al., 1977)
Decrease need for episiotomy (Stiles, 1980)
Lessen pain (Frazer, 1978; Cyriax, 1980)
Decrease edema (Cyriax, 1980)
Improve mobility (Wakim, 1985)
Improve varicose ulcers (Cyriax, 1980)
Induce sleep (Bauer & Dracup, 1987)
Facilitate communication (Bauer & Dracup, 1987)

USES

Massage is commonly used to relieve tension and produce relaxation. Table 23.1 lists conditions for which massage has been used. While physical therapy assumes prime responsibility for the use of massage for treating these conditions, nurses also may find massage a valuable intervention to use for persons with these or similar conditions. A discussion of the use of massage in four areas—relief of tension, relief of pain, improvement of skin and muscle function, and transport of fluids—will be presented.

Relief of Tension

Previous reference has been made to the use of massage to relieve tension and promote relaxation. Constant high levels of stress have been identified as the largest cause of illness in the industrialized world (Garrison, 1978). Studies also have shown that hospitalization creates high levels of stress for many patients. These high levels of stress and the hospital environment frequently interfere with the patient's ability to sleep. A return to the use of back massages, particularly in critical care units, may do much to reduce stress and induce sleep without having to resort to medications. Bauer and Dracup (1987) reported that only one subject in their study did not find the back rub to be relaxing; six of the subjects fell asleep during the massage or postmassage period.

Decrease Pain

Several factors may contribute to the effectiveness of massage for decreasing pain. Massage improves circulation, which helps to reduce edema. Massage is particularly effective in promoting venous return and the flow of lymph (Wakim, 1985). Secondly, this increased blood flow hastens the removal of waste products in the muscle tissue that may be irritating to nerve endings. Lastly, massage helps reduce muscle spasms and tension in muscles, particularly in the large muscle groups, thus eliminating a source of pain. Perhaps this last factor contributes most to the use of massage for pain relief. The wide use of massage by athletic trainers is indicative of its effectiveness for reducing pain.

Frazer (1978) related use of a massage technique for relieving postsympathetic pain. Massage was as effective as an epidural injection in relieving pain for this group of patients. He suggested that the basis for the success may be that massage served as a counterirritant. Also, because quite vigorous massage was used, the release of enkephalins may have been stimulated, contributing to the decrease in pain.

Improved Functioning of Muscle and Skin

Physical therapists and athletic trainers frequently use massage to improve the functioning of muscles. According to Wakim (1985), massage helps to dissolve soft tissue adhesions that may interfere with muscle functioning.

Stiles (1980) suggested that use of perineal massage would reduce the need for episiotomies. The massaging loosens and softens the muscles and tissues in the perineum. Massage should be begun at least by the eighth month of pregnancy. Perineal massage helps the woman become more aware of the muscles that need to be relaxed during labor.

Transport of Fluids

One usually does not think of chest percussion as a form of massage, but one of the strokes mentioned earlier was vibration. Tapping and clapping are variants of this stroke. Chopra et al. (1977) studied the effects of several therapies on the transportation of tracheal secretions in anesthetized dogs. Chest percussion was the most effective therapy for increasing the tracheal transport of secretions. Percussion was performed for 10 minutes.

Precautions

Some persons may be more sensitive to touch than others. Farber (1982) noted that it is often necessary to use inhibitory techniques to overcome hypersensitivity to touch in persons recovering from head trauma. More gentle strokes may help to decrease sensitivity. Persons may associate sexual intent with massage. Nurses need to be alert to patient reactions that may convey that this is occurring.

Rubin (1978) studied the effects that back massage had on blood pressure, heart rate, and heart rhythms. She noted that many times nurses were reluctant to use back rubs for persons who had had myocardial infarcts because it was believed that back rubs stimulated sympathetic responses. Her findings do not support this fear. The findings of Bauer and Dracup (1987) likewise found no untoward responses to back massage in subjects who were recovering from an acute myocardial infarction.

Adaptations in positioning may be necessary for patients who find it difficult to assume the prone position. Persons with breathing problems, arthritic conditions, and abdominal surgery are among those who will find it difficult to maintain the prone position for a period of time. A foot massage is an alternative to consider for these patients.

Longworth (1982) found significant increases in autonomic activity after the slow-stroke back massage had been administered for three minutes. She stated that this increased autonomic activity was associated with an elevated psychoemotional arousal. Significant changes in autonomic and psychoemotional responses were not found after five minutes of back massage, and a decrease in the initial elevations was noted. This may indicate the need to spend at least five minutes in providing the back massage if the purpose is the reduction of anxiety.

RESEARCH QUESTIONS

Massage has a long history of use as a nursing intervention. However, little documentation exists to support its use for specific conditions or with particular patient populations. This is especially true for foot massage. Massage, including the use of all of the strokes, has the possibility for wider use as a nursing intervention. The following are areas in which research is needed to help provide a more scientific basis for its inclusion in the repertoire of nursing interventions:

1. Little documentation exists on the amount of pressure, the type of stroke(s), and the length of the treatment that would be most effective for a back massage. A number of techniques were addressed in the literature with little basis for the relative benefits of the particular technique. This area is ripe for nursing researchers to explore.
2. The effect of the gender of the nurse and the patient has been alluded to but no data were found to support the need for the therapist to be of the same sex as the patient. Does this really alter the therapeutic effectiveness of the back massage?

3. A seemingly wide variation in the effects back massage had on the autonomic nervous system was found in the articles reviewed. Studies that control for variables are needed to clarify and resolve these differences.
4. The comparative effectiveness of foot and back massage would provide useful information.
5. Massage is a form of touch and therefore it would appear to be useful in persons, particularly the elderly, who have sensory and cognitive deficits. In particular, explorations of the effectiveness of massage in reducing aggressive behaviors in persons with dementia are warranted.

REFERENCES

Barr, J., & Taslitz, N. (1970). The influence of back massage on autonomic functions. *Journal of Physical Therapy* 50:1679–1689.

Bauer, W.C., & Dracup, K.A. (1987). Physiologic effects of back massage in patients with acute myocardial infarction. *Focus on Critical Care Nursing* 14(6):42–46.

Chopra, S., Taplin, Simmons, D., Robinson, G., Elam, D., & Coulson, A. (1977). Effects of hydration and physical therapy on tracheal transport velocity. *American Review of Respiratory Disease* 115:1009–1014.

Cyriax, J. (1980). Clinical application of massage. Pp. 152–169 in J. Rogoff ed., *Manipulation, traction, and massage.* Baltimore: Williams and Wilkins.

Fakouri, C., & Jones, P. (1987). Relaxation RX: Slow stroke back rub. *Journal of Gerontological Nursing* 13(2):32–35.

Farber, S. (1982). *Neurorehabilitation.* Philadelphia: W.B. Saunders.

Francon, F. (1960). Massage techniques. Pp. 44–56 in S. Licht ed., *Massage, manipulation, and traction.* New Haven, CT: Elizabeth Licht, Publisher.

Frazer, F. (1978). Persistent post-sympathetic pain treated by connective tissue massage. *Physiotherapy* 64:211–212.

Garrison, J. (1978). Stress management training for the handicapped. *Archives of Physical Medicine and Rehabilitation* 59:580–585.

Hofkash, J. (1980). Classical massage. Pp. 51–58 in J. Rogoff ed., *Manipulation, traction, and massage.* Baltimore: Williams and Wilkins.

Joachim, G. (1983). How to give a great foot massage. *Geriatric Nursing* 4:28–29.

Lee, H., & Whincup, G. (trans.). (1983). *Chinese massage therapy.* Boulder: Shambhala.

Lidell, L. (1984). *The book of massage.* New York: Simon & Schuster.

Longworth, J. (1982). Psychophysiological effects of slow stroke back massage in normotensive females. *Advances in Nursing Science* 4(4):44–61.

Maanum, A., & Montgomery, H. (1985). *The complete book of Swedish massage.* New York: Harper & Row.

Michaelson, D. (1978). Giving a great back rub. *American Journal of Nursing* 78:1197–1199.

Rubin, M. (1978). Is a back rub hazardous to health? *JAMA* 240:2402.

Stiles, D. (1980). Techniques for reducing the need for an episiotomy. *Issues in Health Care of Women* 2:105–111.

Tyler, D.O., Winslow, E.H., Clark, A.P., & White, K.M. (1990). Effects of a 1-minute back rub on mixed venous oxygen saturation and heart rate in critically ill patients. *Heart & Lung* 19(5, Pt.2):562–565.

Wakim, K. (1985). Physiologic effects of massage. Pp. 256–262 in J. Basmajian ed., *Manipulation, traction, and massage.* Baltimore: Williams and Wilkins.

White, J.A. (1988). Touching with intent: Therapeutic massage. *Holistic Nursing Practice* 2(3):63–67.

CHAPTER 24

BIOFEEDBACK

BACKGROUND

Biofeedback is an intervention of relatively recent origin springing from research on the instrumental conditioning of autonomically mediated behavior. The intervention is based on a holistic perspective of humans. Psyche and soma are not separated, but rather the unification of the two is integral to the treatment modality. The goal of biofeedback is increased personal control over one's functioning. Nursing views human beings in a holistic manner. Many nursing conceptual frameworks identify control as a key concept. Thus, the holistic focus of biofeedback and its focus on helping persons gain more control over their functioning makes the intervention an appropriate one for nurses to use.

Definition

Katkin and Goldband (1980) defined biofeedback as:

> Any technique that uses instrumentation to provide a person with immediate and continuous signals concerning bodily functions of which that person is not normally conscious. [p. 537]

This definition is broader than many of the early definitions which only focused on the control of responses such as heart rate and blood pressure that are mediated by the autonomic nervous system. The definition of Williams et al. (1981) provides a comprehensive view of biofeedback:

> The technique of using equipment [usually electronic] to reveal to human beings some of their internal physiological events, normal and abnormal, in the form of visual and auditory signals in order to teach them to manipulate these otherwise involuntary or unfelt events by manipulating the displayed signals. This technique inserts a person's volition into the gap of an open feedback loop, hence the artificial name of biofeedback. [p. 22]

Biofeedback has been used to control functions related to all areas of the nervous system—cortical activity of the brain, peripheral somatic nervous system responses, and responses of the autonomic nervous system. These responses are monitored and feedback is provided to the patient concerning the degree of achieved control of the particular response, thus enabling the person to eventually control the activity or response without instrumentation feedback.

Scientific Basis

The basis for biofeedback originates from research in the fields of psychophysiology, learning theory, and behavioral theory. For centuries it was believed that responses such as heart rate and respiration were outside of the individual's control. Smith (1954) is typical of the scientists of his era in noting that the autonomic nervous system (ANS) did not interact with the external environment and was a purely motor system. Therefore, learning to control functions of the ANS was impossible by principles of reinforcement. Works of Kimmel and Kimmel (1963), Miller (1969), and Shapiro et al. (1964) indicated that the ANS had an afferent system, and with instrumentation and conditioning, control of the functions mediated by the ANS was possible. Katkin and Goldband (1980) selected the skills acquisition model as the basis for teaching biofeedback. Persons determine the relationship between voluntary muscle actions and their associated ANS patterns or between cognitive activity and ANS functions. The skeletal muscle and the cognitive activity can then be reinforced to achieve control of ANS responses. The signal received from the feedback instrument informs the persons when the established criterion have been achieved; learning is thus reinforced.

INTERVENTION

This chapter provides an overview of biofeedback. Nurses wishing to use the intervention will need to acquire additional information and skills. This information can be gained from a variety of classes and workshops that are available in most locations. The Association for Applied Psychophysiology and Biofeedback is an excellent resource for information on workshops and classes. Nurses planning to use biofeedback as an intervention will profit from personally using the technique and becoming familiar with the instrumentation.

Technique

Instrumentation

Three types of mechanisms underlie biofeedback units: binary, analog, and derivative. Binary denotes an off-on mechanism; the person is informed only if the index being measured increases. Analog instrumentation, on the other hand, presents continuous feedback on the activities being monitored. In derivative instrumentation a high-pitched tone informs the patient that the measurement has increased while a low-pitched tone denotes a decrease in the activity. Instruments frequently incorporate several or all of these forms of instrumentation.

A biofeedback unit consists of a sensor that monitors the patient's physiological activity, and a transducer that converts what is measured into a format that is electronically recorded and displayed to the patient. Amplification of the activity at varying levels is usually possible. Measurements of the activities or responses being monitored are presented to the patient in either visual or auditory displays. The mode chosen depends on the patient's preference and the therapist's assessment of the patient. However, one mode may be more appropriate for use in certain conditions. Auditory is best for persons being taught relaxation; opening eyes and concentrating on the screen interferes with achieving muscle and cognitive relaxation. Visual is believed to be the best form of display for persons with paralysis trying to gain control of muscle function.

Many of the measurements require application of electrodes. Before electrodes are applied, the skin is cleansed with soap and water and wiped with acetone or a similar substance to remove dead skin and skin oils. A conductive gel is applied to improve the recordings.

Much progress has been made in the sophistication of biofeedback units. Compact models that are relatively inexpensive are now being marketed. Persons may purchase these for home use.

Role of the Nurse

The therapist plays a key role in the success of biofeedback. Basic knowledge about the equipment is necessary. This can be learned from the company from which the equipment is purchased (demonstrations and manuals), classes, or workshops conducted by the Association for Applied Psychophysiology and Biofeedback. An understanding of the rationale for the use of biofeedback including the interaction of the ANS with other body systems and the interrelationship of the psyche and soma is needed. Accurate assessment of the patient allows the nurse to choose the type of feedback to use and the reinforcement that will be needed. Interaction with the patient is one of the keys to the success of this intervention. Since practice is of vital importance, the therapist who succeeds in motivating patients to practice will have patients who are successful in achieving their goals.

It is recommended that nurses using biofeedback become certified therapists. Certification is through the Association for Applied Psychophysiology and Biofeedback. In a survey reported by Pace (1984), 5% of the persons certified by the association were nurses. The majority of these nurses were in private practice, with only 15% practicing in hospitals.

Role of the Patient

The patient is the major factor in the success of the modality. Brown (1977) listed four functions for the patient: to learn the technique, to supply experiential information, to become aware that he can perform the activity, and to keep a record of responses.

Procedure

Brown (1977) advocated using 7–12, 30-minute training sessions. The exact number of sessions should be discussed and decided upon by the therapist and the patient prior to the initiation of training. This allows goals to be set and some determination of what accomplishments can be expected by a certain date. However, mastery or control of a function is desired, and if the patient has not achieved this at the end of the agreed upon number of sessions, reasons for failure to meet the goal and the need for additional sessions should be discussed.

The first session is devoted to providing the rationale for biofeedback, the roles of the nurse and the patient, assessment of the patient, obtaining baseline measurements, and initial instruction in the use of biofeedback. This session will be longer than subsequent ones, perhaps lasting one to two hours. Because the content in this session serves as the foundation for using the equipment and monitoring progress, determining if the person has understood the information and answering questions are critical. Instructions on relaxation skills also are provided in the first session. Chapter 6 presents content on progressive muscle relaxation.

The patient is instructed in how to practice biofeedback at home. A portable unit may be used to assist the person with practice at home. Brown (1977) believed, however, that use of a machine at home ties the patient to the machine, and as the purpose of the training is to assist the person to gain self-control over the activity, use of the home unit only delays the learning. Cues are identified to help the person become aware of the activity being monitored. If the aim is to reduce the pulse rate, the person is taught to take his pulse whenever the telephone rings or to use a similar cue. The new technology for monitoring activities is useful in providing cues at established times.

Record keeping is an essential component of the intervention. Recording responses serves two purposes: the patient is made more aware of the bodily activity for which greater control is sought, and the relationship between it and other variables, and the therapist is provided with information on progress. Adherence to practice also may be furthered through frequent recording of progress.

The final sessions focus on integration of the learning into the person's life. The patient is connected to the machine but does not receive feedback while practicing the technique; the nurse monitors the degree of control achieved. Descriptions of life situations that are often stressful are provided, and the person is asked to practice the procedure as if in that situation. Endline measurements are taken. Follow-up sessions at one month and six months are advocated by Williams et al. (1981).

Table 24.1
Parameters Used for Feedback to Patient

Airway resistance	Brain waves	pH of stomach
Blood pressure	Galvanic skin response	Temperature of skin
Blood volume	Heart rate	Tracheal noise
Bowel sounds	Movement	

Measurement of Effectiveness

Table 24.1 lists parameters that have been used in providing feedback to the patient on body activities. Frequently used parameters include heart rate, muscle tension, temperature, and blood pressure.

Baseline measurements are taken before training begins. The initial measurements taken, particularly in stress disorders, may be high due to the nature of the situation. Katkin and Goldband (1980) suggested taking measurements on several occasions before beginning instruction. Obtaining measurement of several indices helps in getting valid baseline data. Because success will be determined by changes from the baseline, it is essential that these be accurate and reflect the true status of the parameter being used.

Continuing control of the function is the aim of the intervention. Obtaining measurements at the follow-up sessions is critical in determining if biofeedback has been helpful in achieving the outcomes that were determined in the first session. The criteria for success vary depending on the outcomes selected. For example, the goal for a post-stroke patient may be for the person to have the strength and movement necessary for performing activities of daily living independently. Not only would the nurse check on the muscle function but also on the person's ability to perform these activities of daily living.

USES

Biofeedback has been used in the treatment of over 50 medical and psychological problems with either greater success than with conventional methods or with equal success (Brown, 1977). Biofeedback is the treatment of choice for Raynaud's disease, spasmodic torticollis, causalgia, certain types of post-stroke rehabilitation, and for intractable tension headaches (Williams et al., 1981). As the intervention continues to be used and evaluated, its use for other conditions will be more specifically verified.

The intervention, providing the person with feedback on a function, is useful in those situations where the person is not able to discern by normal means what the body's response is. These nondiscriminable responses fall into three categories:

1. Normally nondiscriminable responses such as brain waves, peripheral vascular responses, cardiac rate responses, and electrodermal responses.
2. Usually discriminable responses over which the patient functionally has lost control. This category includes many of the conditions related to high-stress levels.
3. Usually discriminable responses over which the patient has lost control due to organic lesions. This category includes paralysis. (Katkin & Goldband, 1980).

The multiplicity of uses of biofeedback is at times overwhelming and prompts the query, "In what conditions isn't it effective or hasn't it been tried?" After reviewing the literature on biofeedback, Hatch (1987) concluded that there is much need for controlled studies, particularly clinical trials, that can determine the effectiveness of biofeedback in treating physiological and psychological conditions. However, research reports do provide evidence of its effectiveness with a variety of conditions.

Table 24.2
Conditions In Which Biofeedback Has Been Used

Anxiety symptoms (Kogan & Beatron, 1984; Scandrett et al., 1986)
Asthma (Janson-Bjerklie & Clarke, 1982; Mussell & Hartley, 1988)
Bowel incontinence (Riboli et al., 1988)
Headaches (Blanchard et al., 1986; Andrasik & Blanchard, 1987)
Hemiplegia (Wolf et al., 1989)
Hypertension (Blanchard et al., 1989; Nagagawa-Kogan et al., 1988; Pearce et al., 1989)
Insulin dependent diabetes (McGrady et al., in press)
Irritable bowel (Radnitz & Blanchard, 1989)
Pain (Empting-Koschorke et al., 1990; Keefe & Hoelscher, 1987)
Peripheral vascular conditions (Surwit & Jordan, 1987)
Urinary incontinence (Middaugh et al., 1989; Taylor & Henderson, 1986)
Weaning from ventilator (Acosta, 1988)

Health promotion and prevention of illness are goals that fall within the domain of nursing. Biofeedback is a useful intervention for achieving these goals (Kogan & Beatron, 1984). Helping persons to become aware of how their body functions and how they may control functions is beneficial in improving health. Biofeedback also gives the person control. It is hoped that as persons see that they can control body activities and responses, they will be prompted to do so and thus compliance with regimens will increase.

Table 24.2 lists conditions in which biofeedback has been used. Its use in tension headache, hypertension, asthma, weaning from ventilators, urinary incontinence, and peripheral vascular conditions will be discussed.

Tension Headache
High levels of stress often result in persons strongly contracting muscles in the scalp, neck, and shoulders; the continuous contracting of the muscles frequently results in tension headaches. Electromyogram monitoring of the frontalis muscle provides the person with information about the tension level of this muscle, which is one of the muscles that is often tensed during times of stress. It is hypothesized that relaxation of the frontalis muscle is indicative of the relaxation of muscles throughout the entire body. Biofeedback has been more successful in the treatment of tension headaches than in the treatment of migraine headaches (Katkin & Goldband, 1980).

Two types of biofeedback have been used with persons having tension headaches: electromyogram (EMG) and thermal. EMG feedback is the most frequently used form. Results from a survey of clinical centers using biofeedback revealed that the majority of centers reported that 70% or more of the clients had positive results from the use of biofeedback (Andrasik & Blanchard, 1987). Holroyd and Penzien (cited in Andrasik & Blanchard, 1987), in their meta-analyses of studies that had used biofeedback in treating tension headaches, found a lower treatment effect—46%. Speculation is that the results may have resulted from a more thorough assessment made of prospective candidates in the clinics as compared to random assignment in the research studies. Age was found to be a significant variable in response to biofeedback training, with persons 35 years and younger having better results (Holroyd & Penzien, cited in Andrasik & Blanchard, 1987).

Hypertension
Westerners noted that yogi and shami in the Eastern religions were able to lower their blood pressure by meditating and relaxing. This prompted research into the use of biofeedback to lower blood pressure. Glasgow and Engel (1987) did an extensive review of studies in which biofeedback had been used with

hypertension. They noted that reductions of 4 to 22 mm. Hg. systolic and 1 to 1–15 mm. Hg. dyastolic had been achieved with biofeedback training. These changes were maintained for periods of 6 to 48 months. The authors concluded that blood pressure can be effectively reduced through the use of biofeedback. Pearce and colleagues (1989) used biofeedback in a geriatric medicine clinic in which the teaching was done by a nurse. Patients were instructed in lowering their blood pressures through feedback from sphygmomanometer readings. Decreases of 13 mm. Hg. from baseline readings in systolic readings were obtained over a 3-month period. However, questions regarding its use in the treatment of hypertension remain.

Various parameters have been used in providing feedback on the level of blood pressure. Electromyogram, Korotkoff z-sound (K-sound), and pulse wave velocity (PWV) have been used. Tension of striate muscle increases peripheral resistance to blood flow and thus increases pressure. Use of EMG feedback in the attainment of overall muscle relaxation contributes to decreases in blood pressure. The PWV form of feedback shows more promise than the K-sound; it is non-invasive and relatively inexpensive.

The pressure reductions that have been achieved with biofeedback have not always been of a magnitude large enough to be therapeutic. These reductions may, however, allow reduction in dosages of antihypertensive medications and these could help to reduce some of the untoward side effects found with many antihypertensive medications. It has been questioned by some whether the lowered pressures occur continuously or are only present when the person concentrates and practices the technique. As with taking medications, the person will need to adhere to practice of biofeedback to maintain the lowered pressures. Biofeedback may be most useful in helping prevent hypertension from occurring in persons who have normal blood pressure.

Asthma

Asthma is another condition in which increased anxiety has a noticeable impact on the severity of symptoms experienced. Janson-Bjerklie and Clarke (1982) used biofeedback with eight persons suffering from asthmatic attacks. The investigators believed that if the persons could learn some degree of control over their airway constriction and wheezing through the use of biofeedback, they would have an alternative technique to use in the management of a condition that is only partially controlled by other therapies. Total respiratory resistance (TRR) served as the feedback measurement. A significant difference was found between the experimental group and the control group in their ability to decrease respiratory resistance. The investigators noted that determination of long-term effects of the training, such as clinic visits and overall health, is needed before the real efficacy of the use of biofeedback can be shown.

A large segment of the American population suffers from chronic conditions that affect the pulmonary system. Nurses in many settings provide care for these persons. Because biofeedback allows persons some control over the symptoms, individuals may be motivated to learn the technique. Significant advances have been made in instrumentation providing better feedback mechanisms for use in the treatment of respiratory disorders.

Weaning from Ventilator

Nurses play a major role in weaning patients from ventilators. The process is often highly stressful for the patient. Acosta (1988) reported that use of biofeedback and progressive relaxation helped to lessen the patient's stress during the weaning process. Heart and respiratory rates were monitored along with arterial oxygen saturation levels. Both rates decreased after the sessions while the oxygen level increased. Although use with only one patient was reported, the results suggest that biofeedback may be effective and additional studies are needed to verify the intervention's use as an adjunct in the weaning of patients from ventilators.

Peripheral Vascular Conditions

Raynaud's disease and vascular headaches are two conditions for which biofeedback frequently has been used. Constriction of blood vessels is the underlying pathology in both conditions. Increasing the temperature of the skin is the feedback mechanism used in treating these conditions.

Surwit and Jordan (1987) reviewed research that has been done on the use of biofeedback in Raynaud's disease. Although their review indicated that flaws exist in many of the studies conducted, there is evidence supporting the efficacy of biofeedback in the treatment of this condition. The exact mechanism for the effectiveness is not known, but it may be from adrenergic activity. Decreases in symptomatology in the studies reviewed ranged from 30–90%; no side effects were noted.

The use of biofeedback in the treatment of vascular headaches, which included migraine headaches, has not been as successful as it has been in the treatment of Raynaud's disease. Persons are usually taught to warm their hands and cool their forehead. Some researchers believe that teaching the person to relax and overcome the initial vasoconstriction prevents the occurrence of symptoms. Blanchard and Andrasik's review (1987) of studies indicated that progressive muscle relaxation and other therapies are as effective as thermal biofeedback in relieving symptoms of migraine headaches. However, thermal biofeedback is probably the most effective in the treatment of childhood migraine headaches.

Urinary Incontinence

Urinary incontinence is a major problem of the elderly. It is one of the major reasons for institutionalizing a person. Interventions that would help to overcome incontinence would have a major impact on quality of life for persons with incontinence and also would significantly reduce health care costs. Biofeedback has the potential for producing beneficial effects. Middaugh and colleagues (1989) studied the effectiveness of sensorimotor biofeedback in reducing urinary incontinence in persons who had suffered a stroke. All four of the subjects who were taught biofeedback achieved and maintained continence over a 12-month period of time. Bladder pressure readings, abdominal pressure readings, and external anal sphincter pressure readings were feedback mechanisms used. Attention was given to improving voluntary bladder control. The authors noted that persons must have the cognitive ability to follow instructions and remember the content of the teaching in order to participate in biofeedback training.

Precautions

Biofeedback should be used cautiously in persons with depression and hyperactive conditions. Williams et al. (1981) believe that persons with rigid personalities are unlikely to find biofeedback useful as they are unwilling to change their mode of functioning. Few studies have examined the characteristics of persons who have not benefited from biofeedback, particularly those who have dropped out of studies. Therefore, ongoing monitoring is needed to detect untoward effects.

Some patients may have multiple symptoms requiring treatment. Training should only address one symptom at a time. The other symptoms can be treated sequentially after mastery of the first one is attained. The patient decides which symptom will be treated first.

Patient safety is a concern when any electrical equipment is used. Electric shock is the greatest hazard. Dangerous levels of current flow may arise from improperly designed equipment, a failure in equipment, or operator error (Katkin & Goldband, 1980). The Association for Applied Psychophysiology and Biofeedback publishes a list of companies whose products have passed their safety code.

Biofeedback is not a miracle intervention. It requires that the therapist be knowledgeable about the intervention and have a sincere interest in the patient's outcome. Considerable time and attention are demanded of the patient if the intervention is to be successful. This should be made very clear to the patient before training is initiated. Biofeedback holds much promise in the treatment of many conditions. Biofeedback, as a nursing intervention, offers promise for the control of problems experienced by many persons.

RESEARCH QUESTIONS

Chapters in the text by Hatch et al. (1987) present an excellent overview on research studies that used biofeedback. The authors provide suggestions for areas in which additional research is needed and methodologies that would produce more unequivocable data. Nurses employing biofeedback as an intervention have the opportunity to further the knowledge base on its appropriateness for specific conditions and for particular patient populations. It is also important to ascertain if results obtained in nursing differ from those obtained in other disciplines. The following are some of the areas in which research is needed:

1. Does the belief of the therapist concerning the success of biofeedback training have an appreciable effect on the outcomes achieved?
2. What are the patient characteristics of persons who benefit most from biofeedback? Middaugh and colleagues (1989) specified abilities necessary in teaching stroke patients biofeedback. Are other abilities also necessary?
3. How many sessions are needed to effectively teach the technique, and when and how many follow-up sessions are necessary?
4. Does the use of biofeedback units for home practice promote or inhibit mastering the function? Brown (1977) viewed use of home units as hindering progress.
5. Does receiving feedback from several sensory modalities increase the speed and degree of learning?
6. Is biofeedback more effective when it is used in conjunction with another relaxation intervention? Numerous studies have combined relaxation strategies, but study designs often have not allowed interactive effects to be determined.

REFERENCES

Acosta, F. (1988). Biofeedback and progressive relaxation in weaning an anxious patient from the ventilator: A brief report. *Heart & Lung* 17:299–301.

Andrasik, F., & Blanchard, E.B. (1987). The biofeedback treatment of tension headache. Pp. 281–321 in J. Hatch, J. Fisher, & J. Rugh eds., *Biofeedback—studies in clinical efficacy.* New York: Plenum.

Blanchard, E.B., & Andrasik, F. (1987). Biofeedback for vascular headache. Pp. 1–48 in J. Hatch, J. Fisher, & J. Rugh eds., *Biofeedback—studies in clinical efficacy.* New York: Plenum.

Blanchard, E.B., Andrasik, F., Appelbaum, K.A., Evans, D.D., Myers, P., & Barron, K.D. (1986). Three studies of the psychologic changes in chronic headache patients associated with biofeedback and relaxation therapies. *Psychosomatic Medicine* 48:73–83.

Blanchard, E.B., McCoy, G.C., Berger, M., Musso, A., Pallmeyer, T.P., Gerardi, R., Gerardi, M.A., & Pangburn, L. (1989). A controlled comparison of thermal biofeedback and relaxation training in the treatment of essential hypertension, IV: Prediction of short-term clinical outcome. *Behavior Therapy* 20:405–415.

Brown, B. (1977). *Stress and the art of biofeedback.* New York: Bantam Books.

Empting-Koschorke, L.D., Hendler, N., Kolodny, A.L., & Kraus, H. (1990). Nondrug management of chronic pain—what today's pain clinics have to offer. *Patient Care* 24(1):165–168.

Glasgow, M.S., & Engel, B.T. (1987). Clinical issues in biofeedback and relaxation therapy for hypertension: Review and recommendations. Pp. 81–121 in J.P. Hatch, J.G. Fisher, & J.D. Rugh eds., *Biofeedback—studies in clinical efficacy.* New York: Plenum.

Hatch, J.P. (1987). Guidelines for controlled clinical trials of biofeedback. Pp. 323–363 in J.P. Hatch, J.G. Fisher, & J.D. Rugh eds., *Biofeedback—studies in clinical efficacy.* New York: Plenum.

Hatch, J.P., Fisher, J.G., & Rugh, J.D. (1987). *Biofeedback—studies in clinical efficacy.* New York: Plenum.

Janson-Bjerklie, S., & Clarke, E. (1982). The effect of biofeedback training on bronchial diameter in asthma. *Heart & Lung* 11:200–207.

Katkin, E., & Goldband, S. (1980). Biofeedback. Pp. 537–558 in F. Kanfer & A. Goldstein eds., *Helping people change.* New York: Pergamon Press.

Keefe, F.J., & Hoelscher, T.J. (1987). Biofeedback in the management of chronic pain syndromes. Pp. 211–253 in J. Hatch, J. Fisher, & J. Rugh eds., *Biofeedback—studies in clinical efficacy.* New York: Plenum.

Kimmel, E., & Kimmel, H. (1963). A replication of operant conditioning of the GSR. *Journal of Experimental Psychology* 65:212–213.

Kogan, H.N., & Beatron, R. (1984). Blending of a conceptual model and nursing practice, pp. 28–67. In *Accomodation of self-determination: Nursing's role in the development of a health care policy* (ANA Publication No. G-153). Kansas City: American Nurses Association.

McGrady, A., Bailey, B.K., & Good, M. (In press). Biofeedback-assisted relaxation in insulin dependent diabetes mellitus; a controlled study. *Diabetes Care.*

Middaugh, S.J., Whitehead, W.E., Burgio, K.L., & Engel, B.T. (1989). Biofeedback in treatment of urinary incontinence in stroke patients. *Biofeedback and Self-Regulation* 14:3–19.

Miller, N. (1969). Learning of visceral and glandular responses. *Science* 163:443–445.

Mussell, M.J., & Hartley, J.P. (1988). Trachea-noise biofeedback in asthma: A comparison of the effect of trachea-noise biofeedback, a bronchodilator, and no treatment on the rate of recovery from exercise- and eucapnic hyperventilation-induced asthma. *Biofeedback and Self-Regulation* 13:219–234.

Nagagawa-Kogan, H., Garber, A., Jarrett, M., Egan, K.J., & Hendershot, S. (1988). Self-management of hypertension: Predictors of success in diastolic blood pressure reduction. *Research in Nursing and Health* 11:105–115.

Pace, E. (1984). Biofeedback. Presentation at the American Nurses Association meeting. New Orleans.

Pearce, K.L., Engel, B.T., & Burton, J.R. (1989). Behavioral treatment of isolated systolic hypertension in the elderly. *Biofeedback and Self-Regulation* 14:207–218.

Radnitz, C.L., & Blanchard, E.B. (1988). Bowel sound biofeedback as a treatment for irritable bowel syndrome. *Biofeedback and Self-Regulation* 13:169–179.

Riboli, E.B., Frascio, M., Pitto, G., Riboa, G., & Zanolla, R. (1988). Biofeedback conditioning for fecal incontinence. *Archives of Physical Medicine and Rehabilitation* 69:29–31.

Scandrett, S.L., Bean, J.L., Breedan, S., & Powell, S. (1986). A comparative study of biofeedback and progressive relaxation in anxious patients. *Issues in Mental Health Nursing* 8:255–271.

Shapiro, D., Crider, A., & Tursky, B. (1964). Differentiation of an autonomic response through operant reinforcement. *Psychonomic Science* 1:147–148.

Smith, K. (1954). Conditioning as an artifact. *Psychological Review* 61:217–225.

Surwit, R.S., & Jordan, J.S. (1987). Behavioral treatments for Raynaud's syndrome. Pp. 255–279 in J. Hatch, J. Fisher, & J. Rugh eds., *Biofeedback—studies in clinical efficacy.* New York: Plenum.

Taylor, K., & Henderson, J. (1986). Effects of biofeedback and urinary stress incontinence in older women. *Journal of Gerontological Nursing* 12(9):25–30.

Williams, M., Nigl, A., & Savine, D. (1981). *A textbook of biological feedback.* New York: Human Science Press.

Wolf, S.L., LeCraw, D.E., & Barton, L.A. (1989). Comparison of motor copy and targeted biofeedback training techniques for restitution of upper extremity function among patients with neurologic disorders. *Physical Therapy* 69:719–735.

CHAPTER 25

PURPOSEFUL TOUCH

BACKGROUND

Purposeful touch is the term chosen to designate the intervention described in this chapter. This intervention is sometimes termed affective nursing touch (Seaman, 1982) or caring touch (Keegan, 1988). It is one of the three types of touch described by Estabrooks (1989). Protective touch, used to physically protect the patient or the nurse, and task or instrumental touch, that which takes place when performing assessments or treatments, are the other two types of touch specified by Estabrooks. Purposeful touch differs from the intervention of therapeutic touch that is presented in Chapter 20. These two interventions possess some commonalities, but are distinct from one another in the methods used in implementation.

Purposeful touch is a commonly used nursing intervention. The picture of a nurse soothing the brow of a patient is an age old depictor of nursing, a view that a large majority of the public still hold. Tobiason (1981) stated that because touch is used so frequently in providing care, nurses rarely consider its therapeutic value. Purposeful touch is a planned nursing intervention that is used with many patient populations and across the developmental cycle.

As nursing seeks to clarify the dimensions of nursing practice, components that are universal and basic to nurse-patient interaction need to be identified (Weiss, 1979). Purposeful touch is one of these basic components. In a study by Barnett (1972), findings revealed that nurses touched patients twice as often as did other health care workers. The most frequently touched areas were the hand, the forehead, and the shoulder. A colleague of the author who has taught a physical assessment course to nurses for many years recently opened the course to pharmacy students. In contrast to nursing students, he found great reluctance on the part of these students to touch the persons being examined, which differed drastically from experiences with nursing students.

Although purposeful touch has been used for centuries, recent attention to its impact on persons has been spurred by sensory deprivation experienced in intensive care units, in failure to thrive syndromes, and in the elderly. Considerable attention has been given to the need for touch in our high-tech world. Studies in child psychology revealed the importance of touch to normal development of infants and children. With increases in the number of elderly in our society, attention to the special needs of this group has shown that touch is vital in promoting their health and well-being (Langland & Panicucci, 1982; Rozema, 1986). Findings from studies of the impact of hospitalization on persons showed that feelings of separation frequently occurred; sensory contact with others could decrease these feelings and aid in recovery. Jourard and Secord (1955) discovered that the experience of touch enlivens the body and brings the person back into it.

Definition

Purposeful touch is defined as an intentional physical contact by the nurse with the patient for the intent of helping. This definition contains the connotations of intentionality and interpersonal interaction

(Schoenhofer, 1989). It does not include the touching that occurs when performing treatments, for example, giving a bath, feeding a patient, or administering a medication, but rather it is a planned intervention on the part of the nurse. Estabrooks (1989) stated that in caring touch the dominant intent is to minister to the psyche of the patient.

Weiss (1979) described six components of purposeful touch: duration, location, action, intensity, frequency, and sensation. Duration of touch is the temporal length of the stimulation from the initiation of the contact to its cessation. Location refers to the area(s) of the body stimulated. Some areas of the body are more sensitive to touch than are other areas. Social and cultural norms also affect the acceptability of the locations touched. Action is the rate of speed used in approaching the body of the other to stimulate it. A rapid approach may cause the other person to tense; the person may perceive that the other is invading his territory. Intensity is defined as the extent of the indentation incurred. Variation in the degree of intensity has the potential for furthering body esteem, securing an accurate perception of one's body, and viewing oneself as sexual and autonomous (Weiss, 1979). Frequency is the overall amount of purposeful touch experienced in everyday life. Sensation is the perceived comfort or discomfort of the stimulus; an intact nervous system is necessary for this to occur.

Scientific Basis

The somesthetic system, which includes receptors for touch, pressure, vibration, pain, and temperature, plays a key role in the use of touch as an intervention. All of these receptors may be used in purposeful touch, but some types of touch use one type to a greater extent than others. Stimuli increase the permeability of the receptor cell membrane generating impulses in the sensory nerve fibers (Lamb et al., 1980). Depolarization of the sensory nerve fiber follows; this is termed the generator potential. The potential varies depending on the strength of the stimulus. Adaptation occurs if the stimulus is applied constantly for a period of time. Impulses from the receptors are transmitted to the brain primarily via the lateral spinothalamic tract and the sensory component of the cranial nerves. The impulses are relayed to the thalamus before terminating in the post-central gyrus of the parietal lobe. The face, hands, and feet have considerably larger areas of representation in the somatosensory area than do other areas of the body; this has implications for areas to touch.

Haptic system is the term coined by Gibson (1966) to refer to the sensibility of the individual to the world surrounding his body through the use of the body. Perception of the meaning of the sensation depends on past experience. Environmental, cultural, and social factors affect the meaning that a particular tactile stimulant has to an individual. Territoriality, the sacredness or privacy of the space surrounding self, is also a factor in how a stimulus is perceived. The skin is viewed as one's last boundary to privacy.

According to Schoenhofer (1989), touch is used to express many feelings and thoughts. She states

> Although touch itself is not an emotion, its sensory elements bring about combinations
> of neural, glandular, muscular, and mental changes that are called emotions, with
> touch experienced not as a simple physical modality, as sensation, but affectively, as emotion.
> [p. 147]

Touch is used to convey love, concern, hate, or dislike. Estabrooks (1989) identifies two factors that are requisite to caring touch: The nurse's motivation must be to help the person, and the nurse must possess sufficient energy. A third factor, reciprocity, may not be present in every caring touch intervention. Characteristics of the person doing the touching profoundly affect the meaning the receiver ascribes to it.

As touch is one of the first senses to develop, it serves as an elemental form of communication (Farber, 1982). The fetus receives tactile stimulation within the mother's womb. Considerable purposeful touch is experienced during the birthing process. Touch is one of the major ways to communicate with an infant. Tracts in the central nervous system for the transmission of tactile sensations are the first to be myelinated;

myelinated fibers transmit impulses more rapidly than unmyelinated fibers. Studies have revealed that touch is the most important factor to the physical and mental growth of an infant (Frank, 1957). Through caring touch the infant develops confidence, trust, and love. Deprivation of touch leads to future speech, cognition, and symbolic recognition problems.

Hospitalization for many persons causes an increase in stress, often to very high levels. Patients who are in intensive care units find themselves separated from familiar sounds and events. Taking another's hand in stressful situations may create a soothing effect, reduce anxiety, and increase a sense of security (Knable, 1981). Schoenhofer's findings (1989) confirmed this. According to Kübler-Ross (1969), a gentle pressure on the hand is the most meaningful communication that a nurse can have with a dying patient.

INTERVENTION

Purposeful touch can take a variety of forms: Handholding; stroking or patting a patient's arm, hand, or face; placing one's hand on a patient's shoulder; circling one's arm around the patient's shoulder; or hugging the person. Tactile stimulation, another form of purposeful touch, is more forceful in nature and is used to achieve arousal in persons with decreased levels of arousal. Two techniques, handholding and stimulation, will be discussed. Personal characteristics of the nurse, the patient, and the specific situations necessitate individualizing the intervention.

Technique

The perception of touch by the patient greatly influences the success of the intervention; careful assessment of the patient is necessary before using this intervention. When greeting the patient the nurse notes if the person extends his or her hand or if the person tends to withdraw. What does the handshake feel like? Do members of the family or significant others often use touch? Farber (1982) noted that many members of our society are reluctant to touch and be touched; hence, those patients in need of touch are often hypersensitive about it. As the patient becomes familiar with the nurse, touch may become more acceptable.

Handholding

In our Western culture, a handshake is a mode often used in establishing a relationship with another person. Extending a hand is seen as a sign of friendship; for example, after an argument a handshake is a sign of accord. This mode of communicating is very acceptable in Western cultures. It does not involve the touching of more private areas of the body. Extending one's hand also does not invade the other's territoriality as much as other forms of touch, such as an embrace. The other person has more of an opportunity to withdraw or reject the handshake.

In handholding, the nurse sits down next to the patient and places her hand on top of the patient's hand. The length of time a hand should be held was not indicated in any of the studies reviewed (Copstead, 1980; Knable, 1981; McCorkle, 1974; Pollack & Goldstein, 1981; Schoenhofer, 1989; Tobiason, 1981). Walleck (1982) stroked the patient's hand and face for two minutes each. Her intent was to calm the patient in an effort to reduce intracranial pressure. Burnside (1973) advocated using an unhurried handshake in greeting and bidding farewell in each encounter with an elderly person. The amount of pressure to be applied was not indicated. A gentler handshake is given to a person with rheumatoid arthritis.

Schoenhofer (1989) differentiated patting and stroking. She defined patting as "rhythmic intermittent contacts delivered to a single location of the body" (p. 149). Stroking was described as "contact that is extended from one point to another in a continuous motion and may be continued in a rhythmic back-forth pattern" (pp. 149–150). Often a combination of handholding, patting, and stroking is incorporated into a single intervention.

Table 25.1
Categories of Tactile Movement

Fine Touch
   Delicate, light, with slight tension, buoyant, sensitive

Sustained
   Slow smooth, legato, lingering, prolonged, indulgent of time, unhurried

Flexible
   Indulgent of space, roundabout, plastic, wavy, generous in attitude toward space

---

Source: Adapted from J. Pratt & R. Mason (1981). *The caring touch.* Copyright 1981 by John Wiley & Sons, Ltd. Reprinted by permission of John Wiley & Sons, Ltd.

The area of the body touched is very significant. Pratt and Mason (1981) stated that the lower arms and back are the most commonly used areas of contact for expressing understanding and sympathy. Schoenhofer (1989) found that the hand and shoulder were the areas most frequently touched by intensive care nurses.

The force of the stimulus is important. Pratt and Mason (1981) noted that the qualities of weight, time, and space affect the perception of the touch. A stimulus may incorporate any combination of these qualities; a change in one quality alters the meaning of the stimulus. Table 25.1 lists these qualities and their modifiers. A difference in meaning is noted when the touch is firm, sudden, and direct as opposed to a firm, lingering, and direct touch.

Territoriality has much relevance to the intervention of touch. Sudden invasion of one's space is seen as more threatening than a gradual intrusion. In the initial encounter touch is usually of short duration. One rarely embraces or hugs a person until rapport has been established. It is as if permission is obtained for the invasion of the other's space.

Knable (1981) studied the effects purposeful handholding had on critically ill patients. Adult patients who had been in an intensive care unit for at least eight hours were studied. Nurses chose two times within a four-hour period to hold the patient's hand. Physiological responses (blood pressure, heart rate, and respiratory rate) to the handholding were mixed, with some increases and some decreases occurring. However, both nurses and patients reported positive psychological responses to the experience. The investigator noted that after the nurse had terminated the interaction the patient sometimes re-initiated the handholding. In another situation the patient moved his hand next to the nurse's hand, but she did not grasp it. One patient, who was asked if she enjoyed having the nurse hold her hand, stated that it was not done often enough. Nurses noted that both appropriate timing and serious intent were necessary for handholding to be therapeutic.

A caring, empathetic touch by the nurse is an important element of nursing. Patients sense insecurity and reluctance to touch on the part of the nurse. Schoenhofer (1989) examined nurse and patient variables that promoted the use of touch. The type of person the nurse is, the degree of energy, current personal or family variables, and the context of the unit are factors that affect a nurse's use of touch. Patient factors that tend to influence the use of touch include presence of confusion, agitation, pain, anxiety; reciprocation from the patient; and, unfortunate victims, ones with a poor prognosis or those who have been through a difficult procedure. Deterrents to touching include patients with behavioral problems, those presenting a risk to the nurse, and those who are culpable for their current condition.

Tactile Stimulation

In neurorehabilitation, touch is used early in the treatment program as tactile input stimulates arousal (Farber, 1982). Touch may be either inhibitory or facilitory. Inhibitory techniques are used first to normalize hypersensitive skin; this is followed by facilitory techniques.

Inhibitory techniques include maintained pressure with the finger in the perioral region; light, constant pressure to the abdomen; and pressure maintained on the soles of the feet or the palms of the hand. The nurse's finger is placed horizontally above the patient's lip while the other fingers are clenched to keep them out of the field of vision. Constant monitoring is done to determine the patient's response; if sympathetic responses occur, the other areas should be stimulated. The palm of the hand is placed on the patient's abdomen and held in place for a period of time. (Be sure the hand is warm!) The exact length of time that this should be done is not known (Farber, 1982). One method for applying inhibitory touch to the palms is to have the nurse place both palms over those of the patient and hold them in place for a period of time.

Facilitory touch techniques include a moving stimulus as opposed to the constant pressure applied in inhibitory techniques. An example is the nurse moves her forefinger caudally from under the patient's nose to the tip of the chin. This movement is repeated a number of times with a short rest period provided between each movement sequence. If the patient appears to be hypersensitive, inhibitory techniques should again be instituted (Farber, 1982).

Measurement of Effectiveness

The purpose for which purposeful touch is used determines the indices for measuring its effectiveness. Indices that have been used include vital signs, interaction, comfort, self-appraisal, intracranial pressure, and cognitive ability. Nurses need to choose parameters that will give sufficient information on the effectiveness of the intervention and also be usable in the clinical situation.

Drescher et al. (1980) studied the effect touch had on heart rate. They found that the heart rate decreased when the person was touched. Neither differences in sex nor presence of another person affected the findings. In Knable's (1981) study, mixed responses in vital signs were found when patients were touched. If a decrease in anxiety is desired, a decrease in heart rate and blood pressure could be indicative of the response to touch.

Improved self-image can be determined by the Jourard-Secord Self-Cathexis Scale and other psychological tests. Observable measures include the person's grooming, facial expression, and degree of interaction with others. The gleam in the eyes and the smile on the face are ready indicators of improved self-appraisal and well-being.

USES

Purposeful touch is widely used in nursing. Examples for which it has been commonly used include:

1. To communicate with a person; it enhances verbal communication, or it may be the chief mode for interacting.
2. To comfort a person who has experienced a loss or is facing a difficult decision.
3. To calm or quiet a person who is highly anxious or restless.
4. To reassure a person that someone is there and cares about him or her.
5. To encourage a person to do something or that life is worth living.
6. To apply pressure to specific points in the body for healing (acupressure).
7. To increase alertness in persons with lowered levels of arousal.

Purposeful touch can be used with many patient populations. It does, however, have particular efficacy for certain conditions. Two groups for whom it has been used extensively are the very young and the elderly. Other populations for which it is beneficial include immobilized persons, those with deficits in other

Table 25.2
Uses of Touch

Decreases in intracranial pressure (Walleck, 1982)
Communication (Hollinger, 1980; McCorkle, 1974)
Orientation (Burnside, 1973)
Reawakening of perceptual abilities (Hollinger, 1980)
Increase in self-appraisal (Copstead, 1980)
Human development (Farber, 1982)
Decrease in anxiety (Triplett & Arneson, 1979)
Emotional support (Knable, 1981; Schoenhofer, 1989)
Establish rapport (Knable, 1981)
Encouragement (Schoenhofer, 1989)

sensory modalities, those who have suffered a loss, persons who are highly agitated, persons who are disoriented, and those who have a reduced level of consciousness. Table 25.2 lists conditions in which purposeful touch has been used as a nursing intervention.

Elderly

The need for tactile stimulation does not increase or decrease with age. Reports by Barnett (1972) and Tobiason (1981) revealed that nurses touched the elderly less or felt less inclined to touch the elderly than they did persons in other population groups. Barnett found in her study that the 66–100-year-old group received the least amount of touching of all age groups. Student nurses in Tobiason's study used less positive words to describe tactile and affective feelings after touching the elderly than after touching newborns.

Copstead (1980) studied the effect touch had on self-appraisal. She compared two groups of patients: One who was frequently touched and the other who was rarely touched. Self-appraisal was measured by Jourard and Secord's Self-Cathexis Scale (1955). Her findings revealed that those who were touched frequently had a significantly more positive self-appraisal than did those who were touched infrequently. Copstead stated that this clearly demonstrated that the experience of being touched (albeit even for a brief, structured moment) apparently had an impact upon subsequent self-appraisal.

Losses contribute to the need for touch for the elderly. Loss of loved ones with whom touch and intimacy were exchanged is experienced. Vision and hearing senses are frequently diminished. Mobility problems also reduce sensory input. All of these contribute to social withdrawal, cognitive impairments, confusion, and seemingly inappropriate behavior.

Purposeful touch enhances visual information and thus the person is better able to understand the surroundings. Purposeful touch also assists the person to become more involved with himself. Touch can help reawaken the person's remaining perceptual capacities. Interactions of persons in wheelchairs can be furthered by grouping chairs closely, thus allowing persons to make physical contact with each other.

Anxiety

The soothing effect that touch has on persons demonstrating increased anxiety has been observed by most nurses. Holding a crying child does much to dispel fear. One can feel muscles relax during painful procedures when a hand is held or an arm touched. McCorkle (1974) and Knable (1981) have reported its benefits with seriously ill patients. Triplett and Arneson (1979) found verbal and tactile stimulation reduced distress in hospitalized children.

Several studies have shown that purposeful touch has contributed to decreases in intracranial pressure. Walleck (1982) used purposeful touching of the face and hand of patients with increased intracranial pressure. Her findings revealed that pressure decreases occurred; greater decreases were found when the face was stroked than when the hand was stroked. Pollack and Goldstein (1981) noted pressure decreases of 5–10mm Hg in patients with Reyes syndrome following gentle touching; an auditory stimulus also was used. Whether the effect was due to a decrease in anxiety which resulted from the touching or from some other effect is not known. High intracranial pressure has the potential to cause irreparable damage; incorporating nursing interventions to decrease it can have an impact on the patient's ultimate outcome.

Orientation

There are many causes of confusional states: head injuries, electrolyte imbalances, cerebrovascular conditions, dementia, and drugs are common causes. Persons who are confused are a threat to both their own and others' safety. Ways to "reach" the person are sought. Perhaps no intervention is more helpful in orienting this population than touch. Touching conveys acceptance and a trusting relationship is furthered. Touching brings the person into contact with the outside environment. For patients with decreased levels of arousal from head injuries, the use of tactile stimulants is added to the use of touch. Rancho Los Amigos uses a wide variety of tactile stimulants—textures, feathers, light touch, pressure—for unresponsive and confused patients who are recovering from head injury. The International Coma Recovery Institute has reported almost miraculous recoveries from coma when extensive stimulation was used (LeWinn & Dimancescu, 1978).

Precautions

Adequate assessment of the person is essential to the effectiveness of purposeful touch. Because the nurse is comfortable with touch and likes to be touched should not be equated with these properties being possessed by the patient. The nurse needs to be cognizant of cultural differences in relation to the use of touch. Although many times touch is used to help establish a relationship with a patient, in some situations it can only be used effectively after a trusting relationship has been established through other means.

Touch is a learned behavior (Tobiason, 1981). The comfort of the nurse in using purposeful touch has a great impact on the success of the intervention. Faculty should not assume that students know about touch and its use, but rather include content and practice in the curriculum.

RESEARCH QUESTIONS

Although touch is widely used in nursing, in both purposeful and instrumental actions, few studies have been done to determine its effectiveness and to provide parameters for its use. Much research is needed in order to provide direction for prescriptive intervening. In the study of touch, nurses need to provide clear and precise definitions of the intervention being used. The following questions include suggestions made by Weiss (1988) and Schoenhofer (1989) who have reviewed nursing research on touch.

1. Does the perception of purposeful touch vary across the life span? Are prevading aspects found in all age groups?
2. What are the qualities of touch that are most effective in bringing about the desired change? How long should a person hold the patient's hand or touch the person? Is a softer and more gentle touch better in certain situations than a firmer and more intense touch?
3. Do patients with lower self-esteem have a greater need for touch?
4. Does the sex of the nurse affect the outcome of the touch? Does this differ across age groups? Lane (1989) found differences in effects based on gender.
5. Does touching of the patient by the nurse increase the degree to which family members touch and interact with the patient?

6. What effect does reduction in other sensory modalities have on the perception of touch?
7. Do nurses incorporate purposeful touch as part of carrying out procedures and assessments?
8. Are there specific types of touch that should be avoided in persons who are critically ill?

REFERENCES

Barnett, K. (1972). A survey of the current utilization of touch by health team personnel with hospitalized patients. *International Journal of Nursing Studies* 9:195–209.

Burnside, I. (1973). Touching is talking. *American Journal of Nursing* 73:2060.

Copstead, L. (1980). Effects of touch on self-appraisal and interaction appraisal for permanently institutionalized older adults. *Journal of Gerontological Nursing* 6:747–752.

Drescher, V., Gantt, W., & Whitehead, W. (1980). Heart rate response to touch. *Psychosomatic Medicine* 42:559–565.

Estabrooks, C.A. (1989). Touch: A nursing strategy in the intensive care unit. *Heart & Lung* 18:392–401.

Farber, S. (1982). *Neurorehabilitation*. Philadelphia: W.B. Saunders.

Frank, L. (1957). Tactile communication. *Genetic Psychological Monographs* 56:211–251.

Gibson, J. (1966). *The senses considered as perceptual systems*. Boston: Houghton Mifflin Co.

Hollinger, L. (1980). Perception of touch in the elderly. *Journal of Gerontological Nursing* 6:741–745.

Jourard, S., & Secord, P. (1955). Body-cathexis and personality. *British Journal of Psychology* 46:130–138.

Keegan, L. (1988). Touch: Connecting with the healing power. Pp. 331–355 in B. Dossey, L. Keegan, C. Guzzetta, & L. Kolkmeier eds., *Holistic nursing—a handbook for practice*. Rockville, MD: Aspen.

Knable, J. (1981). Handholding: One means of transcending barriers of communication. *Heart & Lung* 10:1106–1110.

Kübler-Ross, E. (1969). *On death and dying*. New York: Macmillan Publishing Co.

Lamb, J., Ingram, C., Johnston, I., & Pitman, R. (1980). *Essentials of physiology*. London: Blackwell Scientific Publications.

Lane, P.L. (1989). Nurse-client perceptions: The double standard of touch. *Issues in Mental Health Nursing* 10:1–13.

Langland, R.M., & Panicucci, C.L. (1982). Effects of touch on communication with elderly confused clients. *Journal of Gerontological Nursing* 3:152–155.

Le Winn, E., & Dimancescu, M. (1978). Environmental deprivation and enrichment in coma. *The Lancet* ii:156–157.

McCorkle, R. (1974). Effects of touch on seriously ill patients. *Nursing Research* 23:125–132.

Pollack, L., & Goldstein, G. (1981). Lowering of intracranial pressure in Reye's syndrome by sensory stimulation. *The Lancet* i:732.

Pratt, J., & Mason, R. (1981). *The caring touch*. London: HM & M Publishers LTD.

Rozema, H.J. (1986). Touch needs of the elderly. *Nursing Homes* 2:42–43.

Schoenhofer, S.O. (1989). Affectional touch in critical care nursing: A descriptive study. *Heart & Lung* 18:146–154.

Seaman, L. (1982). Affective nursing touch. *Geriatric Nursing* 3:162–164.

Tobiason, S. (1981). Touching is for everyone. *American Journal of Nursing* 81:728–730.

Triplett, J., & Arneson, S. (1979). The use of verbal and tactile comfort to alleviate distress in young hospitalized children. *Research in Nursing and Health* 2:15–23.

Walleck, C. (1982). Effect of touch on intracranial pressure. Speech at the American Association of Neurosurgical Nurses, Honolulu, Hawaii.

Weiss, S. (1979). The language of touch. *Nursing Research* 28:76–80.

_____. (1988). Touch. Pp. 3–27 in J. Fitzpatrick, R. Taunton, & J. Benoliel eds., *Annual review of nursing research*, vol. 6.

SECTION 5

SOCIAL INTERVENTIONS

CHAPTER 26

TIMING AND RHYTHMS

BACKGROUND

Nurses manipulate the environment of patients as they assist them to improved well-being. Timing of activities is an aspect of care that nurses manipulate. Underlying the concept of time is its subjective nature and the endogenous and exogenous rhythms that control many human functions. The field of chronobiology has begun to identify the presence of many rhythms and the relationship of these to health. Luce (1973) stated that timing is an integral part of humans and central to well-being. He viewed health as the state in which rhythms are integrated into certain phase relationships. Nurses have many opportunities to evaluate and help bring these rhythms into harmony. According to Newman (1986), considerable evidence exists that temporal patterns are highly individualistic; these patterns have an impact on person's responses to other people and their receptivity to therapy and ability to learn new tasks. This chapter will explore aspects of time and how nurses can employ this information in planning interventions.

Definition

Many definitions of time and rhythms exist that vary depending on the perspective and discipline of the author. Einstein (cited in Grubb, 1980) believed that the perception of time was relative for each individual. According to Grubb (1980):

> Although the individual's perception of time involves his external world, the actual perception of time, including what is perceived, how it is decoded and the affective response, is quite subjective in nature. [p. 277]

Newman (1982) focused on subjective time and not clock time in studying expanded consciousness and health. Time, according to Piaget (1969), is intimately related to change, particularly the rate of change.

Piaget (1969) divided time into physiological and psychological components. Physical time was defined as the relationship between distance traveled and given speed. He saw psychological time as the relationship between the quantity of work accomplished and the effort the person expended (work divided by power). Hall (1984) characterized temporal patterns as being either monochromic or polychromic. Monochromic time is linear and compartmentalized, whereas interactions with people and transactions rather than adherence to schedules characterizes polychromic time. The former type is typical of Western life, and the latter type is found in Eastern cultures.

In addition to temporal or linear time, periodicity or rhythms are an integral part of living. Minors and Waterhouse (1981) defined a rhythm as "a sequence of events that repeat themselves through time in the same order and at the same interval" (p. 2). Changes in the length of the cycle may occur in rhythms. The rhythms studied in chronobiology are based on clock or calendar time. Endogenous rhythms, those originating within a person, and exogenous rhythms, dependent on something external, both have a

Table 26.1
Definitions of Frequently Used Rhythm Terms

Rhythm: any regularly oscillating process
Period: time occupied by a cycle
Exogenous rhythm: dependent on some external periodicity; this can be from environment or personal habit
Endogenous rhythm: originates from within the person and continues in the absence of any external influence
Zeitgeber: dominant periodic influence or synchronizer in the environment that affects a rhythm
Phase: any particular point in the cycle
Circadian rhythms: approximately 24-hour periods
Ultradian rhythms: occurring between 1 and 19 hours
Infradian rhythms: between 29 hours and 5 days
Circaseptan rhythms: 6–8 days
Circavigintan rhythms: 17–23 days
Circannual rhythms: about 1 year

considerable impact on a person. Table 26.1 presents definitions for a number of the rhythms that have been identified.

Temporality, as defined by Fitzpatrick (1980), incorporates rhythmicity. She defined temporality as:

> A manifestation of holistic man's sense of time characterized by non-linearity, identified by rhythmic patterns which are evidenced throughout the developmental process. [p. 150]

Her definition is based on Rogers' theory (1970) of unitary being. Rogers postulated that humans move from slower to faster rhythms and eventually to timelessness. Time moves slowly for children, it flies for adults, and some elderly experience a sense of timelessness.

Scientific Basis

Time

Time dragging, time flying, and time expanding are terms frequently used in common parlance. Investigators have attempted to discover the variables affecting these perceptions. Because these varying perceptions have been linked to the health status of an individual, they are of concern to nurses.

According to Feifel (1957), a normal sense of time assists the person in making adjustments and is an important contributor to establishing contact with and controlling one's environment. Past, present, and future are critical elements of the concept of time, but each is relative for the individual. The three form a whole of the person's life, but at a given time a person focuses more attention on one of the elements rather than the others. Aaronson (1972) used hypnosis to explore the meaning and impact of past, present, and future orientations. Subjects in his study were happy in the present, but if the anchors of past and future were eliminated the person felt adrift. When present time was eliminated, the subjects expressed a feeling of unbeing. Aaronson concluded that the present represents reality to the person, and the person must live in the present to be healthy.

A generalization often heard is that elderly persons live in the past. Whereas this does not apply to many elderly, retreat to memories of the past may offer a safer haven than the present or the future. Reduction in the physical activity of many elderly also may precipitate rumination over past accomplishments. Whitbourne and Dannefer (1986) reported that older men were more past-oriented than were younger men. Several investigators have found that subjective happiness, excitement in life, and future orientation in elderly persons were positively correlated with time passing more rapidly (Kuhlen & Monge, 1968; Lemon & Bengston, 1972). Melillo (1982), however, found no relationship between increased social activity and the perception of time passing quickly. She hypothesized that these findings may have resulted because subjects were pressured to participate in activities rather than choosing to interact.

Factors affecting the perception of the passage of time include stimulus complexity (Grubb, 1980; Schilder, 1981), emotions (Langer et al., 1961), temperature (Hoagland, 1933), gender (Bull, 1973), and mobility (Newman, 1982; Tompkins, 1980). Schilder noted a discrepancy in the literature regarding the effect that stimulus complexity has on perception of time. She concluded that a common sense observation is that the more actively we process environmental stimuli, the more rapidly time passes. When a person experiences fear, time seems to pass very slowly (Langer et al., 1961); in times of sadness or depression, the passage of time also is perceived as being slowed. Hoagland (1933) investigated the effect of body metabolism on perception of time; subjects overestimated time when their body temperature was elevated (time drags). He suggested that variations in metabolism accounted for the differences in perception of time experienced by children and elderly; the child's metabolic rate is faster. Divergencies in perception of time between males and females was reported by Bull (1973); females demonstrated a greater sense of subjective time than did males.

Several nursing studies have looked at the relationship of mobility and perceived time (Newman, 1982; Tompkins, 1980). Newman's findings revealed that persons have a more accurate perception of time when they are walking than when they are sitting. In Tompkin's study, findings supported the premise that the perceived duration of time is shortened (time drags) in persons experiencing restricted mobility.

Cultural backgrounds affect perception of time (Hall, 1984). The Oriental perspective on time is toward timelessness; they do not have, therefore, a cultural need to accomplish everything at once. In contrast, in Western cultures, especially American culture, there is an urgency to get things done.

Rhythms

Although the majority of scientific work relating to rhythms has been done in the past quarter century, humans have been aware of internal and external rhythms since the beginning of history. Bunning, in the eighteenth century, studied biological rhythms in botany. More recently, the studies of Halberg and colleagues have contributed significantly to the understanding of human rhythms. However, much remains to be known about biological rhythms. Synchronization of rhythms is necessary for health (Luce, 1973).

Attention has focused on establishing whether a particular rhythm is endogenous or exogenous. If the rhythm is exogenous, the phase of the rhythm can be altered by changing the length of external periodic influences on it (Minors & Waterhouse, 1981). Endogenous rhythms are more difficult to change as the transmission process between the clock and the overt rhythm would need to be altered. A rhythm is termed endogenous if:

1. It persists even when rhythmic influences most likely to affect it are absent.
2. Its period is not precisely 24 hours when the zeitgeber is excluded.
3. It maintains an approximate 24-hour cycle despite habit and environment adapting another rhythm.
4. Its phase does not change immediately when habit or environment are altered.
5. When it has become entrained to a new phase, as in #3 or #4, it does not revert to its previous phase even when former habits or environment are restored (Minors & Waterhouse, 1981).

Rhythms of various phases are found in humans and in the universe. Long and short rhythms are thought to have an overall integration. According to Luce (1973):

Certain rhythms are clearly determined by a creature's physiological characteristics. For instance, heart rate depends upon an animal's size, his surface-to-volume ratio, and circulatory efficiency. But whether the rhythm is as rapid as a discharge of nerve cell, or as slow as the menstrual cycle, various types of rhythmic phenomena are bound to interact and to influence one another. They are also bound to be influenced by a person's habits. [p. 435]

Circadian rhythms have been studied more extensively than other types of rhythms. Minors and Waterhouse (1981) stated that no sole and sufficient link between any two circadian rhythms could be found pointing to the fact that the link is not single, unidimensional, or immutable. They postulated that the hypothalamus, reticular-activating system, and autonomic nervous system serve as internal control mechanisms. These interact with each other and with some circadian rhythms; control mechanisms of the systems and rhythms are influenced by these interactions. The impact of the external environment on circadian rhythms also must be considered in studying these phenomena.

INTERVENTION

Timing is an important variable for nurses to consider before implementing specific nursing interventions. The time chosen for implementing an intervention may affect the outcome. For example, teaching done when the metabolic rate is slowed may not be as effective as if it were done when a person's metabolic rate were higher. No particular technique for timing exists, but rather the nurse assesses the person and uses knowledge about subjective time and rhythms in determining when it would be most efficacious to intervene.

Instruments for determining a person's perception of time will be discussed. A number of instruments exist: Time Reference Inventory (Roos & Albers, 1965), Time Opinion Survey (Kuhlen & Monge, 1968), Time Metaphor Test (Knapp & Garbutt, 1958), and Money Game (Cottle, 1976). In addition, parameters that provide data on circadian rhythms will be presented.

Instruments for Assessment

One instrument that has been used to gain information on a person's perception of time is the Time Reference Inventory (TRI), developed by Roos and Albers (1965). The 30-item instrument measures the relative direction of the person's time orientation (past, present, future). The scale includes 10 items that are affectively positive, 10 affectively negative items, and 10 affectively neutral statements. The person assigns past, present, or future reference to each of the items. The more often a person chooses one category of time, the less the other two time frames can be chosen. Foulks and Webb (1970) reported that the instrument had high validity and reliability.

Another instrument is the Time Opinion Survey (TOS) designed by Kuhlen and Monge (1968); this instrument measures the individual's attitudes on the passage of time and the consequences. Table 26.2 presents selected items from the TOS. Scores are generated for five areas: Speed of time passage, future orientation and achievement, feelings of time pressure, ability to delay gratification, and current life situations. Kuhlen and Monge reported face validity for the instrument.

Rhythms

Knowledge about rhythms is becoming an increasingly integral part of clinical therapeutics. All body functions are believed to be influenced by various circadian cycles such as sleep, temperature, blood pressure, and enzyme production. Drew (1989) details the importance of cardiac rhythms in determining patient responses. Obtaining accurate measurements of various parameters assists in establishing an

Table 26.2
Sample Questions Contained in the Time Opinion Survey

How rapidly does time seem to pass for you now?
    4 Extremely rapidly
    3 Fairly rapidly
    2 Neither rapidly nor slowly
    1 Fairly slowly
    0 Extremely slowly

How fast does time seem to be passing now compared to 10 years ago?
    0 Much more slowly
    1 Somewhat more slowly
    2 About the same
    3 Somewhat more rapidly
    4 Much more rapidly

Do you have a feeling that "time is running out" or that there is a certain urgency with respect to time in the achievement of any major goals or hopes?
    3 Yes, very much so
    2 Yes, somewhat so
    1 Yes, but only slightly so
    0 No

Source: From R. Kuhlen & R. Monge (1968). Correlates of estimated rate of time passage in adult years. Reprinted by permission of *The Gerontologist/Journal of Gerontology* 23:432–433.

individual's circadian rhythms. Nurses are instrumental in securing these measurements, often through the use of sophisticated instrumentation.

Measurement of Effectiveness

Timing is a variable that has an impact on the effectiveness of other interventions. It is important that studies on interventions be designed so that the effect of time on the outcome of an intervention can be evaluated. These data will assist nurses in planning care for patients. To date, few studies have explored the impact that timing has had on outcomes.

USES

Numerous patient situations and patient conditions could be discussed in relation to time and rhythms.

Alterations in Time Perception in Persons with Disabilities

Newman (1982) noted that persons use their walking pattern for gauging their learned relationship to clock time. Persons who have restricted mobility perceive duration of time as shortened as compared to when they are able to walk in their usual manner (Tompkins, 1980). Tompkins concluded that the slowing of perceived time found in persons with restricted mobility may be useful in preserving system integrity. Nojima and colleagues (1987) found that persons who had greater difficulty in performing activities of daily living had higher consciousness index scores than did those with lesser problems. Nurses need to be aware of the alteration in time perception in planning activities for persons with physical disabilities; a slower pace for activities may be beneficial.

Confusional states found in patients who are on prolonged bed rest is not an uncommon finding. This is particularly true for elderly persons who have been active and suddenly find themselves hospitalized. Although the use of clocks and calendars has been advocated in nursing literature, little evidence exists that supports their effectiveness in lessening confusion. Instituting some rhythms in the person's environment may assist in decreasing the degree of confusion experienced. Regularly occurring activities, music, and exercise may help to compensate for the rhythms the person had experienced and that served to orient him to time and person.

Teaching Patients

Few studies on patient teaching have considered the impact that the variable time of day has on the acquisition of knowledge and skills. Numerous authors recommend that teaching take place when the person is rested. When to teach the patient, in relation to stress levels that occur following an illness diagnosis, has been discussed by some investigators but little definitive data exist to provide guidance for teaching patients.

Schilder (1981) stated that nurses need to be more aware of the patient's time focus (probably present- rather than future-oriented) when planning teaching and care. Patients may feel that their concerns are being ignored if the nurse focuses on another timeframe. This may contribute to noncompliance with therapeutic regimens. Assessing patients to determine their time perspective will provide guidance to the nurse in teaching strategies to employ.

Administration of Medications

Multiple studies have been conducted on the effects obtained when specific medications are administered at various times throughout the day. If therapeutic effects can be maximized by administration at specific times, lower dosages can be used, helping to decrease the toxic effects of many medications. Side effects of the medications also may be lessened (Minors & Waterhouse, 1981). Scheving (1979) noted the following alterations in drug effectiveness when the time of administration was changed:

Sleep cycles after administration of pentobarbital at different times during the 24-hour cycle varied from 104-43 minutes.

When cytosine arabinoside was given at one phase 72% of mice died as opposed to only 15% when it was given at another phase of the circadian cycle.

Amphetamines given at one time of the circadian cycle resulted in only 6.6% of the mice surviving as compared with 77.6% when it was given at another time.

These examples point to the profound effect that the time of administration has on the pharmacokinetics of drugs. DeScalzi et al. (1986) found wide variability in the peaks of diastolic and systolic blood pressures at various times of the day; they recommended individualizing the times antihypertensive medications are taken based on a person's rhythm spectrum. Members of the International Union Against Cancer were unanimous in stating that experimental chemotherapy should not be done without attention to principles of chronobiology. Implantable, programmable drug infusion pumps now allow for chemotherapeutic agents to be given at specific times (Lanning et al., 1990).

Nurses frequently are responsible for establishing the times for administration of medications. In addition to maximizing the therapeutic effects of the drug, timing affects other areas that are of particular concern to the nurse. Moore (1982) explored the influence that the time of administration of cis-platinum, a drug used in cancer chemotherapy, had on nausea and vomiting. She believed that hormonal levels may affect the vomiting center and, thus, altering the time of administration would reduce vomiting. Although her findings were not conclusive, she found that patients who had more sleep before receiving chemo- therapy reported less vomiting.

Health Promotion

Knowledge of an individual's rhythms has many implications for teaching the person about ways to improve his health. Scheving (1979) stated that persons can determine what their specific body rhythms are by some quite unsophisticated methods. Measurement of blood pressure, oral temperature, pulse rate, pulmonary function using a flow meter, eye–hand coordination using a simple means, physical strength by grasp, and mental ability by performance of tasks at intervals around the clock will provide the person with vital knowledge about self. This knowledge can be used by the person in choosing the time of the day or the month in which he is most responsive to make decisions that require concentration and care.

Variations in measurement of blood pressure, temperature, and other parameters have been found when taken at various times during the 24-hour cycle. Assessments at varying times are needed to obtain an accurate picture of an individual. Persons with mild hypertension might go undetected if their blood pressure was only measured at one time of day. Rotating times for clinic appointments may aid in detection and early intervention. Findings of Furrario et al. (1982) revealed that intraocular pressure readings varied with the circadian rhythm. Thus, early indications of glaucoma could be missed if the person's measurements were taken at only one time frame. DeScalzi et al. (1986) found variation in the times for peaks of systolic and diastolic blood pressures. Hoskins (1981) noted that little attention is given to the fact that a person's greatest susceptibility to fear is early in the morning when corticosteroids are at their peak. Avoiding stress at this time may be extremely beneficial to the patient.

RESEARCH QUESTIONS

Research on timing and biologic rhythm research has much relevance to nursing practice. Determining ways that nurses can control forces that cause desynchronization or intervene to assist the person in returning to normal functioning will help persons in achieving health (Felton, 1987). Research on timing is relevant for nurses in many practice realms, but it has particular importance to critical care nurses for whom synchronization of rhythms in patients is a major concern. The following are a few of the areas in which nursing research is needed.

1. Does inclusion of cultural differences on the perspective of time in the planning of care affect patient outcomes?
2. Does assessment and diagnostic measurements at varying times lead to earlier detection of pathology?
3. What are ways in which nursing actions can help promote the synchronization of internal and external rhythms of the patient? Does this result in less confusion in patients?
4. Can the side effects of certain medications be decreased by changing the time the medication is administered?
5. What is the relationship between expanding consciousness and the overall health of elderly persons?

REFERENCES

Aaronson, B. (1972). Behavior and the place names of time. Pp. 405–436 in H. Yaker, H. Osmond, & F. Cheek eds., *The future of time*. Garden City, NY: Anchor Books.

Bull, D. (1973). Effects of aging on temporal experience. *Dissertation Abstracts International* 34:2921-A.

Cottle, T. (1976). *Perceiving time*. New York: John Wiley & Sons.

DeScalzi, M., DeLeonardis, V., Fabiano, F.S., & Cinelli, F. (1986). Circadian rhythms of arterial blood pressure. *Chronobiologia* 13:239-244.

Drew, B.J. (1989). Cardiac rhythm responses: 1. An important phenomenon for nursing practice, science, and research. *Heart & Lung* 18:8-15.

Feifel, H. (1957). Judgments of time in younger and older persons. *Journal of Gerontology* 12:71–74.

Felton, G. (1987). Human biologic rhythms. Pp. 45–77 in J. Fitzpatrick & R. Taunton eds., *Annual review of nursing research*, vol. 5. New York: Springer.

Ferrario, V., Bianchi, R., Giunta, G., & Roveda, L. (1982). Circadian rhythm in human intraocular pressure. *Chronobiologica* 9:33–37.

Fitzpatrick, J. (1980). Patients' perceptions of time: Current research. *International Nursing Review* 27:148–153, 160.

Foulks, J., & Webb, J. (1970). Temporal orientation of diagnostic groups. *Journal of Clinical Psychology* 26:155–159.

Grubb, C. (1980). Perceptions of time by multiparous women in relation to themselves and others during the first postpartal month. *Maternal-Child Nursing* 9:225–331.

Hall, E. (1984). *The dance of life.* Garden City, NJ: Anchor Books.

Hoagland, H. (1933). The physiological control of judgment duration: Evidence for a chemical clock. *Journal of General Psychology* 9:267–287.

Hoskins, C. (1981). Chronobiology and health. *Nursing Outlook* 29:572–576.

Knapp, R., & Garbutt, J. (1958). Time imagery and the achievement motive. *Journal of Personality* 26:426–434.

Kuhlen, R., & Monge, R. (1968). Correlates of estimated rate of time passage in adult years. *Journal of Gerontology* 23:427–433.

Langer, J., Wapner, S., & Werner, H. (1961). The effect of danger on time experience. *American Journal of Psychology* 74:94–97.

Lanning, R.M., Von Roemeling, R., & Hrushesky, W.J. (1990). Circadian-based infusional FUDR therapy. *Oncology Nursing Forum* 17:49–56.

Lemon, B., & Bengston, V. (1972). An exploration of the activity theory of aging: Activity types and life satisfaction among inmovers to a retirement community. *Journal of Gerontology* 27:511–523.

Luce, G. (1973). Biological rhythms. Pp. 421–444 in R. Ornstein ed., *The nature of human consciousness.* New York: Viking Press.

Melillo, K. (1982). Informal activity involvement and the perceived rate of time passage for an older institutionalized population. *Journal of Gerontological Nursing* 6:392–397.

Minors, D., & Waterhouse, J. (1981). *Circadian rhythms and the human.* Bristol: John Wright & Sons Ltd.

Moore, J. (1982). The influence of the time of administration on cis-platinum induced nausea and vomiting. *Oncology Nursing* 9(3):26–32.

Newman, M.A. (1982). Time as an index of expanding consciousness with age. *Nursing Research* 31:290–293.

———. (1986). *Health as expanding consciousness.* St. Louis: C.V. Mosby.

Nojima, Y., Oda, A., Nishii, H., Fukui, M., Seo, K., & Akiyoshi, H. (1987). Perception of time among Japanese inpatients. *Western Journal of Nursing Research* 9:288–300.

Piaget, J. (1969). *The child's perception of time.* New York: Ballantine Books.

Rogers, M. (1970). *An introduction to the theoretical basis of nursing.* Philadelphia: F.A. Davis.

Roos, P., & Albers, R. (1965). Performance of alcoholics and normals on a measure of temporal orientation. *Journal of Clinical Psychology* 21:34–36.

Scheving, L. (1979). Chronobiology and its relation to developing a knowledge base for regulatory decisions in health and prevention. *Chronobiologica* 6:45–52.

Schilder, E. (1981). On the structure of time with implications for nursing. *Nursing Papers* 13(3):17–23.

Tompkins, E. (1980). Effect of restricted mobility and dominance on perceived duration. *Nursing Research* 29:333–338.

Whitbourne, S.K., & Dannefer, W.D. (1986). The "life drawing" as a measure of time perspective in adulthood. *International Journal of Aging and Human Development* 22:147–155.

CHAPTER 27

STORY-TELLING

BACKGROUND

Only recently have articles on the use of story-telling as a nursing intervention begun to appear in the literature. The dearth of reports on use of story-telling does not mean that nurses have not used stories or metaphors in varying ways as an intervention. Rather, the absence of articles more likely reflects difficulties encountered in verifying the therapeutic effectiveness of the intervention. Larkin and Zahourek (1988) noted that qualitative reports documenting the multidimensional value of story-telling are beginning to accumulate.

Story-telling played an important role in primitive societies. The master story-teller held a high place of honor in tribal society. Some cultures, such as the Irish, continue to value and honor master story-tellers. The art of story-telling is again emerging, not only as a specific therapeutic intervention but also as an entertainment form. Garrison Keillor is an example of a story-teller who has entertained vast audiences. Almost everyone constructs and tells stories. These include relating to a neighbor the calamity that occurred when a cup of coffee was spilled or embellishing a happening. Because persons are familiar with story-telling, use of the intervention does not introduce something that is new or foreign to them.

The intervention story-telling can take several forms. One method is asking the patient to tell her or his own story related to a specific problem. Coles (1989), a psychiatrist, details the value of eliciting stories from patients. Bornstein (1988) noted that patients naturally tell their stories when nurses obtain health histories. A second method is reading a story to an individual or group, with the story serving as the stimulus for the person to explore a topic. Using the metaphor is another variation of story-telling that has been used in health care (Welch, 1984). Metaphors have been used extensively in psychotherapy to assist persons in resolving past conflicts.

Definition

Simply, story-telling is the oral narration of fact or fiction (Gustafson, 1988). Stories may be ones the patient is asked to construct or ones that have been constructed by others and related to the patient. Stories may be very short in length or extend over a considerable time frame.

Metaphors are extensively used in storytelling. A metaphor is

> a figure of speech in which a word or phrase literally denoting one kind of object or idea is used in place of another to suggest a likeness denoting an analogy between them. [*Webster's Ninth New Collegiate Dictionary,* Mish (ed.) 1989:746]

Kopp (1971) defined a metaphor as a way of speaking in which one thing or situation is expressed in terms of another. This bringing together of the two ideas casts light on the nature of what is being described. Metaphors, according to Gordon (1978), can be used to help persons change their ideas or behaviors.

Scientific Basis

Use of a story can serve three functions: change time and place for persons, stimulate strong emotions, and encourage communication (Gotterer, 1989). The story helps the person/group make the transition from the day-to-day routines to another world. Stories frequently initiate active imaging. The imagery may result in strong emotions being manifested; these may assist the person in resolving conflicts and moving forward. According to Barker (1985), for psychotherapeutic interventions to achieve quick changes, the right hemisphere of the brain must be involved. Metaphors or stories are one of the interventions that are classified as right brain.

Wallis (1985) noted that stories work because persons bring the story into the framework of their own experience. Attempts are made to make sense of the story in relation to their lives. Wallis stated

> And although the content of the story is a metaphor which evokes but does not literally reproduce the actual circumstances of client's lives, they can accept what the story seems to imply about their problems and consider new solutions within the framework of their own lives. [p. 5]

Because stories deal indirectly with persons' problems and have meanings that are often veiled, they may be less threatening to persons than dealing with the problems directly (Barker, 1985). The various meanings that are presented become part of the unconscious level where they are interpreted and used. Stories may provide ideas for the resolution of a problem.

Telling one's own story may assist persons in resolving problems. This is similar to life review which is discussed in Chapter 14.

INTERVENTION

The technique of using a constructed story will be presented. Persons interested in having persons construct their own stories will find the discussion of reminiscence and life review in Chapter 14 helpful.

Technique

Creating an atmosphere for story-telling is important, whether this be on an individual or group basis. Persons need to be comfortable. Using a simple, short relaxation technique will help set the mood for receptivity to the story. Bornstein (1988) suggests telling persons who appear to be anxious about hearing a story to just sit back, relax, and listen.

Selecting the story to use is critical to the success of the intervention. Therefore, the nurse wishing to use this story-telling technique must have knowledge about a wide variety of stories and literature. Gotterer (1989), in working with the elderly, selected short stories from a wide variety of sources. Native American stories, Hasidic tales, Chinese folklore, and stories by contemporary authors were used. Bornstein (1988) describes the value that fairy tales have in psychotherapy. She noted that fairy tales and stories are experienced as external to the person; thus persons are not likely to react defensively. Table 27.1 lists sources for stories that may be used in story-telling.

Stories may be used with an individual or with a group. Metaphors are most often used on an individual basis. This allows for more intimate exploration of personal meanings of the metaphor.

Gotterer (1989) used stories in a once-a-week, 90-minute session for 10 weeks with a group of elderly women. The sessions were structured with a beginning story that would stimulate discussion. A second story was used to conclude the session; this story was used to knit together the day's session and provide a closure. The length of time to use for each session and the number of sessions used will depend on the purpose for which story-telling is being used and the characteristics of the population. For persons with

Table 27.1
Sources for Stories to Use in Storytelling

Chase, R. (1943). *The jack tales.* Boston: Houghton Mifflin.

Clarkson, A., & Cross, G.B. (1980). *World folktales: A Scribner resource collection.* Chicago: Scribner.

Dorson, R.M. (ed.) (1975). *Folktales told around the world.* Chicago: University of Chicago Press.

Glassie, H. (ed.) (1985). *Irish folk tales.* New York: Pantheon Books.

Lankton, C.H., & Lankton, S.R. (1989). *Goal-oriented metaphors for adults and children in therapy.* New York: Brunner/Mazel.

Lobel, A. (1980). *Fables.* New York: Harper & Row.

Wallis, L. (1985). *Stories for the third ear.* New York: W.W. Norton & Co.

low energy levels, a much shorter time would be used. Other activities, such as writing poetry or doing artwork, can be included in story-telling sessions.

Reading a story to an individual or an audience requires that the reader make the story come alive. This requires background reading about the story to enable the reader to have knowledge about the author and the context in which the story was written. Pre-session reading of the story and timing the story are needed. Nonverbal communication is used to convey meaning or to emphasize a particular part of the story (Bornstein, 1988). Pauses and repeating phrases are other strategies for drawing attention to a specific passage. Although visual prompts may be used to add color to the story, use of too many prompts may hamper the audience in developing their own images.

An important component in the use of stories is providing time for the patient to digest the story and to respond to it. Many persons need time to think about the story before being ready to express themselves and the relation the story has to her/his life. The storyteller must be attentive to the nonverbal cues being displayed. Emphasizing that stories are very rich in meaning and that individuals have very different interpretations may assist persons in responding to the story.

Measurement of Effectiveness

Depending on the purpose for which story-telling is being used, various parameters can be used to measure the effectiveness of the intervention. Instruments that measure decreases in anxiety or depression could be used when improvement in mood is desired. Comparisons of before and after patterns of communication and social interaction would be appropriate for determining the effectiveness of story-telling in achieving improved social interaction. Subjective reports of improved functioning also would be appropriate in determining the effectiveness of story-telling.

USES

Story-telling has been used with a number of patient populations and to achieve a variety of goals. Bornstein noted that nurses could use stories in explaining procedures, in evoking hope for a successful outcome of a diagnostic procedure, in obtaining information about the patient, and in helping persons resolve conflicts.

Coles (1989) details the use of literature of all types in teaching medical students and working with patients. Story-telling is one of the teaching strategies included in the *Teacher's Desk Reference* (Gustafson, 1988). This author has found that novels and autobiographies assist nursing students to gain an appreciation of the impact that a chronic condition has on a person's life. These examples point to the use story-telling may serve in patient education and in helping persons adapt to life changes.

Stories and metaphors have been used extensively in psychotherapy. Milton Erickson, the father of modern hypnosis, employed metaphorical stories to assist persons in resolving their conflicts. Welch (1984) provides an excellent overview on the use of metaphors in psychotherapy.

Story-telling has been used in health teaching in transcultural nursing. Werner and Bower (1982) detail the use of stories in doing health teaching in Third World cultures. Stories assist persons in identifying local problems and discovering answers to these problems.

Precautions

Because stories may elicit very powerful responses, nurses must be prepared to deal with the feelings that may be evoked. In addition to having adequate knowledge about the patient, only nurses who have training in psychotherapy should utilize story-telling for patients with psychological problems. However, even when stories are used with patients to achieve other outcomes, nurses need to be aware that diverse reactions may be displayed and be ready to assist the patient.

RESEARCH QUESTIONS

Nurses have used stories and metaphors for many years, but they have not documented their effectiveness in achieving patient outcomes. A variety of techniques relating to story-telling has been used. Therefore, it is imperative that the technique being used be fully described so that comparisons can be made across studies and among the various techniques. The following are several of the many areas in which research on story-telling is needed:

1. What are the conditions/situations for which the various story-telling techniques would be most appropriate?
2. What methodologies would be most appropriate for studying the effectiveness of persons telling their own story?
3. What are stories/metaphors that practicing nurses have used?

REFERENCES

Barker, P. (1985). *Using metaphors in psychotherapy.* New York: Brunner/Mazel.

Bornstein, E.M. (1988). Therapeutic storytelling. Pp. 101–118 in R. Zahourek ed., *Relaxation and imagery: Tools for therapeutic communication and intervention.* Philadelphia: W.B. Saunders.

Chase, R. (1943). *The jack tales.* Boston: Houghton Mifflin.

Clarkson, A., & Cross, G.B. (1980). *World folktales: A Scribner resource collection.* Chicago: Scribner.

Coles, R. (1989). *The call of stories.* Boston: Houghton Mifflin.

Dorson, R.M. (1975). *Folktales told around the world.* Chicago: University of Chicago Press.

Glassie, H. (ed.) (1985). *Irish folk tales.* New York: Pantheon Books.

Gotterer, S.M. (1989). Storytelling: A valuable supplement to poetry writing with the elderly. *The arts in psychotherapy* 16:127–131.

Gustafson, M. (1988). *Teacher's desk reference,* vol. 2. Unpublished manuscript, University of Minnesota, School of Nursing, Minneapolis.

Lankton, C.H., & Lankton, S.R. (1989). *Goal-oriented metaphors for adults and children in therapy.* New York: Brunner/Mazel.

Larkin, D.M., & Zahourek, R.P. (1988). Therapeutic storytelling and metaphors. *Holistic Nursing Practice* 2(3):45-53.

Lobel, A. (1980). *Fables.* New York: Harper & Row.

Mish, F.C. (ed.) (1989). *Webster's ninth new collegiate dictionary.* Springfield, MA: Merriam-Webster Inc.

Wallis, L. (1985). *Stories for the third ear.* New York: W.W. Norton.

Welch, M.J. (1984). Using metaphor in psychotherapy. *Journal of Psychosocial Nursing* 22(11):13-18.

Werner, D., & Bower, B. (1982). *Helping health workers learn.* Palo Alto, CA: Hesperian Foundation.

CHAPTER 28

PRESENCE

Susan Diemert Moch, RN, PhD and Carol C. Schaefer, RN, BS

BACKGROUND

Presence is central to nursing, yet little development of the concept has been completed. Although often considered a given for the nurse–patient relationship in nursing theoretical formulations, explicit delineation of the concept is yet to be accomplished.

Convinced of the importance of presence for nursing practice, use of the concept in nursing continues despite the lack of an agreed-upon definition (Gadow, 1980; Paterson & Zderad, 1976; Watson, 1985). For the purpose of this discussion, presence is a process of being available with the whole of oneself and open to the experience of another through a reciprocal interpersonal encounter. This definition is a modified version of the definition proposed by Paterson and Zderad (1976).

Scientific Basis

Definitions

A scientific base for presence is limited, due in part to the difficulty in defining the concept and isolating the variable. Some definitions of presence, in addition to the definition of Paterson and Zderad (1976), have more recently been proposed. Gardner (1985) defined presence as "the nurse's physical 'being there' and the psychological 'being with' a patient for the purpose of meeting the patient's health care needs" (p. 317). Presence, according to Gardner is operationalized 1) through the cognitive domain by verbal communication; 2) in the affective domain through a generation of positive regard, trust, and genuineness; and 3) in the physical domain through being physically available.

Liehr (1989) identified true presence as "genuinely engaging with another" (p. 7). According to Liehr, the nurse uses extreme sensitivity to grasp the other's anger, joy, fear, or pain. For true presence to occur, the nurse must bring her or his own humaneness and acceptance of self to the encounter.

Despite limited empirical evidence, validity for the concept of presence can be known through examples from and discussion with nurses in practice. Nurses understand presence in their own personal way and often relate examples of being present to clients. Case studies (Benner & Wrubel, 1989; K. Cohen, 1987; L. Cohen, 1987; Liehr, 1989; Rawnsley, 1982; Swanson, 1990), essays about nursing (Chenitz, 1984), and poetry on the nursing experience (Krysl, 1989) depict presence in action.

Knowledge about presence may evolve through modes of knowing and research methods that are unrelated to the scientific or empirical way of knowing. Carper (1978) proposed four modes of knowing in nursing: empirics, esthetics, ethics, and personal knowing. The aesthetic and personal knowing modes may be most appropriate for the development of knowledge related to presence. The esthetic or the artistic mode is "the comprehension of meaning in a singular, particular, subjective expression" (Chinn & Jacobs, 1987:9). Esthetic knowing involves the artistic aspect of the nursing act through which meaning is perceived and acted upon in a creative, expressive manner. Knowledge development may also take the form of personal knowing which is discovery of self-and-other arrived at through reflection, synthesis of perceptions, and connecting with what is known (Moch, 1990a). Personal knowing emerges through interpersonal processes, life and clinical practice experiences, and through one's own intuition.

Knowledge in practice as proposed by Lather (1986) and expanded upon for nursing by Newman (1990) may also serve to enlarge the body of knowledge on presence. Through this method the researcher engages with the subject in a process of negotiation, reciprocity, and empowerment toward mutual insight of the phenomenon being studied. Knowledge in practice, or "research as praxis," on presence would involve data collection of the experience of the subject and the nurse and/or the researcher engaged in an experience of presence.

Definitions of Nursing

Definitions of nursing underscore the significance of presence for nursing. The interpersonal nature of nursing as portrayed in many definitions demonstrate(s) the essential nature of presence to the nursing experience. According to Travelbee (1966), nursing is an interpersonal process through which nurses often help patients find meaning. Describing nursing as "an experience lived between human beings" (p. 3) or a lived dialogue of authenticity in which presence is essential (Paterson & Zderad, 1976) confirms this interpersonal focus. Another description by Gadow (1980) identifies nursing as:

> the nurse's participation with the patient in determining the unique meaning which the experience of health, illness, suffering, or dying is to have for that individual. [p. 81]

Participation "with" involves presence.

Theoretical Foundations

Paterson and Zderad (1976) recognize presence as integral to their theory of humanistic nursing. Presence implies an openness, a receptivity, readiness, or availability on the part of the nurse. Many nursing situations require close proximity to another person, but that in itself does not guarantee presence. In order to experience the lived dialogue of nursing, the nurse responds with an openness to a "person-with-needs" and with an "availability-in-a-helping-way" (p. 28). A reciprocity and a mutuality often emerge through the dialogue as the nurse can also gain through the interpersonal encounter as was evident in a study of cross-cultural caring (Butrin, 1990).

According to Benner and Wrubel (1989), the nurse's ability to presence oneself, or "to be with a patient in a way that acknowledges your shared humanity" is basic to nursing practice (p. 13). Using case studies that describe situations in which expert nursing is practiced, presencing is depicted. In one situation a nurse says:

> I came, through caring for this woman for several weeks, to both admire and respect her quiet strength and dignity and to love her as a person. I wanted for her what she wanted for herself—a quiet and peaceful end with those she loved in attendance. [p. 90]

In the situation the nurse was able to be an advocate by having a "Do Not Resuscitate" order written, as through presence, she truly understood the wish of the patient. Another nurse described through example how presencing is not "walking out" when you come through the door to a patient's room (p. 15); presence is being there and not running away.

Vaillot (1966) describes the role of the nurse as helping the patient become an authentic person through the illness experience by being "presences" to patients. Ferlic (1968) says the nurse is a presence to the patient. This implies closeness, perception, awareness, and involvement.

Presence is an aspect of the caring theory of Watson (1985). The nurse is a co-participant in the caring process and caring is related in part to the nurse's self-knowledge and knowledge of one's power and transaction limitations. "A truly caring nurse/artist is able to destroy in the consciousness of the recipient the separation between him or herself and the nurse" (p. 68). The union or total presencing that happens through the experience leads to healing, discovery, and finding meaning.

Anderson (1979) encourages nurses to move beyond surface interpersonal encounters and to accept the presence responsibility.

> Every nursing situation carries within it the artistic potential for creating. If the nurse is fully and authentically present with her whole being, and open to her client as a presence, she becomes an artist who sees the forms of health and growth within the other person. [p. 48]

Through this process a change is brought about both within the nurse and the patient.

INTERVENTION

Preparation for Presence

Presence involves a conscious attention to readying the nurse to engage in the process. For the nurse to be available with the wholeness of oneself and to be open to the experience of another, the nurse must focus on self as the instrument. Thus the nurse consciously attends to the moment by centering self so that being available to the other is possible. This process may involve a period of quiet attention to self before a planned encounter. The nurse may simply take a deep breath and close his or her eyes in order to center self and detach from other distractions.

This centering process promotes the nurse's openness and readiness for caring which are essential to interpersonal presence. The attitude of openness and readiness may be the most important criteria for presence to occur. Possessing an attitude of compassion, sympathy, empathy, and risk also facilitates presence (Schaefer, 1990). A desire to help and to become involved in compassion, sympathy, and empathy pushes the nurse toward taking the necessary risk for being totally present to the other. Without a willingness to risk on the part of the nurse, presence cannot occur. The risk involves a choice on the part of a nurse as one nursing student said in reflecting on presence:

> We are always present, in some way, with other people. But are we *really* present with them? By really present, I mean are we there by chance or by choice? I think the only way to be present is to choose to allow the real you to be there for someone at a given time. [Kelcher, 1990]

The skills needed by the nurse in order to engage in presence are centering, listening, seeing (observing), and feeling (Schaefer, 1990). Listening is an active process of searching for meaning. Listening also requires the ability to be silent and to be truly open to the other person. Through silence, the feelings of acceptance and caring can be portrayed.

Excellent observation or seeing skills are essential to the presence experience. As nurses listen, they use their trained observation skills to look for subleties in expression and communication. Feeling skills are also used in this observation as the nurse listens to his or her own self to really hear or to really see what the patient is saying. Often the nurse feels what the patient is saying through his/her unspoken words.

Technique

The technique involves: openness, unknowing, attention, and connectedness. Openness has been proposed as essential to the process. If the nurse is open, he or she can be available with the wholeness of self. Openness can be likened to Travelbee's use of transcendence or "the ability to get beyond and outside of self in order to perceive and respond to the human being in the patient" (1966:47). It involves cutting through the facades of role, title, position, or status in relating to another.

Unknowing is approaching another with a question (Sarosi, 1986), a desire to know more coupled with the confidence that the other person will be the teacher; a position of knowing that there is much more for you to know about the situation. It opens one to vulnerability—as if the nurse is the learner juxtaposed with the patient–teacher in the encounter.

Presence demands the attention of the nurse. Attention is focusing completely on the other person, especially the sensations, emotions, cognitions, and spiritual elements in the other's experience and the sensations, emotions, cognitions, and spiritual elements of the nurse that arise through the interaction with the other person (Sarosi, 1986).

Through the experience of presence a connectedness with the patient emerges. Both the nurse and the patient experience a sense of union or joining for a moment in time. In describing one such connection experience a nursing student identified how she immediately connected with a patient. The patient was talking about how he wished he could have the opportunity to ask his deceased parents some questions. The student knew what he was talking about as her parents had also died. She said, "I was truly touched because I really understood" (Vorwald, 1990).

Measurement of Effectiveness

Effectiveness is difficult to measure in an objective manner as the experience of presence is felt more subjectively by both the nurse and the patient involved in the presence experience. Questions related to presence are difficult to formulate and questions related to abstract concepts such as presence are difficult to answer in words. Presence may be most appropriately measured in a nonverbal or artistic manner as discussed earlier.

Since presence is considered a reciprocal interaction, presence may appropriately be measured through descriptions of the experience by the nurse involved. Presence on the part of the nurse creates within the nurse: knowing of another, awe and respect for the other, and awareness of self (Moch, 1988). Measuring whether those three aspects occurred in a nurse–patient encounter may be one way to evaluate whether presence occurred.

Describing and attempting to measure the experience of the patient in the presence encounter is appropriate. This may be done by considering the degree of connectedness felt by the patient. Another measure may be the degree to which the patient felt the nurse was open to his or her experience. Identifying whether the nurse engages in behaviors which reflect centering, openness, unknowing, attention, and connectedness may be appropriate.

Chenitz (1984) eloquently describes the difficulty in measuring presence in the nursing interaction. She says:

> My kind of creativity vanishes as soon as the interaction is over. It doesn't get recorded on tape, disc or paper. It's fleeting, hard to define. Almost impossible to recreate. But in its finest form, no matter how brief, it is elegant and transcending. [p. 286]

In these elegant and transcending interactions, the creativity may not really vanish, but since difficulty exists in trying to capture what actually happens, it seems to vanish.

USES

Presence can be used in any nursing situation. Persons struggling with an illness are especially in need of moments of presence. The "being with" aspect of presence within a caring context has been identified as central to the nursing of persons who experienced a miscarriage (Swanson-Kaufman, 1986) and parents whose child has been hospitalized in a Newborn Intensive Care Unit (Swanson, 1990). A psychosocial intervention involving presence has also been identified as important to the nursing care of women diagnosed with breast cancer (Moch, 1990b). Presence is especially indicated with patients experiencing a high level of anxiety and with persons coping with a loss.

Precautions

The major precaution is the necessity for taking the cue from the patient and not forcing a presence encounter on an unwilling person. A true presence encounter does, however, consider the wants and the needs of the patient. If the nurse is "available with the whole of oneself and open to the experience" of the patient, as the definition states, the nurse will be following the experience of the patient and will thus act in accordance with his or her wishes.

RESEARCH QUESTIONS

Initially, research on presence will need to focus on concept development and operationalization of the concept for measurement purposes. Attentive listening to nurses reflecting on their practice may be the key to uncovering knowledge related to presence. Some possible research questions include:

1. What is an operational definition for presence?
2. How do we know when presence occurred?
3. What tools or techniques adequately measure presence?
4. What nurse behaviors are correlated with presence experiences?
5. Does the nurse's experience of presence determine that presence was achieved for the patient?
6. What is the experience of presence for the patient?

REFERENCES

Anderson, N.D. (1979). Human interaction for nurses. *Supervisor Nurse* 10:44–50.

Benner, P., & Wrubel, J. (1989). *The primacy of caring: Stress and coping in health and illness.* Menlo Park, CA: Addison-Wesley Publishing.

Butrin, J.E. (1990). *The experience of culturally diverse nurse–client encounters.* University of Minnesota: Unpublished doctoral dissertation.

Carper, B.A. (1978). Fundamental patterns of knowing in nursing. *Advances in Nursing Science* 1(1):13–23.

Chenitz, C.W. (1984). Someday, when I grow up... *American Journal of Nursing* 84:286.

Chinn, P.L., & Jacobs, M.K. (1987). *Theory and nursing: A systematic approach.* St. Louis: C.V. Mosby.

Cohen, K.J. (1987). At the carousel. *American Journal of Nursing* 87:998.

Cohen, L.J. (1987). A modern parable. *American Journal of Nursing* 87:1043.

Ferlic, A. (1968). Existential approach in nursing. *Nursing Outlook* 16:30–33.

Gadow, S. (1980). Existential advocacy: Philosophical foundation of nursing. Pp. 79–101 in S. Spiker & S. Gadow eds., *Nursing images and ideals.* New York: Springer.

Gardner, D.L. (1985). Presence. Pp. 316–324 in G.M. Bulechek, J.C. McCloskey, & M. Adelotte, eds., *Nursing interventions: Treatment for nursing diagnosis.* Philadelphia: W.B. Saunders Co.

Kelcher, T. (1990). Course journal. Unpublished document.

Krysl, M. (1989). *Midwife and other poems on caring.* New York: National League of Nursing.

Lather, P. (1986). Research as praxis. *Harvard Educational Review* 56(3):257–277.

Liehr, P.R. (1989). The core of true presence: A loving center. *Nursing Science Quarterly* 2:7–8.

Moch, S.D. (1988). Health in illness: Experiences with breast cancer. Doctoral dissertation, University of Minnesota, Minneapolis, MN.

____. (1990a). Personal knowing: Evolving research and practice. *Scholarly Inquiry for Nursing Practice: An International Journal* 4:155–165.

____. (1990b). Health within the experience of breast cancer. *Journal of Advanced Nursing* 15:119–123.

Newman, M.A. (1990). Newman's theory of health as praxis. *Nursing Science Quarterly* 3(1):37–41.

Paterson, J.G., & Zderad, L.T. (1976). *Humanistic nursing.* New York: John Wiley.

Rawnsley, M.M. (1982). Brief psychotherapy for persons with recurrent cancer: A holistic practice model. *Advances in Nursing Science* 5:69–76.

Sarosi, G.M. (1986). An experiment in understanding: The nurse is the laboratory. Unpublished paper, University of Minnesota, Minneapolis, MN.

Schaefer, C.C. (1990). Concept clarification of presence. Unpublished paper, University of Wisconsin-Eau Claire, Eau Claire, WI.

Swanson, K.M. (1990). Providing care in the NICU: Sometimes an act of love. *Advances in Nursing Science* 13(1):60–73.

Swanson-Kauffman, K.M. (1986). Caring in the instance of unexpected early pregnancy loss. *Topics in Clinical Nursing* 8(2):37–46.

Travelbee, J. (1966). *Interpersonal aspects of nursing.* Philadelphia: F.A. Davis.

Vaillot, M.C. (1966). Existentialism: A philosophy of commitment. *American Journal of Nursing* 66:500–502.

Vorwald, J. (1990). Class journal, unpublished document.

Watson, J. (1985). *Nursing: Human science and human care, a theory of nursing.* Norwalk, Connecticut: Appleton-Century-Crofts.

The first author gratefully acknowledges the "Presence Group" of fellow doctoral students at the University of Minnesota, School of Nursing for contributing greatly to the ideas presented. Members were Melissa Avery, JoAnn Butrin, Ann Kelly, Marilyn Loen, and Margot Nelson.

CHAPTER 29

GROUPS

BACKGROUND

Nursing literature is replete with the use of groups for a variety of purposes. Groups were used as an intervention strategy as early as 1907. Dr. Pratt (cited in Phipps, 1982a) established groups in tuberculosis sanitariums; he believed that educational aims could be better accomplished through a group milieu. Positive and encouraging results were obtained. Groups became an integral part of psychiatric settings during the 1940s when shortages of personnel necessitated new approaches for treating the large number of soldiers requiring mental health care. In the 1960s encounter groups became popular. Recently, consumer consciousness has resulted in the establishment of a large number of self-help support groups; the largest number of these are for persons with chronic conditions or persons dealing with crisis situations. Thus, many persons have experienced the therapeutic effects resulting from involvement in a group.

Use of groups as a nursing intervention is congruent with nursing's concern for individuals, families, groups, and communities. In many instances groups are established to help persons become more independent, either by learning new behaviors or acquiring knowledge in order to adapt to a condition. Fostering independence is a goal of many of the conceptual frameworks in nursing. Groups also are used for health promotion and prevention of illness, again in agreement with goals of nursing. According to Phipps (1982a), nurses have frequently viewed health care in the context of society. Groups, as an intervention, are congruent with this focus as they are a microcosm of society.

A mammoth amount of literature on groups, group process, types of groups, and uses of groups exists. This chapter will present an overview on groups, with the focus specifically on their use in providing support for persons and for persons learning new behaviors. Texts and articles that contain a more in-depth presentation on groups and their use for other purposes can be found in the reference list.

Definition

Phipps (1982a) defined a group as:

> An interdependent association of two or more persons united by a common interest, whose actions are interrelated so that each person influences and is influenced by other persons.
> [p. 3]

A group is more than an aggregate or collection of persons. The focus is on the total group and not on the individual. Participants gain a sense of shared awareness, of belonging together, and of how the behavior of one member affects all members of the group. Interdependence results from a common purpose, a shared attribute, or a pattern of interaction that is mutually established (Sampson & Marthas, 1981). Some structure is necessary to facilitate and maintain this interdependence. The type and degree of structure is dictated by the purposes of the group.

Loomis (1979) classified groups according to their use: support, task accomplishment, socialization, learning or changing behavior, human relations training, and psychotherapy. Support groups are helpful in assisting persons to monitor and/or maintain their health status. In task accomplishment groups, the group provides a vehicle for maximizing the problem-solving skills of the members in accomplishing complex tasks. Health professionals have used groups for socialization of patients; groups have helped persons adapt to and comply with the demands imposed by their health condition. Human relations training promotes interpersonal competence that can be transferred to the person's daily living environment. Psychotherapy groups assist persons in gaining insight into their own behavior and learning ways to change behaviors. Loomis's classifications are not mutually exclusive; for example, a person may derive support and learn new behaviors while participating in a group. However, a group usually has only one main focus.

Other systems for classifying groups exist. Groups may be categorized by the number of participants such as dyads, triads, etc. The theoretical basis underlying the use of the group is another method for classifying groups; gestalt, systems, interaction, and psychoanalytical are examples of theories used as the basis for conducting groups.

Scientific Basis

Humans are social beings. The collective effort of the group, whether it be supplying support, assisting in identifying factors that help persons in gaining insight, or providing a vehicle for interaction, relates to a human being's social orientation. Yalom (1985) identified 11 curative factors that are possible outcomes of groups. Some of these also are outcomes from the use of groups for other purposes: instillation of hope, universality, imparting information, altruism, development of socialization techniques, imitative behavior, learning interpersonal skills, group cohesiveness, and catharsis.

Sampson and Marthas (1981) used Lewin's systems theory as the theoretical basis for the use of group process for changing behaviors and/or maintaining changes. An individual's attitudes and behaviors do not exist in isolation but are greatly influenced by significant others — family, friends, teachers, etc. Cultural and group norms have an impact on a person's behaviors. Rewards, acceptance, or rejection have a profound influence on attitudes and behaviors. If a person deviates greatly from these norms, he or she can expect sanctions, hostility, or expulsion. The behaviors are frozen within these supportive group settings; if behaviors are to be changed, an unfreezing needs to occur. Sampson and Marthas (1981) stated that the individual's dependence on the normative group in which the old behavior is frozen must be lessened or that group's standards changed. After a new behavior has been acquired, a group context that will help support the behavior is needed. Refreezing can then occur.

Groups assist persons with chronic health problems to cope with their condition and make needed adaptations in their lives. Persons with chronic illnesses frequently feel inferior and view themselves as helpless victims of a disease process that is out of their control (Cole et al., 1979). Cobb (1976) stated that social support can protect persons in crisis situations from experiencing pathological states. Numerous studies have validated the effectiveness of groups in improving adherence to prescribed regimens. Peer pressure and insights gained from other group members assist persons in continuing difficult regimens.

INTERVENTION

Groups established for the purpose of support and behavioral change will be discussed. Establishing, running, and terminating a group requires specific knowledge and skills. Organizing the group; determining the criteria for membership, the number of sessions to be held, the group process to use, and the role of the leader; and terminating the group will be addressed. Groups have been used in many settings and with persons with diverse problems.

Technique

It is difficult to describe a particular technique for the intervention, group. Important factors will be provided that will enable practitioners to choose the strategies that are the most practical and usable in their specific situations.

Formation of the Group

Loomis (1979) listed five questions that the nurse should ask when considering the use of a group. These are:

1. What are the client's needs I am attempting to meet?
2. Can these be met in a group?
3. What are the nurse's own objectives for the proposed group?
4. What are the expectations of the system?
5. Is there a discrepancy or conflict to questions 1–4? [pp. 18–20]

Heiney and Wells (1989) included a list of planning questions for nurses who are considering the use of groups. Questions focus on the structure of the group (frequency of meeting and type of group), functions of group (goals, rules), and responsibilities of the leader(s). Table 29.1 provides an outline developed by Heiney and Wells that can guide nurses in organizing a group.

Table 29.1
Planning Questions for Group Leaders

Group Structure

What will be the schedule for meetings?
   Weekly/monthly
   Day/hour
What type of group will be established?
   Open versus closed
   Inpatient versus outpatient or combination
   Structured versus unstructured

Group Functioning

What are the goals of the group?
What are the ground rules of the group?
What is the maximum number that can be handled?
Who will start the group?
How will the group be processed?
How will negative group processes be handled?

Leader Responsibilities

What kind of records will be maintained?
When and how will periodic evaluations be done?
How many leaders are needed?
What kind of schedule or rotation is needed to prevent burnout?
What is the backup plan for absent leaders?
How will potential publications be handled?

From S. Heiney & L. Wells (1989). Strategies for organizing and maintaining successful support groups. *Oncology Nursing Forum* 16:804. Used with permission.

A contract is useful for elaborating the goals of the group, the individual's responsibilities, and the leader's responsibilities (Loomis, 1979; Marvin, 1982). (See Chapter 17 for details on contracting.) A contract helps eliminate misunderstandings persons may later have about the purpose of the group. Loomis (1979) stated that a preparatory session in which the contract is explained and discussed contributes to the success of a group. Heiney and Wells (1989) suggested the development of a mission statement for the group; this is shared with all participants.

Although studies have shown groups to be an effective intervention in many situations, a careful initial assessment will help in determining if a group would or would not contribute to the achievement of patient outcomes in a specific situation.

Using a group to accomplish the intended outcome should not be viewed as second class (Marvin, 1982). Although Loomis (1979) listed economics as one of the advantages for using a group, this is not the primary reason for selecting this intervention. It is necessary to convey to the prospective members that a group is deemed the most satisfactory way to achieve the desired outcome.

Membership

A group is defined as two or more persons interacting. The minimum and maximum number of members for a successful group has been debated (Sampson & Marthas, 1981). According to Loomis (1979), groups should not be smaller than five or six nor exceed ten or twelve. The type of persons who will be participating in the group dictates the number of members in a group. Burnside (1976) recommended groups of only six–eight members when participants are elderly persons with cognitive deficits.

If the group size is too small, interaction and gain from others is lessened. Absences or dropouts interfere with the functioning of extremely small groups. One member may feel very excluded if several of the other members band together.

When the group becomes too large, subgroups tend to form which mitigates against the cohesiveness of the total group. Therapeutic exchange also is lessened in large groups as there is less time for each member to speak. The more timid member is often ignored. It is difficult for the leader to keep track of all members when the membership exceeds seven (Sampson & Marthas, 1981). Hare (1952) reported decreased member satisfaction in large groups. However, large groups usually provide for much diversity and the pooling of many resources. If it appears that the number of participants will be too many for one group, division into two groups should be done before the first session. Waiting until after the first session creates confusion for the members and may result in persons dropping out.

Homogeneity of membership is another factor to be considered in the selection of members. No conclusive evidence exists on the particular mix a group should have to be successful (Loomis, 1979). The goals established for the group guide the development of criteria for participants. Kriegsman and Celotta (1981) reported significant success in a group that included women with a wide range of disabilities in addition to diversity in age, marital status, economic background, and stage of development. They felt that the common threads of womanhood and of having a disability bound the group together. Similarly, Hartings et al. (1976) opened the group to any person with multiple sclerosis irrespective of the extent of the pathology or the person's acceptance of this condition. It appears that success is attained even when group membership is rather heterogeneous.

Another issue to consider is whether or not attendance at sessions is mandatory for members. Mandatory attendance insures that sufficient members will be present for interaction and support. Cohesiveness of the group also is enhanced by mandatory attendance. This prevents the individual from being a "fair weather friend" and attending only when he or she feels the need of the group, but with little concern about the needs of other members of the group.

Thought needs to be given to whether membership will be open or closed. Some types of groups allow new members to join at any point. The meetings of Alcoholics Anonymous are structured to facilitate new members joining at any time. Many of the support groups established for families of patients in intensive care units also allow new members to join at any time. The membership is in a constant flux with some members leaving and others joining at each session. Groups that have definite objectives to be accomplished in a predetermined time would find it difficult to function as an open group.

Determining and publicizing membership policies will help to avoid problems and questions that may arise as the group progresses. In some instances the group itself may have a major input into these policies. Cronenwett (1980) was surprised that women in a postpartum support group did not elect to have their husbands attend the group meetings. Reasons members gave included feeling that men would dominate the group and being more comfortable expressing concerns with only women present.

Sessions

The number of sessions needed varies according to the purpose for which the group was established. Many psychotherapy groups extend over months and even years. In the rehabilitation group Segev and Schlesinger (1981) established for patients who had experienced myocardial infarctions, patients stayed in the group as long as they desired. They found that after the first year patients began to gradually drop out with about 50% continuing to attend the group sessions held in the third year. By the fourth year the majority of the patients no longer attended the group meetings.

It is more common, however, to schedule 6–12 sessions. Marley (1980) held six sessions to assist elderly to become more comfortable with the demands of aging. In the Creative Coping Group for women with physical disabilities, Kriegsman and Celotta (1981) offered eight sessions. Group consensus was, however, that the group had only begun to work on valuable points when the sessions ended.

Several authors (Baker & McCoy, 1979; Rancour & Moser, 1980) reported using only four sessions. Rancour and Moser focused on helping persons cope with chronic illnesses. Even though four group meetings were scheduled, the authors noted that group members continued to meet on an informal basis after the formal sessions had ended. Baker and McCoy stated that patients generated topics for subsequent sessions and felt that additional sessions for sharing emotions would have been helpful.

Although single-session groups are used infrequently, Lonergan (1982) believed that they do have value, particularly for enhancing self-esteem. One positive group experience can bring temporary healing to a person suffering from depression or guilt. Halm (1990) frequently found that family members of patients in critical care units attended only one group session. Single sessions have been used successfully for preoperative teaching and for other teaching purposes.

A variance was also found for the length of each session. One hour to two hour sessions were common. Because it takes time for the group to feel as one, sessions shorter than one hour may fail to accomplish established goals. If persons have to travel to attend the meetings, they may feel that short sessions are not worth their effort. One and a half-hour sessions were used by Rancour and Moser (1981) and Kriegsman and Celotta (1981). Inattentiveness and restlessness are likely if the session exceeds two hours. It is important that the participants know the length of each session with the expectation that they will remain until the end of the session. Beginning and ending on time is critical.

Process

Jasonik (1982) divided the group process into three phases: initial or inclusion phase, the middle or work phase, and the final or termination phase. Members get acquainted with each other and the leader in the initial stage and make a decision on whether or not to continue in the group. Power ploys are prominent in this phase. The majority of the group work is accomplished in the middle phase. Tasks that focus on attaining the group's goals and maintaining the group are performed. The termination phase is as difficult, in many instances, as the initial phase because of the interdependence that has developed.

Cohesiveness is a critical factor in the effectiveness of a group. Festinger (1968) defined cohesiveness as the result of all forces acting on members to keep them in the group. It's the glue that holds the group together. A number of factors affect the degree of cohesiveness in a group: goals of the group, established norms, and the role of the leader (Loomis, 1979). Realistic goals that are clearly delineated help to unite the group. Group rules, made known in the first session, provide members with expectations regarding behaviors expected and the sanctions that will be imposed if these are violated. Unspoken norms may evolve, particularly in long-term groups. The leader has an important role in making the goals and the rules known to the members and in seeing that they are adhered to.

Group work includes dealing with both external tasks that encompass group goals and internal tasks that are concerned with maintenance of the group. Tasks related to group goals are more obvious; keeping content focused on the group outcomes is an example of an external task. Members may be asked to come to group meetings with a list of questions and concerns in an attempt to help the group complete its stated work. It is easier to identify external tasks for some types of groups, such as support groups, than for other types of groups such as self-help groups.

Maintenance tasks are more elusive. Loomis (1979) stated that every group is unique and develops a process specific to it. Although the main burden for group maintenance lies with the leader, group members also have to assume responsibility for maintaining the group. Creating a climate in which there is respect for each member's contribution is essential. If a member is absent, the structure of the group changes and maintenance of the group may be threatened. Members assume a specific role in the group, and this role defines and regulates the person's behavior. Behavioral expectations regarding the role of participant evolve (Phipps, 1982b). Role conflicts interfere with group maintenance, and strategies are necessary for avoiding and resolving conflicts.

Leader

The leader's behavior and skills have a profound effect on the group process. According to Janosik (1982), the leader creates and maintains the group as a whole while attending to the individual member's needs. Functions include establishing norms that facilitate interpersonal relatedness, participation, careful self-disclosure, nonjudgmental acceptance; rules concerning feedback; and receptivity to change. Greater emphasis is placed on specific functions at various times in the group development. Creating an accepting climate is of utmost importance in the formative stages of the group, whereas attention to change is needed later in the group process.

Loomis (1979) delineated four functions for the group leader: emotional stimulation, caring, meaning-attribution, and executive. To fulfill the emotional stimulation function the leader shares feelings and encourages members to do likewise. Creating an accepting and supportive climate are integral elements of the caring function. In the meaning-attribution function the leader assists members in understanding their feelings. Organizational tasks and establishing boundaries are included in the executive functions of the leader. According to Loomis (1979), the effective leader is one who gives moderate attention to the emotional stimulation and executive functions and greatest focus to the caring and meaning-attribution functions. However, specific types of groups or the composition of a group dictate the amount of attention a leader devotes to each function.

In some instances the use of co-leaders is advantageous. Having co-leaders allows one person to lead the group while the other leader records the content and interaction of the group. Another format is for a senior leader to work with a junior person who is learning group process techniques. The more common form is for the co-leaders to assume equal responsibility for the group. Co-leadership provides for continuity if one person is ill or unable to be present. However, some persons find this type of leadership very trying and a special effort is needed to avoid rivalry between the co-leaders. Members may become attached to one leader rather than another and try to place the co-leaders in conflict with each other. Considerable planning is needed if co-leadership is to be used.

Measurement of effectiveness will be discussed in each of the subsections of the uses section.

USES

Nurses have used groups to accomplish a wide variety of goals with diverse patient populations. Measuring the effectiveness of groups has been difficult because of the many factors involved and the interaction of

Table 29.2
Uses of Groups

Support and Self-Help

Chronic illnesses (Rancour & Moser, 1980)
Caregivers (Dellosega, 1990)
Elderly (Haber, 1983)
Families of brain-injured patients (Mauss-Clum & Ryan, 1981)
Families of open heart surgery patients (Wilson, 1982)
Oncology patients (Maisiak et al., 1981; Rice & Szopa, 1988)
Ostomy patients (Gussow & Tracy, 1976; Trainor, 1982)
Physical disabilities (Dixon, 1981; Kriegsman & Celotta, 1981)
Postpartum mothers (Cronenwett, 1980)
Stroke (Adsit & Lee, 1986; Pierce & Salter, 1988)
Substance abuse (Janosik, 1982)

Socialization

Elderly (Matteson & Munsat, 1982)
Oncology patients (Maisiak et al., 1981)
Psychiatric patients (Yalom, 1985)

Task Accomplishment

Elderly (Janosik & Miller, 1982; Loomis, 1979)

Learning–Changing Behaviors

Coronary heart disease (Baker & McCoy, 1979)
Holistic health practices (Kutlenios, 1987)
Hypertension (Nath & Rinehart, 1979)
Lupus erythematosus (Kroll, 1987)
Learn about medications (Neizo & Murphy, 1983)
Multiple sclerosis (Hartings et al., 1976)
Myocardial infarct (Segev & Schlesinger, 1981)
Parkinson's disease (Mitchell et al., 1987)

Human Relations Training

Assertiveness training
Sexuality

Psychotherapy

---

these factors. In some instances groups have been instituted as the most economical way to perform another intervention, such as reality orientation, rather than for the particular advantages afforded by using a group. Table 29.2 presents specific populations/conditions for which groups have been used; these are grouped according to the categories proposed by Loomis (1979). As noted, the categories are not mutually exclusive. Only the first four categories are addressed.

Support Groups

Within recent years the number of support groups has increased dramatically, especially for persons with chronic illnesses and disabilities. In 1942 only four self-help groups, exclusive of Alcoholics Anonymous, existed. Over 2000 self-help groups were identified by Gussow and Tracy (1976). They stated:

Continued interaction with others provides a reservoir of special information and coping techniques. Aside from instructing new members in specialized skills related to their condition, relations between members frequently provide an avenue for the expression of strong sentiments that if continually dumped on family and relatives would be disruptive of normal relations. [p. 411]

Although support groups serve a social function, their importance extends beyond opportunities for social interaction. These services often focus on health and wellness-promoting behaviors. According to Corbin (1983), self-help support groups help persons adopt a wellness role rather than a sick role.

Members frequently monitor the behavior of group members and seek to provide assistance for needed changes. Alcoholics Anonymous is an excellent example of the type of caring and aid given to a fellow member by other members of the group. Support in coping and adjusting to the condition are quite readily accepted because the individual believes that, "They know what it is all about." Some contend that the health professional should only initiate this type of group and then withdraw to the status of resource person. The health professional's presence may lead to members becoming dependent on the professional rather than on each other.

One area in which support groups have been widely used in nursing is with families of patients in intensive care units. Wilson (1982) initiated a support group for families of patients who had had open heart surgery. The primary purpose for the groups was to lessen the level of stress of family members through discussing their fears and learning ways to cope with this period of uncertainty. The originator also hoped that reducing the anxiety of the family members would also decrease the anxiety of the patient. Wilson noted three elements for the leader to address: dealing with feelings, controlling the group so all have a chance to express themselves, and being a good listener. Halm (1990) used a support group for relatives of patients who had suffered a myocardial infarct. Participants manifested a significant decrease in anxiety following group interactions. The long-term effects resulting from group participation were not examined.

Mauss-Clum and Ryan (1981) established a support group for families of patients in a rehabilitation center who had suffered brain trauma. The uncertainty of the outcome and the altered behavior of the head-injured person create much anxiety for family members. Attendance at group meetings was an expectation but not a requirement. Topics discussed varied with each meeting but frequently included effects and treatment of the brain injury, finances, family reactions, and coping strategies. In a follow-up questionnaire to participants, 59% indicated that participating in a group when the patient was in the intensive care unit would have been helpful.

Support groups have been used extensively for persons with chronic conditions. TOUCH (Today Our Understanding of Cancer is Hope) is a self-help group established for persons with cancer (Maisiak et al., 1981). Members held monthly meetings to discuss both psychological and physiological adjustment problems. After initiating the group, the professional staff served largely as a resource to the group. A support group was used by Rancour and Moser (1980) in helping persons to cope with chronic disease. They stated:

The group can provide the social context for giving hope to newly diagnosed clients coming into contact with "veterans," and provide the veterans with an opportunity to feel needed by sharing their skills with the "rookies." [p. 117]

Kriegsman and Celotta (1981) organized a support group for women with physical disabilites regardless of the cause. Eight sessions were scheduled; the initial sessions focused on the building of relationships with problem-solving occupying later sessions. An evaluation of the outcomes of the intervention was performed using the Coping-Ability scale developed by the investigators. Findings showed that the women felt more comfortable discussing their disability, were more accepting of the disability, had an improved self-image, reported a greater acceptance of others, and had less fear of rejection by others.

Reports from support groups related the importance of members assuming a leadership role in the group. Trainor (1982) found that persons enrolled in the United Ostomy Association who served as visitors demonstrated a greater level of acceptance of their ostomy than those who did not serve in this capacity. Similar findings were reported by Maisiak et al. (1981) from their evaluation of an oncology support group. A larger percentage of the counselors reported improvements in dealing with their cancer and in adjustment to life than those members who had not become counselors.

These studies point out the need for formal evaluation of the effects of the group. Because many support groups have rather broad goals, precise measurement is often difficult. Outcomes of groups include sharing of hopes and despairs, improving self-esteem, increasing motivation to continue with rehabilitation, becoming more independent, changing life style, increasing socialization, and lowering levels of stigmatization (Kriegsman & Celotta, 1981).

Socialization

Socialization is frequently one of the goals of a support group, but it is not necessarily the main outcome desired. Conditions in which groups may be established with the primary intent being increased or improved interaction include persons who have suffered a loss, depressed individuals, persons who are isolated and lonely, and individuals who recently have been discharged from mental institutions (Loomis, 1979). The group provides a safe and certain place to meet other persons without the fear of rejection. Maisiak et al. (1981) stated that TOUCH was probably more socially oriented than many support groups in that it sponsored biannual parties and other special gatherings for its members. Numerous groups for the aged have socialization as a primary goal. The increased interaction has a profound effect on the psychological and physical well-being of group members.

Task Accomplishment

Groups established to accomplish a particular task are commonly used with elderly persons and with persons in long-term care facilities. In addition to the performance of the task, other outcomes, such as increased social interaction, may occur. A group in a nursing home or daycare center may be charged with organizing and supervising a party for a holiday. The group disbands after the event, but ties with the other members are often lasting. Loomis (1979) stated that a group maximizes the problem-solving skills of the members and thus more complex tasks can be attacked. Social action projects also may be the focus of a group.

Learning or Changing Behaviors

Development and modification of health-related behaviors and acquisition of knowledge and skills are areas in which nurses focus considerable time and attention. Groups have been used effectively in helping persons acquire needed knowledge and skills (Kutlenios, 1987). Group pressure has been shown to have a positive effect on individuals adhering to a diet or continuing not to smoke. Some persons find it easier to learn in a group. Teaching preoperative patients about their surgery and what is expected has been done in a group setting.

Neizo and Murphy (1983) used a group format to teach patients in an adult psychiatric unit about their medications. They believed that this would lead to greater adherence with the prescribed medications by providing an opportunity for the patients to verbalize their fears and hopes related to the medications. Four sessions were held. Evaluation of the outcomes of the groups was done through an 18-item scale that addressed didactic, affective, and socialization aspects. Findings showed that 60% had increased information about their medication, 65% responded that they were more positive about their medications, and 74% stated that the sessions enhanced their social skills.

Mitchell and colleagues (1987) used a group format to help persons with Parkinson's disease become involved in an exercise regimen. Positive results were obtained, with improvements noted in objective mobility and overall subjective functioning. The generalizability of the study findings are limited because only seven subjects were included in the study.

Adsit and Lee (1986) used art within a group context to facilitate communication in persons who had suffered strokes. Use of a media other than verbal communication was needed as many patients who have had strokes are dysphasic. Participants found that using the art media in a group provided an opportunity for communicating and resolving problems.

Other studies have compared the differences in learning that occurred in groups as opposed to gains in learning from individual sessions. Nath and Rinehart (1979) compared the effects on blood pressure in persons with hypertension who had been taught progressive relaxation individually and in a group. No difference in the decreases in blood pressure were noted between the two methods. Few research studies have explored the characteristics of persons who learn best in groups.

Precautions

Although groups have been widely used, the intervention, group, should not be used with everyone (Dixon, 1981). Loomis (1979) and Adrian (1980) stressed the importance of doing an adequate assessment of the person before recommending that the person become a member of a group. Some persons need extensive one-to-one interaction before they can benefit from group interaction. Not only initial assessment, but ongoing assessment is also necessary to determine if the person is benefiting from participation in the group.

The termination period of the group process can be a traumatic time for some persons. Cole et al. (1979) stated that a successful group is one in which the member leaves after a limited and defined time period. Some persons need to have these limits enforced. They suggested having the person join an "alumni club" that meets less frequently. Of course, the purpose of the group may be for it to be ongoing, in which case termination is not a concern.

Loomis (1979) identified a number of disadvantages of groups. A group may be too large for the purpose of the group, and the members may become dissatisfied because they are unable to meet their goals for joining the group. Leading a group requires specific knowledge and skills. Too often groups are begun without the leader(s) having the requisite basic skills, particularly in knowing how to resolve problems that may arise. Planning the environment and the number, length, and content of sessions is critical to the success of the group (Heiney & Wells, 1989). Preplanning takes time, but is rewarded in the end by the success of the group.

RESEARCH QUESTIONS

Little definitive data exist on the use of groups even though the intervention has been widely used in nursing. Most of the available research on groups is found in the social sciences. Clinical research is needed to examine, specify, and expand the use of groups in nursing. Often other interventions, such as imagery, music, or dance, are used within the context of a group; the interactive effects frequently have not been examined. The questions that follow suggest wide areas in which further research is required:

1. What are the characteristics of persons who will benefit most from participation in a group? Dixon (1981) stated that a comparison of assessment variables for assignment to groups should be compared with random assignment to determine if a clinical assessment protocol is effective in determining the effectiveness of the group for an individual.
2. What are the effects that membership in a group has on a person over time? Few longitudinal studies have been done; Segev and Schlesinger (1981) examined the effects that a group over a period of years had on persons who had suffered a myocardial infarction.

3. What is the number of sessions needed to produce optimum results? Some articles on the use of groups suggested that the number they had used was not sufficient.
4. The effects that the personal qualities of the leader have on the group process and the group outcomes have not been established. What are the characteristics of a successful group leader? How can nurses best learn the techniques necessary for being a good group leader?
5. What guidance and involvement on the part of the nurse is best for self-help groups? Movement toward independence is often sought, but when and to what extent the nurse should bow out of the group remain.
6. What mix of persons is best for a group? Kriegsman and Celotta (1981) found that persons with physical disabilities from various etiologies functioned effectively in a group. Is this true for other conditions, and is there an age mix which is optimum?
7. Groups are used extensively with the elderly. However, other interventions are frequently used in conjunction with groups. Studies are needed that examine the effects of these interventions both within the context of the group and alone.

REFERENCES

Adrian, S. (1980). A systematic approach to selecting group participants. *Journal of Psychiatric Nursing and Mental Health Services* 18(2):37–41.

Adsit, P.A., & Lee, J. (1986). The use of art in stroke group therapy. *Rehabilitation Nursing* 11(5):18–19.

Baker, K., & McCoy, P. (1979). Group sessions as a method of reducing anxiety in patients with coronary artery disease. *Heart and Lung* 8:525–529.

Burnside, I. (1976). Formation of a group. Pp. 197–204 in I. Burnside ed., *Nursing and the aged.* New York: McGraw Hill.

Cobb, S. (1976). Social support as a moderator of life stress. *Psychosomatic Medicine* 38:300–314.

Cole, S., O'Connor, S., & Bennett, L. (1979). Self-help groups for clinic patients with chronic illness. *Primary Care* 6:325–340.

Corbin, D. (1983). Self-help groups: What the health educator should know. *Health Values: Achieving High Level Wellness* 7(3):10–14.

Cronewett, L. (1980). Elements and outcomes of a postpartum support group program. *Research in Nursing and Health* 3:33–41.

Dellosega, C. (1990). Coping with caregiving: Stress management for caregivers of the elderly. *Journal of Psychosocial Nursing* 28(1):15–22.

Dixon, J. (1981). Group-self identification and physical handicap: Implications for patient support groups. *Research in Nursing and Health* 4:299–308.

Festinger, L. (1968). Informal social communication. Pp. 182–191 in D. Cartwright & A. Zander eds., *Group dynamics.* New York: Harper & Row.

Gussow, Z., & Tracy, G. (1976). The role of self-help clubs in adaptation to chronic illness and disability. *Social Science and Medicine* 10:407–414.

Haber, D. (1983). Promoting mutual help groups among older persons. *The Gerontologist* 23:251–253.

Halm, M.A. (1990). Effects of support groups on anxiety of family members during critical illness. *Heart & Lung* 19:62–71.

Hare, A. (1952). Interaction and consensus in different-sized groups. *American Sociological Review* 17:261–267.

Hartings, M., Pavlou, M., & Davis, F. (1976). Group counseling of MS patients. *Journal of Chronic Disease* 29:65–75.

Heiney, S.P., & Wells, L.M. (1989). Strategies for organizing and maintaining support groups. *Oncology Nursing Forum* 16:803-809.

Janosik, E. (1982). Aspects of group development. Pp. 75–92 in E. Janosik & L. Phipps eds., *Life cycle work group in nursing.* Monterey, CA: Wadsworth Health Sciences Division.

Janosik, E., & Miller, J. (1982). Group work with the elderly. Pp. 248–265 in E. Janosik & L. Phipps eds., *Life cycle group work in nursing.* Monterey, CA: Wadsworth Health Sciences Division.

Kriegsman, K., & Celotta, B. (1981). A program of group counseling for women with physical disabilities. *Journal of Rehabilitation* 47(3):34–39, 80.

Kroll, C.J. (1987). Lupus clients assisting one another: A model for supportive services. *Rehabilitation Nursing* 12:239–241.

Kutlenios, R.M. (1987). Healing mind and body: A holistic perspective. *Journal of Gerontological Nursing* 13(12):9–13.

Lonergan, E. (1982). *Group intervention.* New York: Jason Aronson.

Loomis, M. (1979). *Group process for nurses.* St. Louis: C.V. Mosby Co.

Maisiak, R., Cain, M., Yarbro, C., & Josof, L. (1981). Evaluation of TOUCH: An oncology self-help group. *Oncology Nursing* 8(3):20–25.

Marley, M. (1980). The making of a group. *Journal of Gerontological Nursing* 6:275–279.

Marvin, L. (1982). Group organization: Selection criteria, member preparation, contractural issues. Pp. 117–130 in E. Janosik & L. Phipps eds., *Life cycle group work in nursing.* Monterey, CA: Wadsworth Health Sciences Division.

Matteson, M., & Munsat, E. (1982). Group reminiscing with elderly clients. *Issues in Mental Health Nursing* 4:177–189.

Mauss-Clum, N., & Ryan, M. (1981). Brain injury and the family. *Journal of Neurosurgical Nursing* 13:165–169.

Mitchell, P.H., Mertz, M.A., & Catanzaro, M.L. (1987). Group exercise: A nursing therapy in Parkinson's disease. *Rehabilitation Nursing* 12:242–245.

Nath, C., & Rinehart, J. (1979). Effects of individual and group relaxation therapy on blood pressure in essential hypertensives. *Research in Nursing and Health* 2:119–126.

Neizo, B., & Murphy, M. (1983). Medication groups on an acute psychiatric unit. *Perspectives in Psychiatric Care* 21:70–73.

Phipps, L. (1982a). Group work: history and overview. Pp. 3–15 in E. Janosik & L. Phipps eds., *Life cycle group work in nursing.* Monterey, CA: Wadsworth Health Sciences Divsion.

____. (1982b). Group dynamics: Leadership roles and functions. Pp. 155–176 in E. Janosik & L. Phipps eds., *Life cycle group work in nursing.* Monterey, CA: Wadsworth Health Sciences Division.

Pierce, L.L., & Salter, J.P. (1988). Stroke support group: A reality. *Rehabilitation Nursing* 13:189–190, 197.

Rancour, P., & Moser, T. (1980). Group synergy or how to multiply health potential in persons coping with chronic disease. *Health Values: Achieving High Level Wellness* 4:117–118.

Rice, M., & Szopa, T. (1988). Group interventions for reinforcing self-worth following mastectomy. *Oncology Nursing Forum* 15:33.

Sampson, E., & Marthas, M. (1981). *Group process for the health professions.* New York: John Wiley & Sons.

Segev, U., & Schlesinger, Z. (1981). Rehabilitation of patients after acute myocardial infarction—an interdisciplinary, family-oriented program. *Heart and Lung* 10:841–847.

Trainor, M. (1982). Acceptance of ostomy and the visitor role in a self-help group for ostomy patients. *Nursing Research* 31:102–106.

Wilson, L. (1982). How to develop a support group for families of open heart surgery patients. *Dimensions of Critical Care Nursing* 1:108–116.

Yalom, I. (1985). *The theory and practice of group psychotherapy.* New York: Basic Books.

CHAPTER 30

FAMILY SUPPORT

Michaelene Mirr, PhD, RN

BACKGROUND

Inclusion of families in nursing care has occurred since the beginning of the nursing profession. However, this focus has had varying priorities within the profession over the centuries. Only recently, during the 1970s, has nursing experienced a resurgence of the family as a priority in nursing care (Bomar et al., 1989). Currently, standards of care developed by three professional organizations (ANA, AACN, AORN) include families. The emphasis on family nursing has been primarily through community health nursing, midwifery, and psychiatric nursing. Individual patients frequently remain the primary, if not the single focus, of nursing care in acute care settings. It is now time for all facets of nursing to recognize the importance of families in the care of the patient. Support of the family as a nursing intervention is one mechanism that can bridge the gap between nursing care of the patient and the family. This chapter will define family support within the context of nursing and demonstrate how family support can be incorporated into daily nursing care resulting in positive outcomes for the patient, family, and nurse.

Definition

A single definition of family support is not universally accepted because family support is a fairly new concept within nursing. Family support is defined as assistance provided by nurses to patients and families. Family support is a family intervention that assists the family in realistically assessing the impact of the event on the patient and family (Rosenthal & Young, 1988). Family support as a nursing intervention focuses on family members in relation to their effect on the patient. Although family support can mean support within the family unit, the emphasis of this intervention focuses on how nurses can support families rather than using families to give support to patients. Family support includes the concept of presence as an underlying component.

The term "family" needs to be defined. Family is usually defined as the individual's closest biological relations or spouse. However, broader interpretations include whomever the individual is closest to (Buchanan & Brock, 1986). This broader definition of family should guide the nurse in offering support to "family."

Family support should not be confused with family therapy. Family therapy is a formal therapeutic approach involving treatment of the entire family unit for problems that are disruptive to family functioning. Family therapy is an ongoing process with a qualified and licensed therapist. Family therapists require special skills such as interviewing families in conflict, assisting in resolving the conflict, supporting one family member against another, and facilitating change when resistance is strong (Gilliss et al., 1989). Family support includes the family as a unit, but is more episodic and informal in structure. All professional nurses should be qualified to provide family support.

Scientific Basis

A review of nursing literature indicates an increasing number of manuscripts describing concerns and needs of families during periods of stress, crisis, developmental changes, and hospitalization (Caine, 1989; Cray, 1989; Meijs, 1990; Richmond & Craig, 1986; Stanik, 1990). Although the recognition of concern and care for families is becoming more apparent, research demonstrating the effect of nursing interventions such as family support is minimal.   Several investigators have examined various aspects of family coping and family needs (Bedsworth & Molen, 1982; Bouman, 1984; Boykoff, 1986; Breu & Dracup, 1978; Cleveland, 1980; Daley, 1984; Halm, 1990; Jacono et al., 1990; Mathis, 1984; Mirr, 1988; Molter, 1979; Norris & Grove, 1986; Nyamathi, 1987; O'Keefe & Gilliss, 1988; Siegel, 1982; Spatt et al., 1986). These studies have indicated that families need to have hope, need to be close to the injured family member, need to have information, need to know that they will be contacted at any time, and need to know their family member is being cared for.   Although these exploratory studies have identified needs and concerns of families, focus now needs to turn toward nursing interventions to meet these needs.

One of the themes identified by the needs assessment studies is the need for family support during periods of stress such as hospitalization or critical injury (Richmond & Craig, 1986).   Because families are dealing with the stress of injury or illness, family support is often the only form of assistance people use at a time of high stress or crisis (Halm, 1990).   Recent studies of families of critically ill patients confirm this need (Halm, 1990; Mirr, 1988).

Assessment of the need for family support during acute hospitalization or following a situational crisis is often obvious because the families are visibly distressed.   However, one must keep in mind that family support is also needed during chronic illness or developmental changes (Woods et al., 1989).   Often, acute situational crises become long-term situations such as recovery from severe head injury or acute myocardial infarction (Rosenthal & Young, 1988).   Family support may become more instrumental in chronic illness because families continuously deal with stressors without any relief.   The nature of support should be correlated to the demands of the illness or situation (Woods, Yates, & Primono, 1989).   In this respect, family support by professional nurses can take on various dimensions, particularly if caring for families over a period of time. For example, during a period of high stress or crisis, emotional support may be needed by family members. As time progresses, emotional support may be replaced by cognitive support in the form of information sharing.   Depending on the situation, cognitive support may periodically change to material support in finding appropriate resources or finances. In time, organized family support groups may meet some of the needs previously satisfied by professional nurses.   Although family members generally acknowledge the benefits of participating in a support group, studies examining the effectiveness of family support groups have not always demonstrated significant differences between families who attended support groups and families who have not attended support groups (Sabo et al., 1989).

INTERVENTION

In caring for patients in a holistic manner, family support becomes inherent in the care of the patient.   Each patient is entitled to support being provided to his/her family because every patient originates from some type of family unit. Various techniques or methods can be used in providing family support. The following techniques can be used in providing family support.   Careful family assessment is needed to determine which technique best fits the particular family and situation.   The techniques listed below are not meant to be exhaustive.

Techniques

1. Initiate contact with family and introduce self.   Inquire as to how families wish to be addressed and document.   Subsequent contacts should be frequent and build upon previous interactions.

2. Listen for and acknowledge fears, concerns, that families may have. Encourage family participation in resolving these concerns.
3. Provide unsolicited information on patient condition in understandable terms. Repeat information as often as needed.
4. Verify information with family members.
5. Offer information regarding patient's response at each family visit or contact.
6. Provide a comfortable environment for families of hospitalized patients when they are not in patient's room. If patient is critically ill, comfortable furniture in a quiet environment can provide periods of rest while being close to the ill family member.
7. Modify hospital or agency routines to provide normal routines for families as much as possible; i.e. visiting hours, sleeping facilities, or a telephone hotline.
8. Initiate referrals for crisis intervention, family therapy, or other specialized family treatment when needed.
9. Follow-up phone calls to families following discharge from unit and/or hospital.
10. Arrange for periodic relief of caregiving for chronically ill or disabled patients.
11. Provide suggestions to family friends regarding ways to assist the family; i.e. provide a complete meal, mow lawn, care for siblings, etc.
12. Facilitate family contact with other families of similar circumstances for additional support.
13. Provide information on appropriate family support groups if available.

Each of these techniques can be adapted for individual families. For example, in providing information to families (techniques 3, 4, and 5), one nurse should be identified as the primary information provider to a particular family. Information needs to be offered frequently and presented in clear, lay terms. Technical terms, such as surgical or diagnostic procedures, need to be defined clearly and written down for families to use for future reference. Nurses may struggle with what information family members need. Asking families if they have any questions is not adequate because families usually do not know what questions to ask. Offering information such as what the patient did during the day or night provides the background for families to begin asking questions. Families frequently use a literal interpretation of information. Families often define time in terms of hours and minutes whereas health professionals use time more loosely, that is, "one day" may mean approximately 24 hours. Families often set hopes based on their literal interpretation of information. Therefore, in providing information, nurses need to use caution in the use of terms. Validation of the family's comprehension of information also needs to occur frequently because families try to incorporate medical terminology in their discussions yet often use these terms inappropriately.

Measurement of Effectiveness

Current research is underway to determine if family support decreases stress experienced by family members. However, in the interim, patient and family outcomes can be assessed to determine effectiveness of the intervention. Assessments of effectiveness can be validated with families via self-report and documentation. Documentation of outcome is extremely important in evaluating the effectiveness of the nursing intervention. Ongoing family assessment and validation will verify if information is comprehended. Several questions can be asked to assess the effectiveness of family support. For example, do family members seek out the nurses or address them by name? Do family members express their fears and concerns? Are family interactions with patient appropriate and nonstrained? Do families seek out nurses for support? Do verbal and nonverbal messages indicate successful intervention? These examples provide a basis for evaluating family support. Other questions can also be used to assess the effect of family support on the family. Until a valid and reliable tool is available to quantitatively measure family support, the nurse must assume the responsibility for assessing and documenting outcomes.

USES

Family support can be used in a variety of settings in a variety of ways. Family support can be instrumental in situational crises such as acute or critical illness, developmental life changes, chronic illness, and times of stress. Although stress can never be totally eliminated, it is hypothesized that family support can be instrumental in reducing the amount of stress experienced by families. Families are traditionally shy in approaching care providers. Initiation of family support can open the door to meaningful family/nurse relationships. Use of family support in situational crises, developmental life changes, chronic illness, and stressful periods will be discussed separately.

Situational Crisis

Family support is an important nursing intervention, particularly during situational crises. During time of acute or critical illness, families often feel alone in an unfamiliar environment. Feelings of warmth and acceptance by families may make an unpleasant experience less traumatic. Family emotions often resemble a rollercoaster and can benefit from external support. A personal routine that closely resembles the family's can provide less disruption to family life than insistence on conforming to hospital routines. Frequent informational sessions also decrease anxiety regarding the patient's condition. This is particularly true regarding a patient undergoing surgery. Intraoperative reports have been appreciated by families and decrease the intensity of that waiting period (Stanik, 1990).

Developmental Life Changes

Developmental life changes also provide an opportunity for family support. The birth of a child or adjustment to menopause has impact on families. Assistance in coping and adjusting to these changes as a family can lessen any traumatic transition that may occur. Educational opportunities as well as recurrent offerings of assistance can be valuable to families. Post-discharge contact can also be beneficial.

Chronic Illness

Long-term stress associated with chronic illness provides an ideal opportunity for family support. Family relations and interactions can become strained in the daily care and routine of caring for a chronically ill family member. The type and level of family support will change over time, necessitating frequent assessment of family needs. Some families have unique needs and require ongoing assessment and intervention strategies. Kuehne (1989) suggests the development of intergenerational family support services for families of patients with chronic illness. Nurses can facilitate this program by identifying elderly volunteers to care for the chronically ill for short periods of time to relieve family members of caregiving responsibilities.

Stressful Periods

Family support can be beneficial during times of stress. Stress can occur with the hospitalization of a family member, diagnosis of a chronic or terminal illness, or periods of personal adjustment. Recognition of the family need for family support by professional nursing staff can be instrumental in relieving or resolving family stress before reaching a crisis level. Meeting family members' basic needs such as comfort, sleep, and food is often sufficient support at this time. Offering realistic hope is also helpful during this time.

Precautions

One must be conscious of the fine line that may exist between family support and family therapy. Families who need long-term therapy or crisis intervention should be referred to appropriate sources. Strong family assessment skills can be useful in differentiating between the two needs.

One must also become aware of dependency needs. The professional nurse must recognize the point in time when family support is no longer needed and the family's own support systems and resources can take over. One must also respect the wishes of families who do not want family support.

RESEARCH QUESTIONS

Family support as an independent nursing intervention is a fairly new phenomena within nursing. Continuous research efforts in the following areas will provide a solid research base for family support:

1. What methods of family support are most effective? Research efforts need to determine which techniques are most helpful for families.
2. When is family support most beneficial to families? The timing of support is an important component of a positive outcome.
3. What method or tool is most effective for evaluating family support? Evaluation tools are currently not available to effectively evaluate family support as an intervention. Development of a specific instrument to measure support to families is needed.
4. What types of families or situations benefit most from family support? Family support needs to be tested in a variety of settings and with a variety of populations.

REFERENCES

Bedsworth, J.A., & Molen, M.T. (1982). Psychological stress in spouses of patients with myocardial infarction. *Heart & Lung* 11(5):450–456.

Bomar, P.J., McNeeley, G., & Palmer, I.S. (1989). Family health nursing: History and role. Pp. 1–12 in P.J. Bomar ed., *Nurses and family health promotion*. Baltimore: Williams & Wilkins.

Bouman, C.C. (1984). Identifying priority concerns of families of ICU patients. *Dimensions of Critical Care Nursing* 3(5):313–319.

Boykoff, S.L. (1986). Visiting needs reported by patients with cardiac disease and their families. *Heart and Lung* 15(6):573–576.

Breu, C., & Dracup, K. (1978). Helping spouses of critically ill patients. *American Journal of Nursing* 78:51–53.

Buchanan, A., & Brock, D.W. (1986). Deciding for others. *The Milbank Quarterly* 64(supp. 2):17–94.

Caine, R.M. (1989). Families in crisis: Making the critical difference. *Focus on Critical Care* 16(3):184–189.

Cleveland, M. (1980). Family adaptation to traumatic spinal cord injury: response to crisis. *Family Relations* 29:558–565.

Cray, L. (1989). A collaborative project: Initiating a family intervention program in a medical intensive care unit. *Focus on Critical Care* 16(3):212–218.

Daley, L. (1984). The perceived immediate needs of families with relatives in the intensive care setting. *Heart and Lung* 13:231–237.

Gillis, C.L., Roberts, B.M., Highley, B.L., & Martinson, I.M. (1989). What is family nursing. Pp. 64–73 in C.L. Gillis, B.L. Highley, B.M. Roberts, & I.M. Martinson eds., *Toward a science of family nursing*. Menlo Park, CA: Addison-Wesley Publishing Company.

Halm, M.A. (1990). Effects of support groups on anxiety of family members during critical illness. *Heart and Lung* 19(1):62–71.

Jacono, J., Hicks, G., AntZononio, C., O'Brien, K., & Rasi, M. (1990). Comparison of perceived needs of family members between registered nurses and family members of critically ill patients in intensive care and neonatal intensive care units. *Heart and Lung* 19(1):72-78.

Kuehne, V.S. (1989). "Family Friends": An innovative example of intergenerational family support services. *Children's Health Care Journal* 18(4):237-246.

Mathis, M. (1984). Personal needs of family members of critically ill patients with and without acute brain injury. *Journal of Neurosurgical Nursing* 16(1):36-44.

Meijs, C.A. (1989). Care of the family of the ICU patient. *Critical Care Nurse* 9(8):42-44.

Mirr, M.P. (1988). Decisions made by family members of patients with severe head injury. Unpublished doctoral dissertation. University of Minnesota, Minneapolis, MN.

Molter, N.C. (1979). Needs of relatives of critically ill patients: a descriptive study. *Heart and Lung* 8(2):332-339.

Norris, L.O., & Grove, S.K. (1986). Investigation of selected psychosocial needs of family members of critically ill adult patients. *Heart and Lung* 15(2):194-199.

Nyamathi, A.M. (1987). The coping responses of female spouses of patients with myocardial infarction. *Heart and Lung* 16(1):86-92.

O'Keefe, B., & Gilliss, C.L. (1988). Family care in the coronary care unit: an analysis of clinical nurse specialist intervention. *Heart and Lung* 17(2):191-198.

Richmond, T.S., & Craig, M. (1986). Family-centered care for the neurotrauma patient. *Nursing Clinics of North America* 21(4):641-651.

Rosenthal, M., & Young, T. (1988). Effective family intervention after traumatic brain injury: theory and practice. *Head Trauma Rehabilitation* 3(4):42-50.

Sabo, K.A., Kraay, C., Rudy, E., Abraham, T., Bender, M., Lewandowski, W., Lombardo, B., Turk, M., & Dawson, D. (1989). ICU family support sessions: family members perceived benefits. *Applied Nursing Research* 2(2):82-89.

Siegel, R. (1982). A family-centered program for neonatal intensive care. *Health and Social Work* 7:50-58.

Spatt, L., Ganas, E., Hying, S., Kirsch, E.R., & Koch, M. (1986). Informational needs of families of intensive care unit patients. *QRB: Quality Review Bulletin* 12:16-21.

Stanik, J.A. (1990). Caring for the family of the critically ill surgical patient. *Critical Care Nurse* 10(1):43-47.

Woods, N.F., Yates, B.C., & Primono, J. (1989). Supporting families during chronic illness. *IMAGE: Journal of Nursing Scholarship* 21(1):47-50.

CHAPTER 31

ADVOCACY

Margot L. Nelson

BACKGROUND

The role of advocate for the patient or client and the implementation of advocacy as an intervention are integral to the profession and practice of nursing. Although there are various definitions and models of advocacy, there are also conceptual bases.

Definitions

A foundational definition of advocacy in nursing is that it is a "way of being" on the part of the nurse in relationship to another person or group of persons (clients). (The terms "client," "patient," and "consumer" are used interchangeably throughout this chapter to refer to an individual or group who is the recipient of health care in general or nursing care in particular.) Kohnke (1982) describes it as caring, which involves an act of free will and a studied choice to view and position oneself in a particular way in relationship to others. Similarly, Bourassa (in Anderson, 1989) describes advocacy as "an attitude, a certain professional presence..." that is a part of the person of the nurse, not just what he or she does. Some nurse authors deem advocacy as *so* essential as to be the philosophical foundation of nursing (Curtin, 1979; Gadow, 1980a).

Gadow (1980a), in her definition of "existential advocacy," describes advocacy as an essential feature of the nurse–patient relationship whereby the patient is enabled to determine the unique personal meaning of health experiences and, on this basis, exercise self-determination. Curtin (1979), in her discussion of "human advocacy," echoes the nurse's role of assisting persons to find meaning in their living or dying, emphasizing that it is *their* experience and *their* meaning and values, not the experience, meaning, and values of the nurse or anyone else.

Curtin (1979) and Fowler (1989) describe alternative models of advocacy emphasizing different aspects of the above definitions (see Table 31.1):

1. Legal advocacy (Curtin), or the guardian of patient rights model (Fowler), is based upon such legal rights as to be informed, to accept or refuse treatment, and to be protected from incompetent, illegal, or unethical practices. Actions that empower patients in their interaction with the health care system fit within this model of advocacy.
2. Moral–ethical advocacy (Curtin), or the preserver of patient values model (Fowler), is based upon patient goals of values awareness and decision making which is congruent with those values. This type of advocacy occurs within an authentic nurse–patient relationship and requires that the patient desires self-determination and is able to participate in values exploration and decision making.
3. Substitutive advocacy, or the conserver of patient's best interests model (Fowler), emphasizes beneficence and respect for the individual. It is relevant in situations where patients are unable to exercise their rights to self-determination in real time (not prospective or retrospective, but immediate)

Table 31.1
Types of Advocacy: Contrast of Models from Curtin* and Fowler†

Type	Curtin's Typology	Fowler's Model	Underpinnings
Legal advocacy	Legal advocacy	Guardian of patient rights	Individual rights (e.g. to informed consent, to refuse, to competent care and privacy).
Moral-Ethical advocacy	Moral-ethical advocacy	Preserver of patient values	Goal of values awareness and congruent decision making.
Substitutive advocacy		Conservator of patient best interests	Preservation of respect for rights of persons who are unable to speak for themselves.
Political advocacy	Political advocacy	Champion of social justice	Access to "adequate" nursing and health care for everyone.
Spiritual advocacy	Spiritual advocacy		Patient rights to spiritual comfort and counsel in the quest for meaning.

*Curtin, Leah L. (1979). The nurse as advocate: A philosophical foundation for nursing. *Nursing Science* 1:1–10.
†Fowler, Marsha D.M. (1989). Social advocacy. *Heart & Lung* 18(1):97–99.

decision making because of mental incapacity or nonresponsiveness. The less able a person is to protect him/herself, the more vigilant the nurse must be in protecting his/her rights (Curtin, 1979).

4. Political advocacy (Curtin), or the champion of social justice model (Fowler), is rooted in a belief that every person should have access to adequate nursing and health care. It calls for nurses to participate in social criticism and change on behalf of individuals, groups, and society as a whole so that inequities and inconsistencies are identified and corrected.

5. Spiritual advocacy (Curtin) involves the patient's right to spiritual comfort and access to the clergy of choice.

Advocacy, therefore, is the nurse's way of being in relationship with a patient/client, a way of being which respects and promotes the uniqueness of the individual as a total human being in the context of his/her health experience. The goal is to facilitate that individual's exercise of self-determination in decision making related to health and to promote decision making in congruence with who the person is, the level of self-determination possible at a given point in time, and what he/she values. "The goal of advocacy is to preserve the patient's control over his or her own life" (Morrison in Anderson, 1989:66). Advocacy also includes actions which influence the context of health care so that self determination is more possible.

Evolution of Intervention

In order to understand the concept of advocacy and its relevance for nursing and to develop guidelines for its application, one must comprehend its evolution, which parallels the historical evolution of professional nursing. Advocacy in nursing has evolved from a posture of interceding, supporting, or pleading a case for the client to acting as guardian of the client's rights and promoting autonomy and free choice for all health care consumers (Nelson, 1988).

Acting For or On Behalf of Another

Some of the earliest nursing leaders, although they did not use the term "advocacy," viewed the nurse as an actor for or an intercessor on behalf of the patient. Florence Nightingale's definition of nursing in 1859 implies such a role in its emphasis upon manipulating environmental factors "to put the patient in the best condition for nature to act upon him" (Nightingale, 1969:2). On a social scale, Nightingale's actions to improve the quality of care for the wounded during the Crimean War and to reform care of the sick and nursing education in England fit into this definition of advocacy.

Other nurse leaders, including Lillian Wald and Lavinia Dock, also acted as advocates in seeking social and health care reforms. In recent years, however, objections have been raised to this version of advocacy. It clearly implies, according to Leddy and Pepper (1984), an active position for the advocate and a passive role for the client, a "mothering" image, or the vertical nurse over the horizontal patient (Fagin & Diers, 1983).

Loyalty and Obedience

Historically, loyalty and obedience have been strong *counter*themes to advocacy. Advocacy for the client/patient has been given highest priority, *unless* it conflicted with advocacy for the physician or the employing institution. These themes are rooted in Winslow's (1984) military analogy for medicine and health care in the early twentieth century. Medical care was at war with disease, the invading enemy to be combatted and conquered. With this framework for their education, nursing students were steeped in a military protocol of unquestioning respect for higher rank and authority; and it was obvious that nurses were at the lower end of the rank and file of health care providers, with only nursing students beneath them! Perry, in 1906, declared that a nurse should be "trained" by repeated acts to absolute accuracy and skill and obliteration of "herself." In this context of loyalty and obedience, no criticism of hospital or school, fellow nurses, or physicians was allowed.

In 1910, however, some radical questions began to be heard, exemplified in an *American Journal of Nursing* (1910) editorial, "Where Does Loyalty End?" The author acknowledged that she was treading on dangerous ground with such questions as, "Is a nurse required to be untruthful or practice deceit to uphold the reputation of the physician at her own expense or that of the patient?"

Equally radical was the "Suggested Code of Ethics for Nurses," which was presented to the American Nurses' Association Convention in May of 1926. This first version of the code stated that "Loyalty to the motive inspiring nursing should make the nurse fearless to bring to light any serious violation of the ideals (by another nurse)" (American Nurses' Association, page 600, 1926). The assumption was of a larger commitment to the community and the well-being of the patient than to an erring colleague. The "Tentative Code for the Nursing Profession" (still awaiting adoption 14 years later) took an even larger step in the direction of advocacy, calling for mutual understanding and respect between medicine and nursing. Nevertheless, loyalty continued as an overriding theme in the practice of nursing: the nurse should conscientiously follow instructions and build the patient's confidence in the physician, while at the same time using "reason and intelligence in carrying out orders!" (*American Journal of Nursing,* 1940).

Such themes of loyalty were still evident in a 1970s study of nurses' moral reasoning (Murphy, 1983). Loyalty to physician and hospital was found to strongly influence decision making by nurses. Decisions were made more often in accordance with physician advocacy than according to a patient-advocate model.

Nurse as Mediator

Gradually, the advocacy role in nursing evolved to one of mediation, emphasizing coordination of services, explanation to the client of the roles and responsibilities of various health care providers, and clarification of communication by others. Winslow (1984) identified several societal factors which made apparent the need for this kind of advocacy and facilitated the movement of nurses into mediating roles and later into promoting the client's self-determination. One such factor was a loss of confidence in medicine in the 1970s; medicine and the related health care industry came to be viewed as powerful, impersonal, and protected institutions. Additional factors were the increased knowledge base of consumers and better educational preparation of nurses. Together with growing consumerism and feminism, these new ways of thinking challenged the traditionally inequitable distribution of power and expertise. Nursing's first response was to interpret and assist clients to make sense of their health situation. Along with interpreting the client's needs to other members of the health team, this constituted the mediator role.

Nurse as Proponent of Self-Determination

The role of the nurse as promoter of the client's self-determination is a still more radical departure from the initial definition of advocate as "actor for" the patient/client. This most recent version of advocacy represents a shift in emphasis from caretaking and mediation to consideration of the client's rights and autonomy in decision making as the unconditional first priorities. An official declaration in 1973 by the Secretary's Commission on Medical Malpractice, United States Department of Health, Education, and Welfare, concurred with nurses' support of consumers' rights to engage in active decision making about their own health: "...that the interests of health care providers and consumers are best served by effective consumer participation at the decision-making level" (U.S. Health, Education, and Welfare Department, 1973).

A specific vision of the nurse as advocate and the relationship of that role to the client's self-determination was at last reflected, and even termed "advocacy," in the 1985 American Nurses' Association *Code for Nurses with Interpretive Statements:*

> Since clients themselves are the primary decision makers in matters concerning their own health, treatment, and wellbeing, the goal of nursing actions is to support and enhance the client's responsibility and **self-determination** to the greatest extent possible.

> Truth telling and the process of reaching informed choice underlie the exercise of **self-determination** which is basic to respect for persons.

> The nurse's primary commitment is to the health, welfare, and safety of the client. As an **advocate** for the client, the nurse must be alert to and take appropriate action regarding any instances of incompetent, unethical or illegal practice by any member of the health care team or the health care system, or any action on the part of others that places the rights or best interests of the client in jeopardy. (American Nurses' Association, 1985)

INTERVENTION

Technique

Ways of operationalizing advocacy in practice will be discussed with reference to the five advocacy models defined earlier: Legal advocacy, moral–ethical advocacy, substitutive advocacy, political advocacy, and spiritual advocacy.

Legal Advocacy

One basis for this role is the ANA Code for nurses, in which it is stated that nurses are morally obliged to provide patients with information and to do so with "respect for human dignity and the uniqueness of the client, unrestricted by considerations of social and economic status, personal attributes, or the nature of the health problem..." (American Nurses' Association, 1985, p. 2). This statement focuses upon a fundamental patient right, that of adequate information. Adequate information about treatment means that available alternatives have been presented, including a discussion of risks, mortality, and probability of success for all procedures and treatments.

Another way of defining adequate information is through the criteria of informed consent: adequate information to make rational decisions, mental competence on the part of the decision maker, and uncoerced, freely given consent by a nonvulnerable, autonomous person (Grodin et al., 1986). In addition to providing information, the nurse is obligated to ascertain that the client is able to, and indeed does, comprehend the meaning of the information provided and to assure that he/she has been free to choose any of the alternatives presented. To fulfill these obligations, the nurse often must clarify and expand on information presented by physicians and others. In addition, nurses need to assure that information is updated to enable new informed decisions as available knowledge changes.

Other legal rights which the nurse is obliged to protect are that of privacy; the prerogative to refuse any medication, test, procedure, treatment, or care provider; and the freedom to leave an institution which is providing care. Privacy is protected by sharing personal information about clients only in the context of facilitating care provision and expecting other health care providers to treat such information with the same respect. The right to refuse is frequently *not* emphasized by health care providers, and patients and families are often unaware of that right because of the power differential which they perceive between themselves and health care providers. This makes it even more important for the nurse-advocate to make these rights known.

Both to facilitate informed decision making and to make ongoing care available, patient and "family" capabilities must be assessed and appropriate referrals made, either formally or by providing information about resources so that self-referral can occur. Such referrals may involve employment counselors, lawyers, social workers, psychologists, support groups, clergy, government agencies, and others.

The bottom line in legal advocacy is that rights belong to the patient, which means that he or she also has the right *not* to exercise those rights; it also means that patient choices must be accepted and support of the patient continued, even in instances where the nurse disagrees with the choice.

Moral-Ethical Advocacy

According to this model of advocacy, the nurse acts as preserver of patient values, assuring autonomy in decision making and at the same time providing the professional assistance needed to make such decisions. In this type of advocacy, the uniqueness of the person and his/her situation in time are respected, and every decision is viewed within that unique context. In facilitating decision making, nurses often serve as the communication bridge among the health team, the patient, and the family (Copp, 1986).

Gadow (1980b) describes the relationship between nurse and patient within this advocacy model as an existential one with both parties attuned to each other and expressing their wholeness and uniqueness in a clarification and sharing of values. She sets forth a process for information sharing to facilitate decision making: 1) assuring that the patient has relevant information; 2) allowing the patient to select the information desired; 3) disclosing the nurse's view (necessary, according to Gadow, for the nurse to participate in the process as a whole and authentic person); 4) helping the patient identify his/her values; and 5) assisting the patient to determine freely the meaning that health, illness, or dying is to have.

Kohnke (1982) disagrees with the nurse's sharing of personal views or even pursuing a clarification of patient values on the grounds that this may undermine the patient's decisional autonomy. In Kohnke's view, the nurse advocate walks a very fine line between clarification and subtle manipulation, and many times non-action is more desirable in the interest of safeguarding free choice. It behooves the nurse, therefore, to avoid offering conclusions prematurely and to assure that the emphasis is upon the *patient's* values and desires.

Corcoran (1988) outlined a model of self-determination, combining Gadow's model and a process of decision analysis, for patients faced with a decision making situation. Using the illustration of a decision flow diagram, she suggests that the following considerations are necessary to help patients determine the type and amount of information they want and then to choose among options. First, the options or choices in the decision situation must be identified. Then chance events related to the situation (e.g. occurrences such as death, thromboembolism, or infection, which are not under the control of the decision maker but may well affect the outcome) are considered, along with their probabilities of occurrence. Corcoran's rationale for including this dimension is so that patients don't bear the total burden of responsibility for all consequences. Third, possible outcomes resulting from each of the alternative actions plus the chance events need to be identified and the patient given the opportunity to assign values to the outcomes. Corcoran issues a caution that pertains to all decisional support interventions: the nurse must be qualified to provide accurate information. This means he or she must possess appropriate knowledge, communication skills, and rapport with the client.

Another area in which decision-making opportunities arise and in which patient values are significant is education for behavior change. In order to be effective, such teaching must be done in accordance with the values of the learners. In educating about AIDS (Acquired Immunodeficiency Syndrome), for example, teaching programs are most effective when developed in consultation with recipient communities (Anderson, 1989). Education to prevent transmission of the Human Immunodeficiency Virus (HIV) entails an awareness of values associated with addictive behaviors, sexual expression and its control, the effectiveness of condom use in stopping transmission, degree of responsibility for another person's well-being, and vulnerability to illness.

Another useful intervention for nurses dealing with patients of any age or condition is to invite and encourage thinking about values related to life, health, and death prior to a crisis or life-threatening situation (Omery & Caswell, 1989). This may well include the option of an advanced directive (such as a Living Will, which has legal status in numerous states) specifying the kinds of medical intervention and the type of health care experience the person would desire or wish to refuse under certain circumstances. Advanced directives may also include the designation of a proxy decision maker and power of attorney. Early discussion of issues such as resuscitation and life-sustaining therapies is often beneficial to patients, family members, and persons who may be in the position of proxy decision-maker (Grady, 1989).

Substitutive Advocacy

This role has also been referred to as the conservator of patient's best interests and becomes relevant when the patient is no longer able to express his or her own wishes and an identified proxy decision-maker is unavailable to speak on his/her behalf. The underlying principle is the ultimate right of everyone to speak for themselves in determining their own destinies. Authority to speak on behalf of someone, therefore, derives from that person (Batavia, 1989). Furthermore, competence of an adult to speak for him- or herself should be assumed unless there is evidence to the contrary (Veatch & Fry, 1987). Advocacy, as a substitute for the patient's own decision making, is thus not something to be embarked upon lightly.

In instances where mental incapacity or lack of responsiveness clearly preclude the patient's expression of self-determination, it is important that someone serve as a voice for that person's preferences and best interests. This is obviously much easier when discussions with that person have previously occurred. Benner (1981; in DeCoste, 1981b) states that nurses are able to serve as authentic voices for patients because "they stand inside the patient's community in a unique way...mediating between the patient's and family's concerns and health care resources and values" (p. 82).

Another related type of intervention is in advocating for vulnerable populations, by foreseeing and anticipating problems for which certain groups are at high risk (e.g. physical or psychological abuse, chemical substance use, or self-destructive behaviors). When such vulnerable persons are identified, nurses can communicate caution to other health care providers or family members, implement early screening, or intervene by educating and referring in a preventive way (Copp, 1986).

Still another way of implementing this type of advocacy is to apply skill and knowledge to facilitate coping with disease manifestations when they occur. In the case of advanced HIV disease, for example, these manifestations may be fatigue, diarrhea, wasting, and/or dementia. Interventions for maximizing the quality of life in the face of these problems must be individualized and planned with other health care providers in the home or community, with family members, and with patients themselves.

Changes in traditional patterns of care delivery may also be viewed as a kind of substitutive advocacy. For example, some of the acute care practices which were routine early in the AIDS era have been modified to become less restrictive. This includes "family only" visiting; now in many settings it is the patient who identifies those who should be allowed to visit or who constitutes his/her family.

Substitutive advocacy, although not a desirable first option, is sometimes necessary because of circumstances prohibiting patients from acting on their own behalf. Nurses are often in a prime position to serve as a proxy voice.

Political Advocacy

Also referred to as the champion of social justice role, political advocacy is directed at social criticism and change at a policy and legislative level. Historically, nursing has had many role models of political advocacy: Florence Nightingale, who paved the way for formalized nursing education; Lavinia Dock, who addressed the problem of venereal disease through her writings and public health actions; and Margaret Sanger, who provided leadership in meeting the health needs of women and educating the public about birth control options.

Through professional organizations, more effectively than as individuals, nurses can influence changes in such areas as the provision of accessible and affordable health care services. As an example, the American Nurses' Association (ANA) is a member of an even larger organization, National Organizations Responding to AIDS (NORA), which is working for federal changes to promote research, education and prevention, and accessible, nondiscriminatory health care for persons with AIDS/HIV. Other areas where the ANA is attempting to influence change are in promoting health care financing which is responsive to catastrophic illnesses; increasing the availability of long-term care facilities, homes, and apartments for persons with AIDS and other chronic illnesses; and working with the Environmental Protection Agency for solutions to waste management. On a smaller scale, changes are being sought and implemented on local and institutional levels. Collectively, nurses are a large voting block and a potentially powerful lobby to influence changes in health care at a policy and legislative level. According to Fowler (1989), this is an extremely significant advocacy role for nursing, advancing beyond institutional walls to participate in social criticism and social change to rectify inequities and inconsistencies in health care. Alfano (1987) adds, "We have to do more than be critical of systems that don't work; we have to find ways to make them work or change them into systems that will work" (p. 1730).

In order to achieve this kind of influence, nurses must be willing to become more sophisticated politically and to participate in organizations that utilize collective power. This includes membership in professional organizations, supporting nurse membership on health policy-making boards and councils, and seeking opportunities to participate at institutional, local, regional, state, and national levels.

Roy (1990) goes a step further in challenging all health care providers to move beyond even a national arena to advocate for the health of human beings worldwide. He raises the challenge of moral responsibility to fellow human beings across the planet who are more in need of health care services than we are in the United States.

Spiritual Advocacy

This model of advocacy may be a subcategory of the moral–ethical model. The search for meaning is an ethical and spiritual task. Gadow's (1980a) description of advocacy fits into this realm when she discusses the nurse's interaction with the patient to determine the unique personal meaning a health experience is to have for that individual. Through advocacy, nurses communicate sensitivity to personal hopes and values and create an atmosphere of caring and a sense of the possible.

Nurses implement this kind of advocacy when they are able to set aside personal agendas and institutional politics to be present and participate openly with patients in their search for meaning (see Chapter 28 on presence). Nurses also serve as spiritual advocates when they allow and nurture hope, a spiritual endeavor described by Muyskens (1979) as drawn from the innermost aspects of one's being, one's spiritual self. One cannot implement this kind of advocacy without entering the inner world of another human being; such entry is possible only as a caring person, open to and focused upon the uniqueness, the wonder, the now, and the possibility of the other.

Measurement of Effectiveness

Since advocacy includes a significant ethical dimension, pertaining to the good of clients, one approach to its evaluation is through ethical principles as standards. For example, if one uses nonmaleficence (the principle of causing no harm) as a guide, one of the most basic measures of advocacy is that the client not be hurt by advocacy interventions. If beneficence serves as a standard, advocacy should in some way promote the physical, psychological, social, or spiritual well-being of the client. If autonomy is a guiding principle, the client's self-determination must be included in the measure of effectiveness. If justice is a priority, a measure of fairness or equitability in distributing health resources so that the client receives his or her fair share of attention and benefit is in order. Fidelity suggests that one should evaluate fulfillment of obligations, such as commitments to provide care until a satisfactory alternative is found, and the degree to which privacy and confidentiality are honored. The definitions of advocacy supply a more precise framework for posing evaluative questions about whether advocacy behaviors have been effective. Each definition provides somewhat different guidelines and questions.

For legal advocacy, the client's legal rights must be upheld and he or she must be able to verbalize understanding of those rights and resources available to assist with their protection. Specific exemplary rights and questions which may be used to measure effectiveness are:

1. Informed consent: Has the client been given opportunity to obtain the relevant information he/she desires about treatment or other health-related alternatives? Is he or she competent to give consent or been provided the opportunity to identify a proxy decision-maker? Barring this, have earnest attempts been made to determine the substance of previously written or verbalized advanced directives? Does the client feel free to choose or decide without penalty or pressure from health care providers?
2. Acceptance or refusal of treatment: Can the client verbalize understanding of his or her right to refuse? Are the client's expressions of doubt or ambivalence given opportunity for expression and exploration?
3. Protection from incompetent or unethical practices: Are quality assurance measures in place to assure client safety and the competence of health care providers? Are procedures in place and utilized for intervening when there are threats to client safety or rights? Does the client know whom to contact with concerns about the quality of his/her care?

For moral–ethical advocacy, the nurse–client relationship and the client's opportunity to be authentic with himself and a caring other (the nurse) are the focus of evaluation. Has he/she been given the opportunity to explore personal values that are relevant to the present health situation? Have opportunities been provided for considering advanced directives regarding future life, health, and death decisions? Does the client feel he or she has as much control over his/her health planning as he or she desires?

For substitutive advocacy, the major concern is that the best interests of the client are protected when he or she is unable to participate actively in the planning process. Have attempts been made to determine what the client's wishes would be if he/she could express them? Have the safety and dignity of the client been maintained? Has communication through verbalization and touch been maintained despite the client's level of response? Have significant others been allowed and assisted to participate in care and decision making?

For political advocacy, nurses need to participate individually and collectively in actions to promote such goals as a healthy environment and accessible and affordable health care for all. Are nurses visible in community, state, regional, and national organizations and agencies that promote societal awareness of threats to health, seek health-related policy and legislative changes, and strive for resolution of economic and health care inequities?

For spiritual advocacy, clients must be supported as they search for meaning in their health experiences, living, and dying. Is the nurse open and present with the client in such a way that meaningful interchange on a spiritual level can occur? Is there an attitude of caring and hope on the part of the nurse? Are clients' unique personal meanings sought and respected? Are opportunities provided for client contact with the clergy of choice?

Some of these questions can be answered through information in the client's health record, others subjectively by the client, the family, and/or the nurse. Others, such as those pertaining to spiritual advocacy, can only be intuited by an observer or perhaps only by the participants in a nurse–client relationship. Ultimately, however, evaluation of advocacy interventions must occur and modifications be made on this basis.

USES

There are many contexts in which nurses serve as advocates with many different clients (individuals and groups). The nurse may interact only with the client or mediate between client and community resources, client and the health care system, client and other disciplines, client and family (Nelson, 1988).

Since self-determination and well-being of clients are significant goals for all health experiences, advocacy is needed whenever nurses relate to clients. There are particular circumstances, however, in which the needs for advocacy become more glaring. These include situations in which ethical dilemmas arise due to life-sustaining possibilities or allocation of scarce resources. Diseases that were at one time naturally and quickly fatal now are no longer so because of advances in life-support technologies. Patients and families may find themselves involved in a burdensome and prolonged dying process if opportunities have not been provided for advanced directives or discussions of values prior to a crisis (Omery & Caswell, 1989). Examples include people who have experienced head trauma, shock, kidney failure, major surgery, terminal diagnoses, or cardiopulmonary resuscitation.

Another area where the need for advocacy is often evident is with populations who are discriminated against for health-related factors. Such populations include the physically and mentally disabled (Bruce & Christiansen, 1988), people diagnosed with cancer (Hoffman, 1989), persons with HIV infection (Cecchia, 1986; Grady, 1989), and people whose behaviors are typically viewed as deviant (e.g. IV drug abusers and convicted criminals). A related group is persons who typically do not receive an equitable share of health promotional or health care resources: the homeless, the poor, the mentally ill, minorities, women (Gillette, 1988), and the elderly (Nelms, 1989).

Persons who are unable to verbalize their needs or wishes are a group for whom substitutive advocacy is important. This includes infants, people who are mentally incompetent, and dying patients. Another related group are what Copp (1986) terms "vulnerable persons." Vulnerable populations include those potentially vulnerable (e.g. persons with genetic abnormalities which place them at specific risk, adolescent parents, and those with life styles which predispose to cardiac or respiratory disease); the circumstantially vulnerable (because of war, famine, poverty, etc.); the temporarily vulnerable (due to trauma, depression, family disruption, sexual assault, or abuse); the episodically vulnerable (e.g. those with chronic pain, alcoholism, or other recurrent problems); and the permanently vulnerable (due to such things as birth injury, hemiplegia, blindness, and residual damage from diseases such as poliomyelitis).

Precautions

Although advocacy is definitely needed by health care recipients and fits within the domain of nursing, there are hazards for nurses who choose to become client advocates. They may have to "make waves" and become "risk takers" to claim a genuine advocate identity (Kosik, 1972). The Tuma case exemplifies such risk. Jolene Tuma was a nurse who answered a patient's questions about alternatives to cancer chemotherapy. Although the patient chose to continue with the chemotherapy, the physician's suit against Tuma for interfering in a doctor–patient relationship caused her to lose her job and license to practice nursing, although the latter was subsequently restored by the Supreme Court of Idaho. Tuma herself asked a critical question with respect to advocacy in nursing: Do we as nurses have the authority to fulfill responsibility as the patient's advocate? (Tuma, 1977).

Several issues need resolution before nurses can fully embrace a commitment to client advocacy. The traditional public view of the physician or Health Maintenance Organization (HMO) as authority and decision maker in health care is an obstacle to nurses' assuming advocacy roles. This prevalent view and practice also lends support to the *need* for advocacy; physicians have tended to treat patients as their exclusive domain, a stance which effectively blocks advocacy by other providers as well as self-determination for the client. As Leddy and Pepper (1984) point out, there is a definite foundation for this view in the real world, given that the patient's admission, diagnosis, treatment, and discharge from health care agencies are usually physician controlled. In such a scheme, the would-be nurse advocate may be viewed as a troublemaker rather than as a meaningful contributor to patients' welfare.

A related issue is that nurses are not recognized by consumers, by physicians, or often by nurses themselves as active initiators of health care, but rather as caregivers or implementers of the physician's plan of care (Weiss, 1983). Patients and families may be less receptive to the nurse as advocate because the nurse has not been selected by them as such. Nurses may, therefore, find themselves offering a service that has not been chosen and may not be expected. Colleagues may also view client advocacy by the nurse as a problem. Patients who have had a nurse advocate may ask too many questions, want to do things their own way, and even be noncompliant (Kohnke, 1982). Nurses may, with fair accuracy, perceive that they must go against the entire system to function in the role of advocate.

Further, most nurses would identify the client as the first priority, but there continue to be competing loyalties to physicians and employing institutions. The nurse is often cast as a "double agent," attempting to represent both patient and physician (Nelson, 1988).

RESEARCH QUESTIONS

There has been little research related to advocacy in nursing, with the exception of surveys to identify role priorities for physicians and nurses in specific settings. For this reason, research is needed to ascertain nurses' commitment to advocacy roles, ways in which advocacy can be operationalized, and the outcomes of nurse advocacy. A few of the many relevant questions which might be asked are:

1. To what extent do nurses perceive themselves as advocates and for whom (clients, families, communities, institutions, or physicians)?
2. What kinds of advocacy interventions are being utilized by nurses, whether or not they are labelled as such?
3. What are the needs for advocacy in specific groups of patients in specific settings?

4. To what extent do clients expect nurses to serve as their advocates?
5. Does operationalizing advocacy in a specific way (e.g. through use of decision analysis) contribute to client outcomes measured by self-report and/or autonomous behaviors?
6. What is the relationship between advocacy interventions and measures of client stress and coping responses?
7. How do advocacy interventions affect the congruence (fit) between client values and decisions made?

REFERENCES

Alfano, G. (1987). The nurse as a patient advocate. *American Journal of Nursing* 87:1730.

American Journal of Nursing. (1910). Where does loyalty end? (editorial). *American Journal of Nursing* 10:230–231.

American Journal of Nursing. (1940). A tentative code for the nursing profession. *American Journal of Nursing* 40:977–980.

American Nurses' Association. (1985). Code for nurses with interpretive statements. Kansas City, MO: American Nurses' Association.

American Nurses' Association, Ethical Standards Committee. (1926). A suggested code. *American Journal of Nursing* 26:599–601.

Anderson, D. (1989). Advocacy for AIDS patients is helping all patients. *RN* May 1989:65–72.

Batavia, A.I. (1989). Representation and role separation in the disability movement: Should researchers be advocates? *Archives of Physical Medicine and Rehabilitation* 70:345–348.

Banner, P. (1981). Commentary. *American Journal of Nursing* 81:82.

Bruce, M.A., & Christiansen, C.H. (1988). Advocacy in word as well as deed. *The American Journal of Occupational Therapy* 42:189–191.

Cecchia, R.L. (1986). Health care advocacy for AIDS patients. *Quarterly Review Bulletin* August 1986:297–303.

Christy, T.E. (1973). New privileges...new challenges...new responsibilities. *Nursing* 3:8–11.

Copp, L.A. (1986). The nurse as advocate for vulnerable persons. *Journal of Advanced Nursing* 11:255–263.

Corcoran, S. (1988). Toward operationalizing an advocacy role. *Journal of Professional Nursing* 4:242–248.

Curtin, L.L. (1979). The nurse as advocate: A philosophical foundation for nursing. *Nursing Science* 1:1–10.

DeCoste, B. (1981). The many faces of advocacy. *American Journal of Nursing* 81:80–82.

Fagin, C., & Diers, D. (1983). Nursing as metaphor. *New England Journal of Medicine* 309:116–117.

Fowler, M.D.M. (1989). Social advocacy. *Heart & Lung* 18:97–99.

Gadow, S. (1980a). Existential advocacy: Philosophical foundation of nursing. Pp. 79–89 in S.F. Spicker & S. Gadow eds., *Nursing, images and ideals: Opening dialogue with the humanities*. New York: Springer Publishing.

_____. (1980b). A model for ethical decision making. *Oncology Nursing Forum* 7:44–47.

Gillette, J. (1988). Advocacy and nursing: Implication for women's health care. *The Australian Journal of Advanced Nursing* 6:4–11.

Grady, C. (1989). Ethical issues in providing nursing care to human immunodeficiency virus-infected populations. *Journal of Advanced Nursing* 14:513–514.

Grodin, M., Kaminov, P., & Sassower, R. (1986). Ethical issues in AIDS research. *Quarterly Review Bulletin* 10:347–352.

Hoffman, B. (1989). Cancer survivors at work: Job problems and illegal discrimination. *Oncology Nursing Forum* 16:39–43.

Kohnke, M.F. (1982). *Advocacy: Risk and reality.* St. Louis: C.V. Mosby.

Kosik, S.H. (1972). Patient advocacy or fighting the system. *American Journal of Nursing* 72:694–698.

Leddy, S., & Pepper, J.M. (1984). *Conceptual bases of professional nursing.* Philadelphia: J.B. Lippincott.

Murphy, C.P. (1983). Models of the nurse-patient relationship. Pp. 8–24 in C.P. Murphy & H. Hunter eds., *Ethical problems in the nurse–patient relationship.* New York: Allyn and Bacon.

Muyskens, J.L. (1979). *The sufficiency of hope.* Philadelphia: Temple University Press.

Nelms, B.C. (1989). Child advocacy: The need is great. *Journal of Pediatric Health Care* 3:1–2.

Nelson, M.L. (1988). Advocacy in nursing. *Nursing Outlook* 36:136–141.

Nightingale, F. (1969). *Notes on nursing: What it is, and what it is not.* Dover, NY: Lippincott Publications.

Omery, A., & Caswell, D. (1989). Ethical perspectives. *Critical Care Nursing Clinics of North America* 1:165–173.

Perry, C.M. (1906). Nursing ethics and etiquette. *American Journal of Nursing* 6:448–452.

Roy, D.J. (1990). Humanity, the measure of an ethics for AIDS. *Journal of Acquired Immune Deficiency Syndrome* 3:449–459.

Tuma, J. (1977). Professional misconduct (letter). *Nursing Outlook* 25:546.

U.S. Health, Education, and Welfare Department. (1973). *Report of Secretary's Commission on Medical Malpractice, Jan. 16, 1973.* Washington, DC: Department of Health, Education, and Welfare (Publication Nos. [05]73–88,89).

Veatch, R., & Fry, S. (1987). *Case studies in nursing ethics.* Philadelphia: J.B. Lippincott.

Weiss, S.J. (1983). Role differentiation between nurse and physician: Implications for nursing. *Nursing Research* 32:133–139.

Winslow, G.R. (1984). From loyalty to advocacy: A new metaphor for nursing. *Hastings Center Report* 14:32–40.

CHAPTER 32

ACTIVE LISTENING

Muriel Ryden, PhD, RN

BACKGROUND

The therapeutic use of self has long been a primary independent nursing intervention. The ability of the nurse to use her personality consciously and in full awareness in an attempt to establish relatedness was described by Travelbee (1966) as a disciplined intellectual approach, not mere kindly feelings. The potential for nurses to be a healing force was emphasized by Ujhely (1968). Both in the presence or the absence of high technology, the instrument "self" is available to the nurse and helpful to the client. Listening represents one of the essential components in the use of the self as an intervention to bring about desired outcomes for clients.

Listening is a part of the classic communication model, which consists of a sender who encodes a message and transmits it through some medium to a receiver, who must listen and hear to decode the message (Arnold & Boggs, 1989). The independent intervention of listening essentially involves the helper remaining in the role of a receiver, assisting the sender/client to more clearly understand his/her own message. In the words of Davis, "Listening is receiving with nothing to prove" (1984:4).

Definition

The dictionary definition of "to listen" is "to make a conscious effort to hear; to attend closely, so as to hear" (Webster's New Twentieth Century Dictionary, 1983:1055). Because the word has a passive connotation, the term "active listening" has come to be used to refer to a disciplined, skilled interpersonal communication style. Active listening is the skill of understanding what another is saying and feeling, and communicating to that person in your own words what you think he is saying and feeling (Gerrard et al., 1980). Active listening may be demonstrated in the following ways:

1. The receiver attempts to clarify a message that was unclear. Example:

    Client: "Well, I came to the clinic because it seemed like the thing to do. I would really rather not, but you know how it is."

    Nurse: "I am not sure I understand what you are saying about your reason for coming here. Can you explain further what you mean?"

2. The receiver paraphrases the content and/or feeling that the sender has overtly communicated. Example:

    Client: "I am so tired of trying one thing after another and having absolutely no success! I have spent thousands of dollars and I am no better than I was when I started!"

    Nurse: "It is discouraging and frustrating to invest a lot of time, energy, and money and not get the results you hoped for."

3. The receiver responds by putting into words content and/or feelings that the sender has only covertly communicated. Example:

> Nurse to previous client: "I wonder if what you are saying is that you feel very hopeless about ever getting better."

An active listener, like a sounding board, does not employ interpersonal strategies that send new messages. Therefore, changing the frame of reference, using self-disclosure, and providing information—all of which may be useful actions in some situations—would not be part of active listening.

An active listener does not require verbal communication by the sender in order to respond, since all behavior is a form of communication. The nonverbal component of social meaning is estimated by Birdwhistell (1970) to be 65% of the communication. The interpretation of emotion from facial expression and body movement across cultures has been studied extensively by Ekman and Friesen (1969, 1971). Six basic human emotions (happiness, sadness, anger, fear, surprise, and disgust) have been found to be associated with a quite limited range of facial muscle movements that were judged correctly from pictures by subjects from various cross-cultural groups (Ekman & Friesen, 1972). When words contradicted silent messages, Mehrabian (1971) found that communicators relied on nonverbal cues.

A nurse who is actively listening to the messages from a client who is verbally noncommunicative might respond: "It seems that talking about this is not something you are comfortable with doing right now." Or, to a comatose client: "I wish you could tell me how you are feeling; you look uncomfortable in that position. I am going to rub your back and turn you to the other side, and prop you with some pillows to try to make you more comfortable."

In discussing holistic listening, Rowan (1986) describes many levels of listening, from obvious acknowledgement of what the other says to the deepest level of entering into an intuitive relationship with the other person.

Active listening also is called "empathic listening." The definition of empathy by Truax and Carkhuff approximates that of active listening: "Accurate empathy involves both the therapist's sensitivity to current feelings and his verbal facility to communicate this in a language attuned to the client's feelings" (1967:46). Rogers (1957) identified empathy, warmth, and genuineness as three qualities necessary and sufficient for therapeutic change to occur in the other.

Empathy, according to Gerrard et al. (1980), has three components. The affective component is sensitivity to feelings; the cognitive component observes and processes messages; and the communicative component restates in response what the receiver has sensed. These authors assert that active listening is the cognitive and communicative component of empathy.

Scientific Basis

In the nursing literature, listening tends to be addressed in an anecdotal and an exhortatory mode more frequently than in a scientific mode. For example, Magnan and Benner (1989) assert that listening allows nurses to become catalysts for recovery and healing; in the process, the authors assert, nurses are also taught by their clients. Listening is identified by Burnard (1987) as the first and most important aspect of counseling persons in spiritual distress. Texts describing interpersonal communication skills in nursing consistently include listening as an essential skill, but tend not to document the scientific basis for its use.

In the field of counseling, Rogers (1975) asserts that research points strongly to the conclusion that a high degree of empathy in a relationship is possibly *the* most potent, and certainly *one of the most potent* factors in bringing about change and learning in clients (Cartwright & Lerner, 1966; Mullen & Abeles, 1971; Rogers et al., 1967). Mehrabian (1971) found that nonverbal messages (facial expression and tone of voice) were more important than words in determining the impact of a total message. Nonverbal behavior can confirm what is said by the degree of congruence with verbal statements, or it can "leak" messages

(Ekman & Friesen, 1969), since it is not as easily subject to control as are verbal messages. Margulies (1984) suggests that empathy is enhanced by creative imagination which allows the helper to feel himself in the reality of a client's experience.

The research in nursing that relates to listening has been done primarily from an educational perspective, not from a clinical outcomes perspective. Researchers have studied the effectiveness of methodologies designed to increase empathic listening skills in students and practicing nurses (Daniels et al., 1988; Hardin & Halaris, 1983; Norris, 1986; Olson & Iwasiw, 1987). Some studies have suggested that nurses as a group possess low levels of empathy (Friedrich et al., 1985; Lamonica et al., 1976). However, in a comparison of the helping styles of nursing students, psychotherapists, crisis interveners, and untrained individuals, Ryden, McCarthy, Lewis, and Sherman (1991) found that undergraduate junior nursing students were similar to trained psychotherapists in their use of statements reflecting affect and content—in other words, empathic listening.

INTERVENTION

Active listening requires the receiver to be exquisitely tuned to the sender—to vibrate on the same frequency. The metalanguage communicated through the nuances of tone, fleeting facial expressions, hesitancies over words, silences, and telling body language may escape the casual listener. To really *hear* the content of the spoken message takes concentration and an ability to differentiate between what is *actually* said and what one *wants or expects* to hear. If the time and energy of a receiver is focused on planning a response to what is being said, a message may only partially be heard. The active listener is wholly focused on trying to determine what the client is really saying, recognizing themes and patterns, and hearing what is left unsaid. Active listening can be hard work. After listening to some clients, you may feel as exhausted as you do when travelling abroad, where you try to make sense of communications in a language that is foreign to you. With other clients, it may not be so much the challenge of the task of interpreting unclear messages as a problem in really "hearing" the messages of clients you find difficult to relate to (Egan, 1986). It is difficult to listen to what you don't want to hear (Kelly, 1984).

Technique

Since the brain is capable of processing information much more rapidly than the rate at which the average person talks (which approximates 150 words per minute) the listener is left with free brain time (Davis, 1984). Often this allows the receiver to become distracted, or to focus attention on what to say in response, rather than concentrating totally on the other person in an attempt to fully understand the messages and the metamessages being communicated.

Active listening requires at least three different skills: 1) skill in interpreting the verbal and nonverbal messages from the client; 2) skill in assisting the client to communicate a message more clearly; and 3) skill in communicating to a client your understanding of her/his verbal and nonverbal messages.

Being able to really *hear* (observe and listen) and to *read* (interpret the meaning of what you hear) a client message is essential to understanding. Frequently the jumbled turmoil of thoughts experienced by persons under stress is expressed in communication that lacks clarity. The receiver's difficulty in decoding such a message may reflect the sender's own lack of self-understanding. Therefore, the external feedback from a skilled active listener which helps a client to communicate more clearly to others also can be a direct means of helping clarify his/her own thinking. This "sounding board" effect can be achieved by reflecting the essence of what you have understood the client to say, by asking for elaboration, by encouraging specificity and concreteness in place of vague, global statements, and by pointing out discrepancies in communication.

Measurement of Effectiveness

Outcomes of listening as a nursing intervention have not been scientifically measured. Instruments that have been designed to measure the psychosocial constructs of trust, rapport, and client satisfaction offer possible methods of evaluating the effectiveness of listening. Physiologically based indicators of healing and traditional health care indices such as length of stay are other variables whose sensitivity of response to a listening intervention warrant testing.

USES

The purpose of active listening is for the client to better understand self and to experience being understood by another caring person. This experience is likely to lead to a number of positive consequences.

First, energy, which previously was channeled into abortive attempts to be understood, may be released for healing, problem solving, and other priorities of the client. Orlando, in her classic text on the nurse-patient relationship (1961:23), points out that patients frequently are unable to communicate their needs clearly. The responsibility of nurses to prevent depletion of energy resources by eliminating not only physiological but also psychological energy wasters is described by Miller (1983).

Second, trust is enhanced as the client perceives the nurse as someone who cares enough to try to genuinely hear and understand. Bok has said, "*Whatever* matters to human beings, trust is the atmosphere in which it thrives" (1978:31). Experiencing being truly heard is a nourishing experience for the client. Being understood can enable the other to open his/her world and allow the nurse to enter, so she/he can know "whatever matters," and be present as a resource.

A third possible consequence is increased self-understanding, which may empower a client to greater autonomy and independence in health care concerns (Greenberg & Kahn, 1979). The goal of nursing is not to create a continuing need for nursing care by the client, nor to paternalistically make decisions in his/her best interest. Through active listening a client may come to understand self and his/her situation more clearly even though the nurse may only partially comprehend. Such self-knowledge may contribute to self-efficacy (Bandura, 1982), and enable the client to act more independently and authentically to achieve goals or, if physically dependent, may make it possible to be self-determining by directing others to take action on his/her behalf.

A final consequence of listening is a clearer grasp by the nurse of the client's perception of the situation. This provides the nurse with a valid data base to use in determining what health-related goals should have priority and what subsequent interventions might offer the greatest probability of helping the client achieve those goals. This understanding by the nurse can allow for collaborative efforts with the client who can then be an agent for his/her own health.

Precautions

There is a need for a willingness to acknowledge one's limitations. Being a good listener is not equivalent to having the advanced practice knowledge and skills that are requisite for the role of psychotherapist. Knowing when to seek help or refer a client to other health care professionals is essential.

In studies by Ford (1981) and Larson (1984), nurses identified listening as the behavior most representative of their caring for clients. However, rankings of nurses' caring behavior that were made by persons with cancer in Larson's study (1984) showed that clients ranked *competency* behaviors higher than *listening* behaviors as indicative of caring. While listening can at times be *the* independent nursing intervention of choice, more often it has its value as the medium through which direct, hands-on nursing care is given. Listening cannot be a substitute for expertise in other aspects of nursing, but, as Benner (1984) describes, it is an integral part of the professional's development from novice to expert.

RESEARCH QUESTIONS

Within nursing there appears to be such a strong belief in the intrinsic merit of listening that attempts to carry out a controlled study in which a group of clients was deliberately *not* listened to probably would be considered unethical. However, studies of the outcomes of an "enriched" intervention of listening might provide answers to the following questions:

1. What psychological and physiological client behaviors are affected by use of listening as a carefully designed nursing intervention?
2. How do the variables of the time, frequency, and duration of a listening intervention influence client outcomes?
3. Does the effectiveness of listening as a nursing intervention differ for client groups with specific characteristics?
4. To what extent is client satisfaction with health care affected when listening is used as a nursing intervention?

REFERENCES

Arnold, E., & Boggs, K. (1989). *Interpersonal relationships: Professional communication skills for nurses.* Philadelphia: W.B. Saunders.

Bandura, A. (1982). Self-efficacy mechanism in human agency. *American Psychologist* 37:122–147.

Benner, P. (1984). *From novice to expert: Excellence and power in clinical nursing practice.* Menlo Park, CA: Addison-Wesley.

Birdwhistell, R. (1970). *Kinesics and context.* Philadelphia: University of Pennsylvania Press.

Bok, S. (1978). *Lying.* New York: Pantheon Books.

Burnard, P. (1987). Spiritual distress and the nursing response: Theoretical considerations and counselling skills. *Journal of Advanced Nursing* 12(3):377–382.

Cartwright, R.D., & Lerner, B. (1966). Empathy, need to change, and improvement in psychotherapy. Pp. 537–545 in G.E. Stollak, B.G. Guerney, Jr., & M. Rothberg eds., *Psychotherapy research: Selected readings.* Chicago: Rand McNally.

Daniels, T.G., Denny, A., & Andrews, D. (1988). Using microcounseling to teach RN nursing students skills of therapeutic communication. *Journal of Nursing Education* 27(6):246–252.

Davis, A.J. (1984). *Listening and responding.* St. Louis: C.V. Mosby.

Egan, G. (1986). *The skilled helper,* 3rd ed. Monterey, CA: Brooks/Cole Publishing.

Ekman, P. (1972). Universal and cultural differences in facial expression of emotion. In J.K. Cole ed., *Nebraska symposium on motivation.* Lincoln, NE: University of Nebraska Press.

Ekman, P., & Friesen, W.V. (1969). The repertoire of nonverbal behavior: Categories, origin, usage and coding. *Semiotica* 1:49–98.

_____. (1971). Constants across cultures in the face and emotion. *Journal of Personality and Social Psychology* 17(2):124–129.

Ford, M. (1981). Nurse professionals and the caring process. *Dissertation Abstracts International* 43:967B–968B. (University Microfilms No. 81-19278).

Friedrich, R.M., Lively, S.I., & Schacht, E. (1985). Teaching communication skills in an integrated curriculum. *Journal of Nursing Education* 24(4):164-166.

Gerrard, B.A., Boniface, W.J., & Love, B.H. (1980). *Interpersonal skills for health professionals.* Reston, VA: Reston.

Greenberg, L.S., & Kahn, S.E. (1979). The stimulation phase in counseling. *Counselor Education and Supervision* 19:137-145.

Hardin, S.B., & Halaris, A.L. (1983). Nonverbal communication of patients and high and low empathy nurses. *Journal of Psychosocial Nursing and Mental Health Services* 21(1):14-20.

Kelly, C.H. (1984). Listen to what you don't want to hear. *Geriatric Nursing* 5(2):83.

Lamonica, E.L., Carew, D.K., Winder, A.E., Haase, A.M.B., & Blanchard, K. (1976). Empathy training as the major thrust of a staff development program. *Nursing Research* 25(6):447-450.

Larson, P.J. (1984). Important nurse caring behaviors perceived by patients with cancer. *Oncology Nursing Forum* 11(6):46-50.

Layton, J.M. (1979). Use of modelling to teach empathy. *Research in Nursing and Health* 2:163-176.

Magnan, M.A., & Benner, P. (1989). Listening with care. *American Journal of Nursing* 89(2):219-221.

Margulies, A. (1984). Toward empathy: The uses of wonder. *American Journal of Psychiatry* 14(9):1025-1033.

Mehrabian, A. (1971). *Silent messages.* Belmont, CA: Wadsworth.

Miller, J.F. (1983). *Coping with chronic illness: Overcoming powerlessness.* Philadelphia: F.A. Davis.

Mullen, J., & Abeles, N. (1971). Relationship of liking, empathy and therapist's experience to outcome of therapy. *Journal of Counseling Psychology* 18(1):39-43.

Norris, J. (1986). Teaching communication skills: Effects of two methods of instruction and selected learner characteristics. *Journal of Nursing Education* 25(3):102-106.

Olson, J.K., & Iwasiw, C.L. (1987). Effects of a training model on active listening skills of post-RN students. *Journal of Nursing Education* 26(3):104-107.

Orlando, I.J. (1961). *The dynamic nurse-patient relationship.* New York: G.P. Putnam's Sons.

Rogers, C.R. (1957). The necessary and sufficient conditions of therapeutic personality change. *Journal of Consulting Psychology* 21:95-103.

_____. (1975). Empathic: An unappreciated way of being. *Counseling Psychologist* 5:2-10.

Rogers, C.R., Gendlin, E.T., Kiesler, D.J., & Truax, C.B. (eds.) (1967). *The therapeutic relationship and its impact. A study of psychotherapy with schizophrenics.* Madison, WI: University of Wisconsin Press.

Rowan, J. (1986). Holistic listening. *Journal of Humanistic Psychology* 26(1):83-102.

Ryden, M.B., McCarthy, P.R., Lewis, M.L., & Sherman, C. (1991). A behavioral comparison of the helping styles of nursing students, psychotherapists, crisis interveners, and untrained individuals. *Annals of Psychiatric Nursing* 5(3):1-4.

Travelbee, J. (1966). *Interpersonal aspects of nursing.* Philadelphia: F.A. Davis.

Truax, C.B., & Carkhuff, R.R. (1967). *Toward effective counseling and psychotherapy.* Chicago: Aldine Publishing.

Ujhely, G. (1968). *Determinants of the nurse-patient relationship.* New York: Springer Publishing.

Webster's New Twentieth Century Dictionary. Unabridged. (1983). (2nd ed.) New York: Prentice Hall Press.

CHAPTER 33

PRAYER

Marilyne Gustafson, PhD, RN

BACKGROUND

Prayer is an intimate conversation or dialog between an individual and God or a higher being. It is a practice common to all faiths and practiced by persons in practically all societies. In addition to the importance as an element in all organized religions, prayer is one of the oldest forms of healing therapies. For patients, prayer is a potential resource to meet spiritual needs, an activity often used as a spiritual coping strategy.

Spiritual needs of clients have begun to be addressed in the nursing literature. The nursing diagnosis of "spiritual distress" as well as research on spiritual well-being and spiritual needs provide the nurse with information on which to build an approach to the consideration of prayer as an independent nursing intervention.

Definition

Prayer is defined as a solemn and humble approach to Divinity in word or thought usually involving petition, beseeching, supplication, confession, praise, and thanksgiving. In the conversation or dialog with Divinity (or the Almighty or God), there is often the concept of communion or relationship. Relationship is central to many people. Further, this is often described as giving meaning or perspective to life as well as affirmation of the presence and power of God.

Prayer is viewed by many as a natural and necessary result of the spiritual aspect of humankind (Carson, 1989; Fish & Shelly, 1987). Thus, it is viewed as a source of strength to the person and thereby as a positive coping strategy which supports individuals when they are ill (Sodestrom & Martinson, 1987). Another definition of prayer is that it is a set form of words, such as a formula for supplication addressed to God or the object of worship; an example of this is a prayer book.

This chapter will provide a nursing framework in which to view prayer as spiritual support that respects the diversity of belief systems and cultural aspects of individuals. This will assist the nurse as an independent intervenor and/or collaborator with the patient, the family, and others concerned with spiritual needs. Although research studies will be used to document pertinent findings in this area of study, a principle of importance is that "the value of prayers or spiritual rituals to the believer is not affected by whether or not they can be scientifically 'proved' to be beneficial" (Carpenito, 1983:453). Prayer is a practice common to all faiths, however faith is highly personal and generally not examined scientifically. Scientific findings and concepts regarding faith are used to assist the nurse in becoming informed and more comfortable in addressing spiritual needs. Appropriate assessment of spiritual needs, including religious needs and practices, can lead to the promotion, maintenance, and restoration of spiritual wholeness.

Scientific Basis

Prayer, which can be used as a coping strategy to meet spiritual needs, has begun to be studied by nurses. The Stallwood-Stoll model is a conceptual model of the nature of human beings that includes the spiritual component. The spiritual or transcendent component is viewed as distinct from the biophysical and psychosocial components. The authors believe that nursing reflects an awareness that a human being is not simply a biological organism but also a psychosocial and spiritual being. Religion is the institutionalized form of spiritual needs and thus comes under the larger component of spirituality. Spiritual needs are defined as any factors necessary to establish and maintain a person's dynamic personal relationship with God, as defined by that individual. Stallwood and Stoll (1979), stated that each person has a basic need for this relationship by experiencing forgiveness, love, hope, trust, and meaning and purpose in life.

Prayer, in nursing texts, is included under spiritual care (Fish & Shelly, 1987; Shelly, 1982) and spiritual dimensions of nursing practice (Carson, 1989). Numerous journal articles suggest prayer as an effective intervention for a variety of situations and patient populations (Carson & Huss, 1979; Piles, 1990; Stoll, 1979).

The need for prayer was the most frequent response in a study by Hess (cited in Shelly, 1982) to the question "Were you aware of having a spiritual need at any time during your hospitalization?" The patients responses centered around the need to pray personally, to be prayed for, or to pray with another person. Direct statements by the patients included: "I can't pray, my prayers aren't heard"; "I couldn't have gotten along without prayer"; "I prayed constantly because I was sure I was dying" (p. 158).

Spiritual Distress is a nursing diagnosis approved by the North American Nursing Diagnosis Association. In 1973 the category was termed "Alteration in Faith in God." In 1978 it was changed to three categories of spirituality: spiritual concern, spiritual distress, and spiritual despair. In 1980, the Fourth National Conference changed it to spiritual distress. In addition, many others (Carson, 1989; Fish & Shelly, 1987; Messner & Ward, 1989) concur with use of the diagnosis. Spiritual distress is defined as distress of the human spirit—a disruption in the life principle which pervades a person's entire being and which integrates and transcends one's biological and psychosocial nature (Kim et al., 1987). The defining characteristics include those of being unable to participate in usual religious practice, such as praying oneself, meeting to pray with others, and finding others to pray for or with the patient. Discussing principles and rationale for the diagnosis of spiritual distress, Carpenito (1983) states that the value of prayers to the believer is not affected by whether or not they can be scientifically "proved" to be beneficial.

INTERVENTION

The need for a research base for nursing practice is no less important in the use of prayer as an intervention. Research, which includes a study of prayer, is found in the area of the spiritual dimension and is often seen in relationship to several terms such as spirituality, spiritual needs, and spiritual distress. The use of research instruments and good assessment will provide important data on which to plan an appropriate nursing intervention. Ellerhorst-Ryan (1988) reviewed research instruments dealing with spirituality. Moberg, a sociologist, pioneered some of the early work focused on religiosity and spiritual well-being (SWB). Moberg worked with the White House Conference on Aging and has written extensively on religiosity, spirituality, SWB, and the elderly. In Moberg's Indexes of Spiritual Well-Being (1979), one of the questions is "How often do you pray privately?" The spiritual well-being scale developed by Ellison (1983) is a 20-item Likert scale that is less lengthy than the Moberg Index. One of the items is, "I don't find much satisfaction in private prayer with God." Both the Moberg Index and the Ellison and Paloutzian scale have been used in several nursing studies. Stoll, a nurse author, used the Ellison and Paloutzian scale in her research and from that she suggested 13 questions and guidelines specific to the roles of prayer to be used for spiritual assessment (Stoll, 1979).

Carson (1989), Fish and Shelly (1987), and Stoll (1979) all emphasize the need for assessment data to determine the patient's beliefs and values regarding prayer. One of Stoll's questions is, "Has being sick made any difference in your practice of praying?" Carson (1989) suggests observations on nonverbal behavior, "Does the client pray during the day?" and verbal behavior, "Does the client talk about prayer, hope...?" to determine the value of prayer in a patient's life. Since prayer can be very private, the nurse may not be aware of behavioral changes resulting from prayer.

Carpenito (1983) indicates that spiritual distress is related to the inability to practice spiritual rituals. Objective data to support this might be that the patient is unable to say prayers or meditate or cannot assume a normal position for prayer or meditation. Before intervening she suggests assessing causative and contributing factors and limitations related to disease process or treatment regimen (e.g. cannot kneel to pray due to traction, cannot vocalize prayers due to laryngectomy).

Carson (1989) provided four guidelines about prayer for the nurse:

1. Prayer or any spiritual intervention is *never* used out of intuition but follows a careful assessment that reveals the presence of a spiritual need.
2. Prayer is *never* to be used as an activity or substitute for the nurse's time and presence with the client.
3. Prayer is *never* used to meet the nurse's needs but only to facilitate the client's relationship with God.
4. Prayer is not used to communicate a magical view of God that conveys a false sense of hope and expectation. [p. 169]

The Chadwich study (cited in Fish & Shelly, 1987) refers to the awareness and preparedness of nurses to meet spiritual needs. It showed that 75% of the nurses surveyed reported they would feel comfortable either reading the Bible or praying with a patient, but 50% of them had never read the Bible or prayed with a patient. The comfort of the nurse in utilizing this intervention is critical. The nurse planning to use prayer as an intervention will do well to assess the appropriateness of prayer in a given situation by asking if it is meeting the patient's need or her own needs. If it is the latter, it would be better for the nurse to pray privately and not assume this reflects a therapeutic use of self. Thoughtful assessment and concern for the client's needs must be paramount. A difference in religious faiths between the client and nurse is discussed in the section on precautions.

Technique

Prayer may be conversational, spontaneous, silent, spoken, formal, written, memorized, or other forms. Aspects of petition, request, or praise may be included. Prayer may also be part of a ritual and/or related to objects such as a prayer book or a rosary. The patients' wishes regarding prayer need to be ascertained and respected, since the purpose of prayer is to help them in their relationship to God, as they perceive God. Therefore, the form which the prayer takes is not what is important but rather the relationship that is involved. Further, prayer should be viewed as providing strength and peace and not as increasing anxiety or offending the person.

The most appreciated prayers are usually simple, informal expressions of the patient's spiritual needs, hopes, and fears to God and a recognition of God's power. For those accustomed to using more formal prayers, spontaneous prayers may seem disrespectful. In the Christian tradition, the Lord's Prayer is familiar and meaningful to many. Children may have memorized table and/or bedtime prayers which are familiar to them. Roman Catholic patients may appreciate having a nurse of the same faith pray the rosary with them. For Jewish patients, prayers to the God of Abraham, Isaac, and Moses are appropriate.

Luna (1989) described the prayer needs of Arab-Muslims. She suggests that elderly Arab-Muslims place great importance on the performance of obligatory prayer along with the ritual cleansing or ablutions which are required according to Islamic tradition. The nurse would assess the client's wishes regarding prayer and the desired frequency. If prayer is desired, the nurse could use the intervention mode of cultural care accommodation by providing a basin of water and/or finding a quiet place for the client to carry out the ritual. For many Arab-Muslims, observing and performing the religious obligation of prayer is an important cultural expression for maintaining health and preventing illness.

Timing and When to Pray

When the nurse prays with a patient and the timing of the prayer are important. Suggestions from Fish and Shelly (1987) include:

1. Adequate communication in the relationship exists.
2. Clarity about the patient's concern (high anxiety, statements about being separated from the faith or worship community) has been indicated.
3. Prayer is not seen as a way of ending a conversation.

The idea of referring the patient to the clergy is deliberately omitted from this discussion, but at times it may be most appropriate to refer the client. However, too often referral to the clergy has been the immediate and first approach used by nurses without the nurse giving consideration to the use of prayer as a nursing intervention. This does not mean that the nurse should ignore an opportunity to join clergy persons in a group time of prayer (Saylor, 1972).

Measurement of Effectiveness

As stated in the section on the scientific basis, the subjective nature of one's beliefs and faith make finding instruments to measure spiritual distress and the effectiveness of the intervention of prayer difficult but not impossible. The purpose for which the prayer was made will dictate effectiveness to the patient; however, some measures which have been reported have been increased peace or peacefulness, decreased anxiety and less feeling of anger, an increased sense of well-being, and a more positive outlook about life changes (Carson, 1989).

USES

The universalness of prayer needs no further documentation. The general uses of prayer apply to many age groups and many nursing and medical diagnoses. Carpenito (1983) states that "an individual is a spiritual person even when disoriented, confused, emotionally ill, delirious, or cognitively impaired" (p. 452). In a study of stress identification and coping patterns in patients with hemodialysis, Baldree et al. (1982) found that praying was a commonly acknowledged coping strategy. Sodestrom and Martinson (1987) studied patients with cancer and reported that the most frequently used coping strategies were personal prayer and asking others to pray for them. Bearson and Koening (1990) asked 40 adults (ages 65–74) about God's role in health and illness and their use of prayer in response to recent physical symptoms. Most held a belief in a benevolent God but were not clear about God's role in health and illness and over one-half had prayed about at least one physical symptom. Symptoms discussed with a physician or for which drugs were taken were more likely to be prayed about than were other symptoms, suggesting that prayer may be used for symptoms seen as serious. It was further suggested that the use of prayer and seeking medical help were not mutually exclusive.

Referring to the use of prayer for patients with psychiatric and mental health needs, Carson (1980, 1989) and Shelly et al. (1983) suggest that prayer is appropriate with this group of patients. In a study by Carson and Huss (1979), major changes occurred in clients. Increased abilities to express feelings of anger and frustration and to have a more positive outlook about possible changes in their lives, and a decrease in somatic complaints occurred.

Prayer is an appropriate intervention for patients with chronic illness. Referring to chronic illness as a long, unpredictable, and uncertain journey unique to each person, Stoll (cited in Carson, 1989) includes prayer as one of the five practical coping strategies. Prayer was found to be helpful to patients on hemodialysis (Baldree et al., 1982). Populations for whom prayer has been used are found in Table 33.1.

Table 33.1
Uses of Prayer

Cancer	(Sodestrom & Martinson, 1987)
Children	(Betz, 1981; Carson, 1989; Foster et al., 1989; Shelly, 1982)
Chronic illness	(Baldree et al., 1982; Carson, 1989)
Community settings	(Burkhardt & Nagei-Jacobson, 1985)
Coronary care units	(Byrd, 1988)
Death	(Carson, 1989)
Dying	(Amenta, 1986; Carson, 1989)
Elderly	(Bearon & Koening, 1990; Carson, 1989; Moberg, 1979)
Healing	(Shlemon, 1976)

Precautions

Although prayer may be a very natural activity for both the patient and the nurse, it may be viewed by the patient as an unusual activity for the nurse in which to engage.

Because of the highly personal nature of faith, spirituality, religious beliefs, and practices, the nurse must assess the patient's need for prayer as well as her own beliefs and comfort in using this nursing intervention. Carpenito (1983) states that in order to assist people in spiritual distress, the nurse must know certain beliefs and practices of the various spiritual groups found in this country. Carson (1989) and Carpenito (1983) provide excellent observations that capture the essence of the beliefs and practices of many faiths. Knowledge about other faiths/religions is becoming more imperative in a culturally pluralistic society. Prayer used improperly may offend, increase anxiety, or be a threat when it reawakens anger or painfully negative, self-deprecating memories. Again, if it has been used to meet the nurse's and not the patient's need, it is inappropriate.

The nurse should be prepared to have a patient request a prayer that the nurse may view as manipulating God or being magical. The wise nurse must consider her own beliefs about requests that raise questions in her mind. Prayers for healing and for what might be considered "impossible" or miraculous are examples of possible requests which the nurse needs to thoughtfully consider before intervening.

RESEARCH QUESTIONS

The majority of the books and articles on the use of prayer are written from a Judeo-Christian perspective. Many of the instruments used by nurses have originated in sociology and psychology and do not necessarily reflect a nursing perspective. Nurses have studied prayer in their investigations of spirituality. However, the area of spirituality, spiritual needs, and prayer as a coping strategy is just beginning to be studied in nursing.

The following are questions which could contribute to improved use of prayer as a nursing intervention:

1. Evaluating and adapting instruments (from other disciplines) to measure the use of prayer as a nursing intervention are needed.
2. Examining the relationship of spiritual diagnoses indicators (such as defining characteristics) to the use of prayer as an intervention is needed.
3. What are factors that help or hinder nurses in the process of cooperating with patients in the use of prayer?

4. Examining the various aspects of cross-cultural significance of prayer to its use as an intervention is needed since most studies that have been conducted have been done from a Judeo-Christian perspective.

REFERENCES

Amenta, M., & Bohet, N. (eds.) (1986). Spiritual concerns. Pp. 115–161 in *Nursing care of the terminally ill.* Boston: Little Brown and Co.

Baldree, K., Murphy, S., & Powers, M. (1982). Stress identification and coping patterns in patients on hemodialysis. *Nursing Research* 31:107–112.

Bearon, L., & Koening, H. (1990). Religious cognitions and use of prayer in health & illness. *The Gerontologist* 30:249–253.

Betz, C. (1981). Faith development in children. *Pediatric Nursing* 7(2):36–41.

Burkhardt, M., & Nagei-Jacobson, M. (1985). Dealing with spiritual concerns of clients in the community. *Journal of Community Health Nursing* 2:191–198.

Byrd, R. (1988). Positive therapeutic effects of intercessory prayer in a coronary care unit population. *Southern Medical Journal* 81:826–829.

Carpenito, L. (1983). *Nursing diagnosis: Application to clinical practice.* Philadelphia: Lippincott.

Carson, V. (1980). Meeting the spiritual needs of hospitalized psychiatric patients. *Perspectives in Psychiatric Care* 18:17–20.

_____. (1989). *Spiritual dimensions of nursing practice.* Philadelphia: W.B. Saunders.

Carson, V., & Huss, K. (1979). Prayer — an effective therapeutic teaching tool. *Journal of Psychiatric Nursing and Mental Health Services* 17:34–27.

Ellerhorst-Ryan, J. (1988). Measuring aspects of spirituality. Pp. 141–149 in M. Frank-Stromberg ed., *Instruments for clinical nursing research.* Norwalk, CT: Appleton & Lange.

Ellison, C. (1983). Spiritual well-being: conceptualization and measurement. *Journal of Psychology and Theology* 11:330–340.

Fish, S., & Shelly, J. (1987). *Spiritual care: The nurse's role.* Downers Grove, IL: InterVarsity Press.

Foster, R., Hunsberger, M., & Anderson, J. (1989). *Family centered nursing care of children.* Philadelphia: W.B. Saunders.

Kim, M., McFarland, G., & McLane, A. (1987). *Pocket guide to nursing diagnosis.* St. Louis, MO: C.V. Mosby.

Luna, L. (1989). Transcultural nursing care of arab-muslims. *Journal of Transcultural Nursing* 1:22–26.

Messner, R., & Ward, D. (1989). The patient with a spiritual need. Pp. 259–269 in S. Lewis, R. Grainger, W. McDowell, R. Gregory, & R. Messner eds., *Manual of psychosocial nursing interventions, promoting mental health in medical-surgical settings.* Philadelphia: W.B. Saunders.

Moberg, D. (1979). The development of social indicators of spiritual well-being for quality of life research. Pp. 4–6 in D. Moberg ed., *Spiritual well-being sociological perspectives.* Washington, DC: University Press of America.

Piles, C. (1990). Providing spiritual care. *Nurse Educator* 15:36–41.

Saylor, D. (1972). Let us: Pray, work together. *Nursing '72* 2:5.

Shelly, J. (1982). *The spiritual needs of children.* Downers Grove, IL: InterVarsity Press.

Shelly, J., John, S., and others. (1983). *Spiritual dimensions of mental health.* Downers Grove, IL: InterVarsity Press.

Shlemon, B. (1976). *Healing prayer.* Notre Dame, IN: Ave Maria Press.

Sodestrom, K., & Martinson, I. (1987). Patient's spiritual coping strategies: A study of nurse and patient perspectives. *Oncology Nursing Forum* 14:41–46.

Stallwood, J., & Stoll, R. (1975). Spiritual dimensions of nursing practice. Pp. 1086–1093 in I. Beland & J. Possos eds., *Clinical nursing.* New York: MacMillan.

Stoll, R. (1979). Guidelines for spiritual assessment. *American Journal of Nursing* 79:1574–1577.

____. (1989). Spirituality and chronic illness. Pp. 180–216 in V. Carson ed., *Spiritual dimensions of nursing practice.* Philadelphia. W.B. Saunders.

CHAPTER 34

PLAY

BACKGROUND

Play, as a nursing intervention, can be conceptualized in several ways depending on the definition of play selected. Play itself can be the end, just enjoyment, or playful activities can be used to accomplish designated goals. The latter context is often termed play or recreational therapy. Play therapy has been used most frequently with pediatric populations. Recreational therapy is the term more often used when referring to activities for adults. This is due to the fact that our Western culture perceives play as frivolous and childish (Vandenberg & Kielhofner, 1982).

This chapter will focus on the use of play to achieve patient goals. However, teaching persons the importance of incorporating play (recreation, leisure) into their lives also has tremendous value. The serious effects that workaholic habits have on an individual's health are receiving considerable attention in our society. Too often the golf game, tennis match, or concert are only extensions of the person's work life and are not engaged in for the purpose of escape or enjoyment. The author bought a figurine of a little girl jumping rope to remind her of the need to pursue playful activities. Teaching persons about the value of leisure and playful activities is an important nursing activity (Johnson et al., 1989).

Definition

Play is a difficult term to define because it is used in many contexts and interchangeably with other terms. Fantasy, sports, recreation, leisure time activities, and games are terms that are either considered as subsets of play, other terms for play, or closely related entities. A differentiation of these terms will not be made; broader, general descriptions of play will be provided.

Huizinga (1979), a Dutch historian, delineated some of the fundamental characteristics of play:

> Summing up the formal characteristics of play we might call it a free activity standing quite consciously outside "ordinary" life as being "not serious," but at the same time absorbing the player intensely and utterly. It is an activity connected with no material interest, and no profit can be gained by it. It proceeds within its own proper boundaries of time and space according to fixed rules and in an orderly manner. [p.13]

Schmitz (1979) viewed play in a similar fashion. He stated that the world of play transcends the natural world and the world of everyday concerns. Play begins by abandoning the forms of everyday behaviors and immersing oneself into a space and time that are not continuous with usual space and time. According to Schmitz, play can be categorized into four types:

Frolic: This is less formal, usually spontaneous, intense, and brief in nature, and often termed "horsing around."

Make-believe: This category epitomizes creativity and inventiveness; daydreaming and costume parties are activities in this group.

Sporting skills: This is a more formal type of play and requires knowledge, skill, and endurance.

Games: These are very formal with set rules requiring mastery of a skill; games are also termed contests.

The Chinese have no single word for play, but a commonly used word is "wan." It is used to signify to be busy, to enjoy something, to trifle, to romp, to jest, to make jokes, to finger, to feel, to twiddle ornaments, and to enjoy the moonlight. Wan does not encompass the idea of competition; thus sports and games would be excluded from this definition. To many Americans, these defining characteristics would be classified as wasting time. Mannell and McMahon (1982) noted that forms of play often fill brief time periods throughout one's day and need not be viewed as separate and distinct activities. Many of the activities in the Chinese definition can be interspersed throughout one's daily life and can contribute greatly to the quality of the person's life (Csikszentmihalyi, 1975).

Play or recreational therapy focuses on the use of specific modalities to achieve specified goals. The purpose is for the person to have fun in accomplishing the goal. Bost and Brown (1982) defined therapeutic recreation as:

> A process which utilizes recreation services for purposive intervention in some physical, emotional, and/or social behavior to bring about a desired change in that behavior and to promote the growth and development of the individual. [p. 45]

This definition is similar to the one used in play therapy for pediatric populations. It serves as the basis for the interventions presented in this chapter.

Scientific Basis

Play provides human beings with a sense of joy (Fink, 1979). It rejuvenates one's inner vitality. Escaping the here and now via play provides persons with a sense of freedom. Play is something within one's control. One cannot be forced to play. While the forced activity may have the appearance of play, it is not play. Schmitz (1979) viewed play as transcending the natural world and the world of everyday concerns. Fantasy reveals the human capacity to go beyond the empirical world of the here and now. Ability to fantasize is needed for survival (Cox, 1969). Play is intrinsically complete and contains its own rewards (Csikszentmihalyi, 1975).

Developmental psychologists have examined the role play serves in human development. Erikson (1950) described play as a function of the ego and as a means to synchronize one's physical and social processes. According to Vandenberg and Kielhofner (1982), play contributes to the acquisition of skill in tool use, language, and culturally derived social skills.

Numerous studies, particularly studies by the Harlows, have explored animal play. The Harlows (1962) found that social play of young animals was intimately associated with their physical growth and the stages of maternal affection. Young monkeys who do not have the opportunity to engage in play become incompetent adult monkeys (Harlow & Harlow, 1962). Einon (1980) reported that rats who did not play were poorer problem solvers and adapted more poorly to new situations than ones who participated in play activities.

Three propositions related to play were proposed by Vandenberg and Kielhofner (1982):

1. Play is a process that produces new behavior forms.
2. Human beings have evolved so that their makeup requires play for them to function properly.
3. Play generates contexts in which new behaviors can be tried out and practiced without fear of judgment.

Play helps to decrease anxiety and tension, allowing the person's creative capabilities to emerge. Just to be busy is not play; one must be enjoying the activity whether it be playing cards, engaging in a tennis match, watching television, or daydreaming.

Play therapy takes enjoyable activities and uses them to achieve specific outcomes. Bost and Brown (1982) initiated a recreational therapy program on an oncology unit for the purpose of enhancing the general well-being of patients and families and helping them to adapt to the changes precipitated by cancer. Millar (1974) noted that Freud recommended the use of play as a mode to help persons overcome fears. Persons can make choices about pleasant activities in which they wish to participate, thus lessening feelings of dependency. Other outcomes of play therapy include finding constructive outlets for emotions, alleviating boredom, providing opportunities for social interaction, and improving self-esteem (Bost & Brown, 1982). Playful activities can be used in teaching; these often decrease anxiety and lessen inhibitions, producing a more conducive learning environment. Play is holistic; playful activities allow the person to integrate cognitive, physical, spiritual, and social realms (Kolkmeier, 1988).

INTERVENTION

Numerous activities are suitable for use as modalities in play therapy. Creativity and inventiveness suggest modalities that have not been used previously and that may be beneficial. Table 34.1 lists only some of the possible activities that can be used. Selection of the specific activity for a patient is determined by the interests of the patient, the purpose of the activity, and the capabilities of the nurse. Three activities—art, poetry, and puppets—will be detailed.

Technique

Art

A variety of art forms can be utilized for play therapy. Smith and Glickstein (1982) noted that art media allow for the expression of internal states; persons can play, ventilate, explore, and experience themselves in new ways. Collages of pictures allow patients to display their feelings, interests, or goals. Clay is a good medium to use with hyperactive patients as it consumes energy; more gross movements are used so the person does not become frustrated with minutae. Drawing and painting are pleasant activities that provide the opportunity for persons to express their emotions. Felt tip pens and crayolas allow for expression of

Table 34.1
Modalities for Use in Play Therapy

Art	(Rhyme, 1976; Smith & Glickstein, 1982)
Bibliotherapy	(Cohen, 1988)
Collage	(Beard et al., 1978)
Games	(Csikszentmihalyi, 1975)
Gardening-horitherapy	(Riordan, 1983)
Nature walks	(Bost & Brown, 1982)
Painting	(Beard et al., 1978)
Photography	(Beard et al., 1978)
Puppets	(Schuman et al., 1973)
Poetry	(Andrews, 1975; Potenza & Labbancz, 1989)
Serial drawing	(Nickerson & O'Laughlin, 1982)
Social dramatics	(Whetstone, 1986)

many types of feelings and ideas that a patient may or may not wish to share with others. The nature of the setting and the desired goals for the patient will influence the type of art form that is selected.

Poetry

Two techniques for using poetry were described in the literature: reading poetry to patients or having patients write poetry. Andrews (1975) chose reading poetry to patients with mental illnesses as a way to help patients express their feelings. After the poem is read, patients provide their responses. The metaphors that characterize poetry allow patients to transfer their emotions and express them without feeling threatened. Anthologies of poems provide a wide variety of selections from which to choose poems to read. Potenza and Labbancz (1989), in working with patients with dementia, had patients compose poems. This was done as a group project. The leader first read a poem; the participants were presented with a theme that served as the basis for the group composing a poem. For example, a color may serve as a stimulus for the participants; descriptors of the color or what the color means to them are elicited from the participants. The leader writes these words and phrases on a large easel and structures these so that they take the shape of a poem. When the group seems to have exhausted the words and phrases related to the particular topic, the poem is read aloud. Feedback from the group is elicited. Being involved in composing a poem provided cognitive stimulation to the participants in Potenza's and Labbancz's group. Writing poetry can also be done on an individual basis; this would be most appropriate for use with persons who are not cognitively impaired. Persons may or may not wish to share their poetry with others.

Puppets

Many persons may feel that the use of puppets is inappropriate for adult patient populations. However, the universal appeal of Kermit, Miss Piggy, and the other Muppets indicates that many adults are intrigued by these characterizations.

Hand puppets with varying facial expressions, of both sexes, and of different age groups have been used with psychiatric patients (Schuman et al., 1973). A wide variety of puppet characters are needed to meet the moods and interests of patients. If all puppets have a smiling face, it is difficult for patients to use these to express emotions such as fear and anxiety.

Schuman et al. used puppets to help patients acquire knowledge about themselves and to gain confidence in dealing with their feelings and judgments in a social context. Specifically, patients used the puppets to practice expressing negative feelings, asking for help from others, experimenting with different methods for dealing with problems, identifying ambivalent feelings, trying new behaviors, and expressing repressed emotions such as anger. Plots were developed for the patients to act out with the use of puppets. Patients were assigned to play specific characters depending on the experiences that would be most advantageous for that particular patient.

Closed-group sessions, one hour long, were used on a weekly basis; most groups met for 10 weeks. Schuman and colleagues noted that close guidance and direction from the group leader is needed for the sessions to be effective. Puppets could also be used on a one-to-one basis. Plots could be developed or the patient could be given the opportunity to use the puppets to freely express feelings and concerns.

Measurement of Effectiveness

The purpose for which play is used as an intervention dictates the criteria and methods used in evaluation. If promotion of health was the intended outcome, scales of well-being would be appropriate methods for measuring the success of play. Observations of social interaction and subjective reports may be used to measure improvement in psychosocial functioning. Decrease in anxiety is another purpose for which play is used. Scores on anxiety tests and observation of facial and body movements for expressions of anxiety would be appropriate for determining the effectiveness of the intervention. Because play has been used minimally by nurses with adult populations, determination of its efficacy is necessary.

Table 34.2
Uses of Play Therapy

Adapt to condition	(Bost & Brown, 1982)
Assessment	(Sheffer & Harlock, 1980)
Cognitive stimulation	(Mayer & Griffin, 1990; Potenza & Labbancz, 1989)
Decrease dependency	(Bost & Brown, 1982)
Express feelings	(Jack, 1987; Potenza & Labbancz, 1989)
Health promotion	(Mannell & McMahon, 1982; Rettie, 1976)
Improve social interaction	(Andrews, 1975; Beard et al., 1978; Schuman et al., 1973; Whetstone, 1986)
Improve communication	(Schuman et al., 1973)
Learn new behaviors	(Martin, 1978; Schuman et al., 1973)
Life review	(Wadeson, 1982)
Personal growth	(Rhyme, 1976)
Stroke rehabilitation	(Adsit & Lee, 1986)

USES

Play can be used with many patient populations. Table 34.2 lists conditions for which it has been used. The author hypothesizes that play therapy would be an appropriate intervention for additional patient problems that are in the domain of nursing. Two purposes for which play therapy has been used, improving psychosocial interaction and enhancing learning, will be discussed.

Improve Psychosocial Interaction

Vandenberg and Kielhofner (1982) provided the basis for the use of play for persons with psychosocial dysfunction and with physical disabilities. Rigidity and lack of flexibility are characteristics of persons who have difficulty interacting in social situations. Because social interactions demand reaction to unpredictable occurrences, flexibility is needed. Serok and Blum (1979) documented the lack of play in juvenile delinquents. Acquisition of playfulness may be very beneficial to persons who experience difficulties in psychosocial functioning.

Beard et al. (1978) used modalities such as finger painting, clay modeling, puzzles, touch and texture, and building activities to improve the social competence of chronically hospitalized psychiatric patients. Significant differences were found between the experimental and control groups on the NOSIE (Nurses' Observation Scale for Inpatient Evaluation) social competence scale.

Enhance Learning

Persons who have suffered problems resulting in physical disabilities have to acquire new skills in order to function adequately. Paap (cited in Vandenberg & Kielhofner, 1982) reported that patients who had spinal cord injuries needed ways to make their failures in rehabilitation seem less consequential. Playfulness was one mode suggested for handling these difficult experiences. Play is used by children to generate new meaning and behavior forms; it may serve this same purpose for adults who need to acquire new skills.

Playfulness helps to decrease anxiety and thus facilitates learning. Martin (1978) noted that empirical data demonstrate that fantasy play enlarges competencies basic for problem solving, concentration, verbal elaboration, and ability to organize and integrate diverse stimuli. Potenza and Labbancz (1989) used poetry for cognitive stimulation in persons with dementia. Teaching tasks after these sessions was not studied, but it would seem plausible that learning would be enhanced.

Precautions

Although play may seem like a benign intervention, certain cautions are necessary. A nurse who does not have a sense of playfulness would probably find it very difficult to use play as an intervention. Similarly, if staff on a unit are uninformed about the intervention, they will most likely not be supportive of it. Schuman et al. (1978) held an extensive orientation program for persons involved in directing puppet sessions.

Care is needed so that play is not used to avoid conflict or certain situations. Play may be beneficial in getting persons to discuss their condition. The problem can then be addressed without as much distress.

Smith and Glickstein (1982) recommended careful assessment of the client population, art activity, therapist's skills, and group's strength before using any particular art experience. This would be true for any modality selected. Careful planning, including groundwork, is important as play is often considered childish. Patients may believe that the intervention is condescending unless adequate explanations are provided.

RESEARCH QUESTIONS

Documentation on the use of play as a nursing intervention is minimal. Kolkmeier (1988) described the use of play interventions in relation to a number of nursing diagnoses. However, little research is available to substantiate these selections. The following are only a few of the countless research questions for which more information is desired:

1. When is it most advantageous to use play in a group session as opposed to implementing it on a one-to-one basis?
2. When are fantasy and other more passive forms of play more appropriate to use than active forms of play?
3. Jack (1987) states that a balance is needed between play and more complex treatment activities in the rehabilitation of patients with psychiatric conditions. More specificity on the degree of balance of these activities at particular times in the treatment trajectory is needed.
4. Minimal documentation exists on the effectiveness of play in decreasing anxiety, specifically in relation to learning. Testing of its effectiveness as an intervention for this purpose is needed.

REFERENCES

Adsit, P.A., & Lee, J. (1986). The use of art in stroke group therapy. *Rehabilitation Therapy* 11(5):18–19.

Andrews, M. (1975). Poetry programs in mental hospitals. *Perspectives in Psychiatric Care* 13:17–18.

Beard, M., Enelow, C., & Owens, B. (1978). Activity therapy as a reconstructive plan on the social competence of chronic hospitalized patients. *Journal of Psychiatric Nursing and Mental Health Services* 16(2):33–41.

Bost, L., & Brown, E. (1982). Recreation therapy: A humanistic adjunct to oncology treatment. *Oncology Nursing Forum* 9(3):45–49.

Cohen, L.J. (1988). Bibliotherapy. *Journal of Psychosocial Nursing* 26(8):7–12.

Cox, H. (1969). *The feast of fools.* Cambridge, MA: Harvard University Press.

Csikszentmihalyi, M. (1975). Play and intrinsic rewards. *Journal of Humanistic Psychology* 15(3):41–63.

Einon, D. (1980). The purpose of play. Pp. 21–32 in J. Cherfas & K. Lewin eds., *Not work-alone.* London: Maurice Temple Smith Ltd.

Erikson, E. (1950). *Childhood and society.* New York: Norton.

Fink, E. (1979). The ontology of play. Pp. 73–83 in E. Gerber & W. Morgan eds., *Sport and the body.* Philadelphia: Lea & Febiger.

Harlow, H., & Harlow, M. (1962). Social deprivation in monkeys. *Scientific American* 207:137–146.

Huizinga, J. (1979). The nature of play. Pp. 18–21 in E. Gerber & W. Morgan eds., *Sport and the body.* Philadelphia: Lea & Febiger.

Jack, W. (1987). Using play in psychiatric rehabilitation. *Journal of Psychosocial Nursing* 25(7):17–20.

Johnson, S.W., McSweeney, M., & Webster, R.E. (1989). Leisure: How to promote inpatient motivation after discharge. *Journal of Psychosocial Nursing* 27(9):29–31.

Kolkmeier, L.G. (1988). Play and laughter: Moving toward harmony. Pp. 289–304 in B. Dossey, L. Keegan, C. Guzzetta, & L. Kolkmeier eds., *Holistic nursing—a handbook for practice.* Rockville, MD: Aspen.

Mannell, R., & McMahon, L. (1982). Humor as play: Its relationship to psychological well-being during the course of the day. *Leisure Sciences* 5:143–155.

Martin, L. (1978). The role of play in the learning process. *Educational Forum* 43:51–58.

Mayer, K., & Griffin, M. (1990). The play project: Use of stimulus objects with demented patients. *Journal of Gerontological Nursing* 16(1):32–37.

Millar, S. (1974). *The psychology of play.* New York: Jason Aronson, Inc.

Nickerson, E., & O'Laughlin, K. (1982). *Helping through action: Action-oriented therapies.* Amherst, MA: Human Resources Development Press.

Potenza, M., & Labbancz, M. (1989). The use of poetry in a day care center for Alzheimer's disease. *American Journal of Alzheimer's and Related Disorders & Research* 4(1):10–12.

Rettie, D. (1976). Leisure life patterns in the next generation. Pp. 71–73 in T. Craig ed., *The humanistic and mental health aspects of sports, exercise, and recreation.* Chicago: American Medical Association.

Rhyme, J. (1976). The gestalt approach to experience, art, and art therapy. Pp. 477–492 in C. Hutcher & P. Himelstein eds., *The handbook of gestalt therapy.* New York: Jason Aronson, Inc.

Riordan, R. (1983). Gardening as a rehabilitation adjunct. *Journal of Rehabilitation* 49(4):39–41.

Schmitz, K. (1979). Sport and play: Suspension of the ordinary. Pp. 22–29 in E. Gerber & W. Morgan eds., *Sport and the body.* Philadelphia: Lea & Febiger.

Schuman, S., Marcus, D., & Nesse, D. (1978). Puppetry and the mentally ill. *The Journal of Occupational Therapy* 27:484–486.

Serok, S., & Blum, A. (1979). Games: A treatment for delinquent youths. *Crime and Delinquency* 25:358–363.

Sheffer, M., & Harlock, S. (1980). Use of drawings in occupational therapy patient-evaluations. *Journal of Rehabilitation* 46(3):44–49.

Smith, T., & Glickstein, C. (1982). Art as a therapeutic modality for individuals with alcohol-related problems in a milieu setting. *Occupational Therapy in Mental Health* 1(4):33–43.

Vandenberg, B., & Kielhofner, G. (1982). Play in evolution, culture, and individual adaptation: Implications for therapy. *The American Journal of Occupational Therapy* 36:20–28.

Wadeson, H. (1982). History and the application of art therapy. Pp. 16–24 in E. Nickerson & K. O'Laughlin eds., *Helping through action: Action-oriented therapies.* Amherst, MA: Human Resource Development Press.

Whetstone, W.R. (1986). Social dramatics: Social skills development for the chronically mentally ill. *Journal of Advanced Nursing* 11:67–74.

CHAPTER 35

HUMOR

BACKGROUND

The nature of humor and laughter has tantalized humans since ancient times. Four humors—choler, melancholy, sanguine, and phlegm—were identified by the ancients; if these were in balance, one was said to be in good humor. Early Greek philosophers wrote treatises on humor (McGhee, 1979). Plato and Aristotle viewed it as base and degenerate (Chapman & Foot, 1976). Ben Jonson, an English author, purposed that humor served as a social corrective in its use as criticism of human follies (cited in Chapman & Foote, 1976). Freud (1960) suggested that humor allows an adult to abandon the rules of logic and the constraints of rationality and to think again like a child.

Despite the evidence on the use of humor as a healing remedy, modern medicine and health care had largely ignored its use until Norman Cousins (1979) drew attention to the positive results he obtained from using laughter. During the past several years numerous articles on humor have appeared in nursing journals (Bellert, 1989; Henry & Moody, 1985; Pasquali, 1990; Rosenberg, 1989; Ruxton, 1988; Simon, 1990; Sullivan & Deane, 1988; Summers, 1988). Workshops on the use of humor and laughter in health care are available. Research on the effects that humor has on health outcomes, including its effects on the psychoneuroimmunological system, is being conducted.

Perhaps it is incorrect to designate humor itself as an intervention, but rather that certain stimuli are used in an attempt to produce a state of mirth in a person. The physiological effects of laughter are also being explored (Fry, 1986).

Definition

Humor is viewed by some to be a distinguishing characteristic of humans (Berlyne, 1972). Recent research, however, has revealed that chimpanzees and gorillas who have been taught to sign respond to humorous situations (McGhee, 1979). Appreciating humor is held by many to be a basic ingredient of overall well-being.

The terms "humor" and "laughter" are often used interchangeably. They are different, but both are difficult to define. McGhee (1979) provided two definitions of humor. The more basic one is:

> The mental experience of discovering and appreciating ludicrous or absurdly incongruous ideas, events, or situations. [p. 6]

The second definition identifies the attributes of a happening that make us laugh. McGhee states:

> Humor is not a characteristic of certain events (such as cartoons, jokes, clowning behavior, etc.), although certain stimulus events are more likely than others to produce the perception of humor. Humor is not an emotion, although it may alter our emotional state, and we are more likely to experience it in some emotional states than in others. Finally, humor is not a kind of

Table 35.1
Esar's Categorles of Humor

Wisecrack: directed at a particular person
Epigram: ridicules group
Riddle
Cunumdrum: punning riddle; double meaning to word
Gag: definite form of comic dialogue
Joke: short story stripped of detail with a definite setting
Anecdote: interesting or striking event or incident

Source: From E. Esar, *The humor of humor.* New York: Bramhall House, 1952.

behavior (such as laughter or smiling), although specific types of behavior are characteristically related to the perception of humor. [p. 6]

McGhee commented that both definitions are rather circuitous and that humor is something that exists in an individual's mind and not in the real world. This statement is supported by dissimilar things being perceived as humorous by different individuals and that no one item is funny to all humans. An item is not consistently humorous to the same individual over time.

Laughter is often the outgrowth of a humorous situation. Laughter is a physiological reaction to something the person views as funny. It is not, however, restricted to responses to humor and can occur when a person is tickled, embarrassed, or nervous. Nervous laughter is termed "inappropriate." Inappropriate laughter is found in certain disease conditions: Alzheimer's disease, multiple sclerosis, and pseudobulbar palsy.

Humor has been categorized in a number of ways. Gruner's (1978) list includes exaggeration, incongruity, surprise, slapstick, absurd (nonsense), human predicaments, ridicule, defiance, violence, and verbal humor such as jokes and puns. These categories are not mutually exclusive. Esar's (1952) categorizations, presented in Table 35.1, tend to be mutually exclusive. One category lacking from Esar's list is the pun, which is frequently used as a form of humor.

Scientific Basis

Many theories on humor have been explored, and no one theory has won general acceptance (Holland, 1982). Lefcourt and Martin (1986) organize humor theories into three main categories: arousal, incongruity, and superiority. Table 35.2 lists the theories grouped under each of these main categories.

According to the arousal theories, humor is used to relieve tension. McGhee (1979) viewed the action of humor as similar to that proposed by Jacobson (1970) for progressive muscle relaxation. Muscles are tense when a person is anxious. Laughing causes the muscles to relax. A mental image of the relaxed muscles is formed and one associates this feeling with situations that can produce a relaxed state.

According to the incongruity theory, humor arises from disjointed pairings of ideas or situations that are divergent from the customary or logical. Keith-Spiegel (1972) viewed the cause of laughter to be the sudden perception of the incongruity between a concept and the real object that one had thought it to be. Laughter is the expression of this incongruity. Some feel that surprise is necessary to make a situation humorous. Surprise and incongruity both involve an instantaneous disruption of one's usual thought or action. The comedian uses surprise to a great extent in getting audiences to laugh. Dodge and Rossett (1982) suggested the following sequence of elements as the basis for the incongruity theory of humor:

Table 35.2
Theories Proposed for Explaining Humor

Arousal theories
    Psychoanalytic (Freud, 1928)
    Arousal boost (Berlyne, 1972)
    Reversal (Apter, 1982)
Incongruity theories
    Bisociation (Koestler, 1964)
    Incongruity-resolution (Suls, 1972)
Superiority
    Mechanical (Bergson, 1911)
    Misattribution (Zillman, 1983)

1. Humor set: The expectancy that funniness is on the way.
2. Establishment of a schema.
3. Introduction of incongruity or conflict with the schema—uncertainty, surprise, bafflement.
4. The resolution of that conflict.
5. The speed of that resolution—fast resolution leads to a sharp guffaw, a slow dawning resolution more often causes a smile. [p. 12]

Suls (1972) used information processing analysis to gain a better understanding of the basis of humor in situations and cartoons. He suggests two stages for viewing a situation as humorous. In the first stage the expectations about the text are disconfirmed by the ending of the joke or caption on the cartoon; this creates incongruity. In the second stage the perceiver engages in problem solving to find a cognitive rule that makes the punch line follow from the main part of the joke and resolve the incongruity. Humor is derived from experiencing a sudden incongruity which is then made congruous. Motivation plays a role in moving the person to the second stage. The degree of incongruity is directly related to the surprise experienced and this influences the desire to solve the problem. Suls (1972) delineated four factors that determine the funniness of a joke or cartoon:

1. Incongruity of the joke ending; it violates the expectation.
2. The complexity of the problem solving.
3. The time that is needed to solve the incongruity.
4. The salience of the content of the joke.

McGhee (1979) supported Suls' two stage humor process; he believed that jokes and cartoons have two distinct structural dimensions, incongruity and resolution. Rothbart (1976) disagreed; she contended that resolution is not always needed for a person to appreciate a situation as humorous. The person may recognize the incongruity but be unable to determine the ramifications of it.

The third category of humor theories, superiority, dates back to Aristotle and Plato (Lefcourt & Martin, 1986). Humor results from a sense of superiority derived from putting down or disparaging another. The types of humor found in this category are often aggressive or sardonic in nature. It has been suggested that the essential affect of humor is derived from a sense of mastery or ego strength (Lefcourt & Martin, 1986).

Laughter encompasses much more than an automatic physiological response to a stimulus. Not everyone laughs at the same things, nor does one view the same things as funny on repeated exposures (Holland, 1982). Laughter is a universal phenomenon, and the basic elements of what is humorous appear to span cultures. More is not always better; Berlyne (1972) stated that a moderate amount of arousal is more

Table 35.3
Effects of Laughter on Physiological Status

Muscle stimulation: ranges from general muscle exercise to increased production of plasminogen

Muscle relaxation: reduces spasms and pain

Cardiac stimulation: increases heart rate and blood pressure

Respiratory stimulation: increases ventilation, accelerates exchange of residual air, disrupts cyclic breathing, aids clearing of bronchial tree

Stimulates catecholamine production: improves memory and alertness

Compiled from Fry, W.F. (1986). Humor, physiology, and the aging process. Pp. 81–98 in L. Nahemow, K. McCluskey-Fawcett, & P. McGhee eds., *Humor and aging.* Orlando: Academic Press.

enjoyable than extremes. Fry (1986) summarized the benefits resulting from laughter. These are found in Table 35.3.

Although much remains unknown about humor, it is a very important part of the lives of most people. The huge sums of money spent yearly to hear comedians and the large number of comedy movies and television programs produced support this premise. The next section will explore ways in which forms of humor can be used as nursing interventions.

INTERVENTION

Technique

What are techniques and materials to use that will be perceived as humorous and evoke laughter? There are numerous joke books, and hosts of cartoons, situation comedies on television, comedians, and comic films. How can a nurse decide what type of humor or which medium to use for a particular patient or group of patients? Norman Cousins rented a hotel room and viewed old comedy movies for hours upon hours, laughing uproariously at the very funny scenes. Is this use of comedy films a practical mode for a particular patient?

First, assessment of the patient is needed. Pollio et al. (1972) provided the excerpts of works of several comedians to undergraduate students. The investigators found a big discrepancy between what people laughed at, pointing to the need for the nurse to determine the types of humor appreciated by a patient. One person may find some humor offensive while another may find it uproariously funny. Holland (1982) tried to establish a link between the types of jokes amusing to persons and personal traits that characterize these groups. In a study by Wilson and Molleston (1981), females found cartoons to be less humorous than did males. Insults and ridicule are often the basis of humor. However, Wicker et al. (1980) found that over-retaliation on a victim decreased the funniness of jokes.

Pollio et al. (1972) investigated reactions to records of Don Rickles, Lenny Bruce, Bill Cosby, Phyllis Diller, and Godfrey Cambridge; humor of Cosby and Diller consistently produced a larger number of laughs than did the others. The albums used were:

"Best of Phyllis Diller" (Verve, #V-15053).
"Revenge" by Bill Cosby (Warner Brothers #1691).
"Wonderfulness" by Bill Cosby (Warner Brothers #1634).

It is best to select humorous materials that will create moderate arousal for the individual.

Mindess and associates (1984) constructed "The Antioch Sense of Humor Inventory" for exploring individuals' appreciation of humor, ability to create humor, and humor preference. Categories included nonsense, social satire, philosophical humor, sexual humor, hostile humor, demeaning to men, demeaning to women, ethnic humor, sick humor, and scatological humor. The inventory may be used on an individual basis or in groups. Mindness found that men preferred hostile, sick, sexual, and scatological types of humor, whereas women's preferences included sick, hostile/social satire, philosophical/demeaning to men, and sexual/scatological.

Timing of the intervention is very important. People seem to engage in frivolity more in the afternoon and evening than in the morning. Playing humorous tapes in the morning may not appeal to some persons. This author, however, noted that a local radio station presents much humor very early in the day and receives appreciative feedback from the listening audience.

In her discussion on the use of humor with oncology patients, Bellert (1989) suggested a number of ways in which humor can be used on nursing units. These include having patients keep a humor journal, conducting joke-telling sessions, providing patients with joke books or humorous stories, having staff wear costumes for holidays, and arranging for clowns to visit the unit. Much creativity can be used in implementing the intervention of humor.

Measurement of Effectiveness

Relief of symptoms or improvement of the state for which it was prescribed is one method for measuring the effectiveness of humor. If the person was depressed, measurement of the depressive state would be indicated. This could be determined by observing engagement in activities, facial expression, degree of involvement in activities, etc.

The Situational Humor Response Questionnaire (SHRQ) for determining an individual's response to particular types of humor was developed by Lefcourt and Martin (1986). The SHRQ has been used in numerous studies and has been validated as truly measuring humor. The SHRQ comprises 21 items. Lefcourt and Martin (1986) also developed a 7-item humor coping scale that assesses the degree to which a person uses humor in coping with stressors.

Humorists have tried to measure the effectiveness of humor by the amount of laughter generated. McGhee (1979) used a five-point scale with the end points being no reaction and hearty laughter. Studies have explored the relationship between physical laughter, depth and length, and the subjective rating of the funniness of the humor (Holland, 1982). Correlations were not high; therefore, the amount of laughter produced is not necessarily indicative of how funny a joke was to a particular person. Cultural and developmental factors influence the degree of response persons have to humor. Some persons, even though they view a joke as very funny, will only smile whereas others laugh uproariously at any humorous incident. Nurses need to keep these points in mind when determining if particular material is humorous to a patient.

USES

Robinson (1970) listed the following as situations for which nurses can use humor:

1. Establishing relationships.
2. Relieving anxiety and tension.
3. Releasing anger and aggression in a socially acceptable manner.
4. Helping persons avoid feelings that are too painful or stressful to face at a particular time.
5. Facilitating learning.

Promotion of overall well-being and increasing comfort are other purposes for which humor has been used.

Relationships

Humor has been used to decrease social distance between persons (Coser, 1959) as it assists in putting persons at ease. Decrease of anxiety and tension contributes to improved interaction. Release of tension in a new situation allows the person to focus more on the message and the other person and less on one's own feelings. Kubie (1971) stated that skillfully used humor created a relaxed atmosphere that encouraged communication on sensitive areas, assisted in gaining insight into conflicts, and helped overcome stiff and formal social styles. Establishing rapport with patients, which can be promoted via humor, is also important to assure the success of nursing interventions.

Decreasing Anxiety and Tension

Decrease of anxiety was proposed by Goldstein and McGhee (1972) as a theory for the effectiveness of humor. Freud (1960) stated that laughter serves as a release of the psychic energy previously used to block expression of socially or personally unacceptable impulses. If one is laughing from a humorous situation, one cannot be anxious (McGhee, 1979). It seems incongruous that laughter can be indicative of both freedom from anxiety and of anxiety, but the two types of laughter are manifested differently. Humor may be used to relieve the tension of an emotionally charged event. Persons can use humor both prophylactically to prevent high-stress levels and to reduce elevated levels of anxiety. Many authors on humor stated that a sense of humor is indicative of being well adjusted. Lefcourt and Martin (1986) found that humor reduced the impact of negative life events. Adasiak (1989) provided case studies that depicted the effectiveness of humor in persons with Alzheimer's disease.

Releasing Anger and Aggression

Humor assists persons to act out feelings or impulses in a safe and nonthreatening manner (Kubie, 1971). Freud (1960) believed humor served as a substitute for inhibited or repressed sexual behaviors. The sexual undertones of many jokes gives credence to his belief. After studying the social function that humor played on psychiatric units, Kaplan and Boyd (1965) concluded that patients used humor extensively to express hostility. When staff were the basis of the humor, group morale was enhanced. Humor aimed at persons outside the hospital served to decrease the distance between the patients and the outside world. According to Lorenz (1966), humor is one of the best ways for humans to reduce aggression.

Avoiding Painful Feelings

Humor can be used as a defense mechanism to avoid dealing immediately with situations that are too painful (Leiber, 1986). Persons may use humor to avoid the overwhelming impact of a diagnosis or treatment modality. Use in this context is probably based on a diminishment of anxiety and fear. Humor reduces tension, allowing the person to confront and handle the situation (Simon, 1990). However, caution is needed as persons may continue to use humor and thus avoid facing the conflict or painful situation.

Enhancing Learning

Countless numbers of lectures and presentations begin with a joke or cartoon. The humor serves to reduce the anxiety of the presenter. Humor also serves to gain the attention of the audience. Research studies have shown that more learning occurs when high-anxiety levels are reduced. Clabby (1979) found that humorous information was retained at a significantly higher level than nonhumorous information in an intentional learning task. This may be the result from laughter increasing catecholamine production (Fry, 1986); McGaugh (cited in Fry, 1986) reported that an increase in catecholamines improved memory. Patients and/or relatives are often extremely anxious when being taught self-care. Interjecting humor can help to reduce this tension.

Some persons associate certain items with the joke that was used; humor thus serves as a memory jogger. Dodge and Rossett (1982) provide heuristics for including humor in instruction. Use of humor in instruction needs to be carefully planned so that it will contribute to learning.

Well-being

A sense of humor is often associated with persons who rate their overall well-being as high. Simon (1990) found a significant positive relationship between use of humor, morale, and health in a group of older adults. Cogan et al. (1987) reported that persons exposed to laughter had higher discomfort thresholds (experienced less discomfort) as compared to a group who had not received this intervention. Thus, humor could be used for persons who are experiencing pain or who would be experiencing a painful procedure.

Precautions

Timing is essential to the effectiveness of the use of humor as a nursing intervention. Harrelson and Stroud (1967) caution against using humor early in psychotherapy; they believe that if humor is used before rapport is established, it could be destructive. The nurse needs to become more aware of areas about which a patient is sensitive and thus avoid these in choosing types of humor. Mindess (1976) stated that before a person can help others recognize the ridiculous aspects of their predicament, the helper must first recognize those aspects in his or her own life. This points to the need for the nurse to know something about humor and to appreciate humor before using it with others. Watson (1988) detailed methods used to raise students' levels of consciousness regarding humor. As has been noted earlier, because of the wide variation in personal perceptions of humor, it is critical that the nurse determine what a particular patient deems humorous before intervening.

RESEARCH QUESTIONS

Although nurses have used humor informally for many years, few formal studies have been conducted by nurses on the use of humor and laughter as a nursing intervention. Norman Cousins' recent book, *Head First, The Biology of Hope,* (1990) indicates that the health care community is beginning to give greater credence to the power of humor and laughter. Explorations on how these contribute to healing and overall well-being are being initiated. The significant increase in articles on humor that have been published in nursing journals reflects the growing interest that nurses have in humor and laughter as a nursing intervention. The following are some areas on which more definitive data are needed:

1. What types of humor are the most effective with particular patient populations? Wilson and Molleston (1981) found that women and men differed in reactions to varying types of humor. What are the best ways for the nurse to assess the type(s) of humor to use with specific patients?
2. Fry (1986) suggested numerous positive physiological effects from laughter. However, little "hard" data exist to substantiate these effects. Therefore, studies are needed to verify these hypotheses.
3. Is humor more effective when used on an individual basis or in a group? Pistole and Shor (1979) found that individuals rated items funnier when humor was presented on an individual basis rather than in a group.
4. Nurses need to have an appreciation of humor in order to use it. What are methods by which nurses can gain this appreciation?
5. Are the assessment instruments (Lefcourt & Martin, 1986; Mindness et al., 1984) that have been developed useable in clinical areas? Are they feasible to use with persons across the age span?

REFERENCES

Adasiak, J.P. (1989). Humor and the Alzheimer's patient: the psychological basis. *American Journal of Alzheimer's Care and Related Disorders and Research* 4(4):18–21.

Apter, M.J. (1982). *The experience of motivation.* London: Academic.

Bellert, J.L. (1989). Humor—A therapeutic approach in oncology nursing. *Cancer Nursing* 12(2):65–70.

Bergson, H. (1911). *Laughter: An essay on the meaning of the comic.* New York: Macmillan.

Berlyne, D. (1972). Humor and its kin. Pp. 43–60 in J. Goldstein & P. McGhee eds., *The psychology of humor.* New York: Academic Press.

Chapman, A., & Foot, H. (1976). *Humour and laughter: Theory, research and applications.* London: John Wiley & Sons.

Clabby, J. (1979). Humor as a preferred activity of the creative and humor as a facilitator of learning. *Psychology, A Quarterly Journal of Human Behavior* 16:5–11.

Cogan, R., Cogan, D., Waltz, W., & McCue, M. (1987). Effects of laughter and relaxation on discomfort thresholds. *Journal of Behavior Medicine* 10:139–144.

Coser, R. (1959). Some social functions of laughter. *Human Relations* 12:171–182.

Cousins, N. (1979). *Anatomy of an illness as perceived by the patient: Reflections on healing and regeneration.* New York: Norton.

————. (1990). *Head first, the biology of hope.* New York: Dutton.

Dodge, B., & Rossett, A. (1982). Heuristics for humor in instruction. *NSPI Journal* 21:11–14, 32.

Esar, E. (1952). *The humor of humor.* New York: Bramhall House.

Freud, S. (1960). *Jokes and their relation to the unconscious,* New York: Norton. (Originally: *Der Witz und seine Beziehung zum Unbewussten.* Leipzig and Vienna: Durticke, 1905.)

————. (1928). Humor. *International Journal of Psychoanalysis* 9:1–6.

Fry, W.F. (1986). Humor, physiology, and the aging process. Pp. 81–98 in L. Nahemow, K. McCluskey-Fawcett, & P. McGhee eds., *Humor and aging.* Orlando: Academic Press.

Goldstein, J., & McGhee, P. (1972). *The psychology of humor.* New York: Academic Press.

Gruner, C. (1978). *Understanding laughter.* Chicago: Nelson-Hall.

Harrelson, R., & Stroud, P. (1967). Observations of humor in chronic schizophrenics. *Mental Hygiene* 51:458–461.

Henry, B.M., & Moody, L.E. (1985). Energize with laughter. *Nursing Success* 2(1):5–8, 36.

Holland, N. (1982). *Laughing, a psychology of humor.* Ithaca: Cornell University Press.

Jacobson, E. (1970). *Modern treatment of tense patients.* Springfield, IL: Thomas Publishing.

Kaplan, H., & Boyd, I. (1965). The social functions of humor on an open psychiatric ward. *Psychiatric Quarterly* 39:502–515.

Keith-Spiegel, P. (1972). Early conceptions of humor: Varieties and issues. Pp. 4–39 in J. Goldstein & P. McGhee eds., *The psychology of humor.* New York: Academic Press.

Koestler, A. (1964). *The act of creation.* London: Hutchinson.

Kubie, L. (1971). The destructive potential of humor in psychotherapy. *American Journal of Psychiatry* 127:861–866.

Lefcourt, H.M., & Martin, R.A. (1986). *Humor and life stress: Antidote to adversity.* New York: Springer-Verlag.

Leiber, D.B. (1986). Laughter and humor in critical care. *Dimensions of Critical Care Nursing* 5:162-170.

Lorenz, K. (1966). *On aggression.* New York: Harcourt, Brace, and World.

McGhee, P. (1979). *Humor, its origin and development.* San Francisco: W.H. Freeman and Company.

Mindess, H. (1976). The use and abuse of humour in psychotherapy. Pp. 331-341 in A. Chapman & H. Foot eds., *Humour and laughter: Theory, research and applications.* London: John Wiley & Sons.

Mindess, H., Miller, C., Turek, J., Bender, A., & Corbin, S. (1984). The Antioch sense of humor inventory. Unpublished manuscript, Antioch University, Psychology Department, Los Angeles.

Pasquali, E.A. (1990). Learning to laugh: Humor as therapy. *Journal of Psychosocial Nursing* 28(3):31-35.

Pistole, D., & Shor, R. (1979). A multivariate study of the effect of repetition on humor appreciation as qualified by two social influence factors. *Journal of General Psychology* 100:43-51.

Pollio, H., Mers, R., & Lucchesi, W. (1972). Humor, laughter, and smiling: Some preliminary observations of funny behavior. Pp. 211-242 in J. Goldstein & P. McGhee eds., *The psychology of humor.* New York: Academic Press.

Robinson, V. (1970). Humor in nursing. Pp. 129-152 in C. Carlson ed., *Behavioral concepts and nursing intervention.* Philadelphia: J.P. Lippincott.

Rosenberg, L. (1989). A delicate dose of humor. *Nursing Forum* 24(2):3-7.

Rothbart, M. (1976). Incongruity, problem-solving, and laughter. Pp. 37-54 in A. Chapman & H. Foot eds., *Humour and laughter: Theory, research and applications.* London: John Wiley & Sons.

Ruxton, J.P. (1988). Humor intervention deserves our attention. *Holistic Nursing Practice* 2(3):54-62.

Simon, J.M. (1990). Humor and its relationship to perceived health, life satisfaction, and morale in older adults. *Issues in Mental Health Nursing* 11:17-31.

Sullivan, J.L., & Deane, D.M. (1988). Humor and health. *Journal of Gerontological Nursing* 14(1):20-24.

Suls, J. (1972). A two-stage model for the appreciation of jokes and cartoons: An information-processing analysis. Pp. 81-100 in J. Goldstein & P. McGhee eds., *The psychology of humor.* New York: Academic Press.

Summers, A.D. (1988). Humor: Coping in recovery from addiction. *Issues in Mental Health Nursing* 9:169-179.

Watson, M.J. (1988). Facilitate learning with humor. *Journal of Nursing Education* 27:89-90.

Wicker, F., Barron, W., & Willis, A. (1980). Disparagement humor: Dispositions and resolutions. *Journal of Personality and Social Psychology* 39:701-709.

Wilson, D., & Molleston, J. (1981). Effects of sex and type of humor on humor appreciation. *Journal of Personality Assessment* 45:90-96.

Zillman, D. (1983). Disparagement humor. Pp. 85-108 in P. McGhee & J. Goldstein eds., *Handbook of humor research,* vol. 1. New York: Springer-Verlag.

SECTION 6

RESEARCH

CHAPTER 36

RESEARCH STRATEGIES TO FURTHER A SCIENTIFIC BASIS FOR INTERVENTIONS

BACKGROUND

The preceding chapters have noted numerous research studies related to nursing interventions. Research testing of the specific interventions described varies with a significant amount of research having been conducted on some interventions and minimal or no research available on other interventions. These differences may reflect the extent to which certain interventions have been used within nursing or other disciplines. What has been heartening in relation to nursing interventions is the increase in the number of published research reports, particularly studies that have been done by clinical nurse specialists. Many of the clinical journals have special sections devoted to research.

Great variation exists in the rigor of the designs used in research on nursing interventions. Major weaknesses exist in many of the studies. Small sample sizes and the absence of random selection of subjects are two problems frequently found. These weaknesses greatly limit the ability to generalize the study findings.

Another deficit in research on nursing interventions is the lack of research programs devoted to specific interventions. Subsequent studies have not built on previous research, thus hampering the development of an explanatory knowledge base for nursing practice (Moody et al., 1988). If subsequent studies have been done, they infrequently include the suggestions or modifications noted in earlier studies.

Although there has been a considerable increase in research on nursing interventions, much work remains to be done. What can be deduced from the research that has been done? What types of studies are needed to provide a more prescriptive basis for the use of nursing interventions? This chapter will explore some strategies that will promote use of current research findings and propose strategies to be used in studying nursing interventions. Literature reviews, consensus conferences, meta-analysis, clinical trials, appropriate methodologies, and utilization of research findings will be discussed.

REVIEW OF LITERATURE

Reviews of literature on particular therapies and interventions are commonly found in journals of other disciplines. Until recently, such reviews have not been commonplace in nursing literature. The first volume of the *Annual Review of Nursing Research* was published in 1983. Each year extensive reviews are presented on selected nursing topics including nursing interventions. Such reviews allow researchers and practitioners to gain a perspective on the research that has been done in an area. The critique of the studies provides direction for planning and conducting subsequent studies in the area.

Cooper (1989) describes two types of literature reviews: integrative and theoretical. Integrative reviews summarize the studies that have been conducted relative to a specific area and provide overall conclusions that can be drawn from the findings. Important issues that are unresolved are highlighted. Theoretical reviews compare and contrast theories that may explain a particular phenomenon. Key research studies are included in theoretical reviews. Integrative reviews are much more common than theoretical reviews, but both serve important roles in knowledge development.

The guidelines for selecting the studies that are being reviewed need to be specified. Was a literature search done to identify studies? If so, what data base(s) was used? Or, was another method used? Schwartz et al. (1988) specified eight other strategies for identifying research studies:

Abstracts for theses and dissertations.
Indexes that identify papers on a topic.
Ancestry searches in which bibliographies of other articles on the topic are used.
Formal and informal networks such as use of research organizations.
Major publishers on topic.
Major research institutions who have conducted research on the topic.
Fugitive literature in which unpublished studies are identified.
Senior investigators who have conducted research on the topic.

Securing studies to be reviewed is time-consuming, but the comprehensiveness of the articles reviewed determine the usefulness of the review. Unless readers are provided with information on the extent of the literature reviewed, they cannot be assured that all studies in the area were critiqued for inclusion.

Reviews need to include studies that present various perspectives, rather than just including those that support a particular point of view (Moody, 1990a). To be useful, reviews need to critique the studies rather than present solely a narrative of the studies. A critique of this nature demands that the reviewer be familiar with the area, with research methodologies, and be honest in presenting positive and negative aspects of each study.

High quality reviews of nursing interventions provide an excellent source of information for nurses considering use of a particular intervention for a specific population. Inclusion of reviews in clinical nursing journals would be very beneficial to practitioners.

CONSENSUS CONFERENCES

Consensus conferences are sponsored by the National Institutes of Health to review the interventions used to treat a particular disorder. An extensive review of the literature is done by the experts who convene to discuss the findings from these studies. At the conclusion of the conference, the experts arrive at the most appropriate intervention to use for treating the disorder.

The Midwest Nursing Research Society has sponsored conferences similar to the consensus conferences; these are termed "Synthesis Conferences." Nursing experts in a particular area present reviews of relevant studies. After discussions by the experts and conference participants, conclusions are drawn regarding the state of the art in the area and the directions future research should take. The proceedings from these conferences are published by Sigma Theta Tau, International. An example of a proceedings is *Individual, Family, and Community Interventions to Improve Exercise and Nutrition Behaviors* (Lobo & Loveland-Cherry, 1989).

META-ANALYSIS

Meta-analytic techniques have a rather short history in statistical analyses (Glass, 1976). Meta-analysis is defined by Glass (1976) as

Table 36.1
Meta-analysis on Nursing Interventions

Educational interventions for surgical patients (Devine & Cook, 1983; Hathaway, 1986)

Nursing interventions (Smith, 1988)

Pain interventions (Broome et al., 1989; Heater et al., 1988)

Relaxation training (Hyman et al., 1989)

> the statistical analysis of a large collection of analysis results from individual studies for the purpose of integrating the findings. It connotes a rigorous alternative to the casual, narrative discussions of research studies which typify our attempts to make sense of the rapidly expanding research literature. [p. 3]

According to Moody (1990a), meta-analysis transcends the typical literature review as it employs a systematic method of review, and the conclusions arrived at regarding the findings from the studies are empirically based. Doing a meta-analysis on studies related to a particular intervention may provide more direction for use of a specific intervention than can be derived from merely looking at the results obtained from individual studies in the area.

Meta-analyses can only be done on experimental studies. Some who have used meta-analytic techniques have used very stringent criteria for the inclusion of studies. Smith (1988), in her meta-analysis of nursing interventions, only included studies that had utilized random selection of subjects. Moody (1990a) indicates that meta-analysis is appropriate when used to increase the estimates of effect size, to increase statistical power, to resolve uncertainties when differences in results have been obtained in the use of an intervention, and to answer questions not posed when the initial study was conducted. A strength of the meta-analytic technique is the ability to arrive at conclusions about an intervention even though different instruments were used to measure the outcome(s). Meta-analysis also provides direction for future research (Curlette & Cannella, 1985).

Nurse researchers have begun to use meta-analysis to determine outcomes in relation to specific interventions. Table 36.1 lists some of the meta-analyses that have been performed on nursing intervention studies. Sufficient studies have been conducted on other interventions warranting meta-analyses. Reductions in funding for research necessitates that the maximum usage be obtained from studies that have been conducted (Cordray, 1990). Meta-analytic techniques will be useful in achieving this end. However, rigor in selecting studies and in conducting the analyses is necessary.

CLINICAL TRIALS

Medicine has consistently used clinical trials for testing the efficacy of treatment modalities. A clinical trial is a prospective study in which the effects and value of one or more interventions/modalities are compared against a control (Moody, 1990b). A clinical trial is indicated when evidence suggests that a new or infrequently used intervention would be more beneficial, safer, more cost-effective, or less harmful than the intervention that is most commonly being used (Moody, 1990b). Various experimental research designs can be used for clinical trials: parallel, withdrawal, crossover, factorial, group allocation, and equivalent (Friedman et al., 1985). One aspect that is key to clinical studies is the randomization of subjects to treatment/control groups; this helps to eliminate investigator bias and to make groups similar in characteristics.

Before conducting a clinical trial, the investigator needs to consider certain ethical issues. Hatch (1987) has elaborated questions for clinicians to answer in relation to the use of biofeedback in clinical trials. Included were issues related to withholding treatment from the control group or from the experimental groups during the baseline period, having sufficient data about the treatment factors so as not to jeopardize participants, and making a decision on whether current knowledge allows a preferred treatment to be chosen. Thus, extensive knowledge of the area is needed before clinical trials can be conducted.

Although a clinical trial can be done in one agency, many clinical trials are multi-site. This allows for larger sample sizes and collecting the data in a shorter period of time. Key to the success of any clinical trial, but fundamental to multi-site clinical trials, is a well-defined protocol for selection of subjects and the procedure to be used. A specific protocol avoids the introduction of extraneous variables. Even if only one agency is used for the clinical trial, the well-defined protocol will allow others to conduct a subsequent trial.

A well-designed clinical trial provides excellent data regarding the efficacy of a particular intervention with a specific population. An increase in the use of clinical trials in nursing will guide nurses in the selection of interventions for use with particular patients/groups. However, the minimal knowledge base related to some interventions precludes the conduction of clinical trials at this point in time.

APPROPRIATE METHODOLOGIES

The above sections have primarily addressed studies that have used quantitative methods for exploring the variables. However, other methodologies also are needed for studying the efficacy of nursing interventions (Phillips, 1989). In fact, the traditional quantitative methodologies are not appropriate for testing some of the nursing interventions, such as presence, that are included in this text. Many nursing studies now include both quantitative and qualitative techniques for studying nursing phenomena. The study question and the nature of the phenomenon being studied determine the design and methodologies that will be used.

Acceptance of the use of qualitative methods has increased. The use of these techniques requires the same rigor in designing studies as does the use of quantitative methods. Researchers need to ascertain which methods are most appropriate for obtaining data that will answer the question posed. Since many research courses have traditionally included minimal information on qualitative methods, nurses may find recent texts on qualitative methods to be helpful in making decisions regarding methodologies to use (Moody, 1990; Woods & Catanzaro, 1988).

UTILIZATION OF RESEARCH FINDINGS

Nursing is a practice discipline. Therefore, the development of knowledge should serve to advance practice; i.e, improve patient care. Because of the vast differences in educational preparation of practitioners, many nurses providing patient care have a minimal understanding about research. Furthermore, few nurses in clinical areas read the journals in which research reports have traditionally been published. The increase of research findings in clinically-focused nursing journals is assisting nurses in clinical areas to become more familiar with nursing research and the findings from nursing research studies.

Pressures for research-based nursing practice are increasing (Goode et al., 1987). To date, two research utilization projects have been conducted in nursing: Western Interstate Commission for Higher Education (WICHE) Regional Program for Nursing Research Development (Krueger et al., 1978) and the Conduct and Utilization of Research in Nursing (CURN) project conducted under the auspices of the Michigan Nurses' Association (Haller et al., 1979). Publications on research-based practice for 10 nursing problems originated from the latter project; these have had wide use in nursing cirlces.

Before implementing a particular intervention with a specific population, a careful and thorough critique of the research reports in which the intervention has been tested is essential. A number of criteria/questions

Table 36.2
Evaluating a Research Report for Use in Practice

A. Problem studied and literature review
  1. Scientific evaluation
    a. Is problem clearly defined?
    b. Is significance of problem discussed?
    c. Was research justified by literature?
    d. Is relationship to previous research clear?
    e. Was conceptual framework evident? Appropriate?
    f. Is specific purpose of study clear? Are variables defined? Are hypotheses stated and well founded?
  2. Practice evaluation
    a. Is this problem significant to nursing practice?
    b. Does the framework "fit" with what the nurse knows about nursing practice and the phenomenon?

B. Setting and subjects
  1. Scientific evaluation
    a. Is the population described? Sample described?
    b. How were subjects recruited? Sampled?
    c. What were the sources of sampling error?
    d. Is sample size adequate?
    e. Were subjects' rights adequately protected?
    f. What was the setting for the study? Laboratory? Community? Hospital?
  2. Practice evaluation
    a. Are the patients typical? Are they similar to the patients in the nurse's setting? Could differences possibly influence results?
    b. Is the setting typical? In what ways is it similar to and different from the nurse's setting?
    c. Would patients be likely to participate if this was not a study?

C. Design
  1. Scientific evaluation
    a. What type of design was used (e.g., descriptive, correlational, longitudinal, cross-sectional)?
    b. Is design appropriate to answer question asked?
    c. Are appropriate controls included?
    d. Can confounding variables be identified?
  2. Practice evaluation
    a. Would it be possible to measure the same outcomes if findings were applied in the nurse's setting?
    b. Are methods adequately described to permit replication?

D. Instruments and measures
  1. Scientific evaluation
    a. To what extent are measures valid and reliable?
    b. Were reliability and validity tested and reported in this study?
    c. Were measures adequately described to determine their relevance to study purpose and findings?
    d. Could the measures have influenced the findings?

Table 36.2 (continued)
Evaluating a Research Report for Use In Practice

---

2. Practice evaluation
   a. Is there any assurance that these measures would be meaningful and accurate in the clinical setting?
   b. Are these data collection methods feasible in the nurse's setting?

E. Data analysis
   1. Scientific evaluation
      a. How were the data distributed (e.g., frequency distribution)?
      b. Do methods answer the questions posed?
      c. Are statistical tests appropriate and applicable to questions or hypothesis?
      d. Are data presented clearly in tables?
   2. Practice evaluation
      a. Do the data fit the clinical picture?
      b. What are the probabilities that findings are due to chance? Or to some other variable?
      c. Are findings clinically as well as statistically significant?

F. Discussion and conclusion
   1. Scientific evaluation
      a. Are conclusions clearly stated?
      b. Are conclusions based on data presented?
      c. Are limitations and alternative explanations presented?
      d. Are findings related to the original framework and purpose of the study?
      e. Are results generalized to population studied?
      f. Are conclusions appropriate, given a. to e. above?
   2. Practice evaluation
      a. Does the nurse agree with the author's conclusions?
      b. What decision does the conclusion promote?
      c. Should the literature be further examined for more information?
      d. Do the findings replicate previous findings? Suggest innovation or change?
      e. Do the findings increase the nurse's sensitivity to the problem, but not lead to direct action?
      f. Does the nurse need more information from the researcher?

From M.G. Killien. (1988). Disseminating and using research findings. Pp. 479–497 in N. Woods and M. Catanzaro eds., *Nursing research: Theory and practice*. St. Louis: C.V. Mosby. Used with permission.

have been developed for guiding nurses in critiquing studies for their use in the clinical setting (Fawcett, 1982; Jacox & Prescott, 1978; Killien, 1988; Stetler & Marram, 1976). The questions posed by Killien (1988) are presented in Table 36.2. A review of the questions indicates that the person doing the critique needs to be very knowledgeable about research. Clinical nurse specialists are in a prime position to review research reports to determine the soundness of the study and the feasibility of using the findings in a specific clinical setting (Gaits et al., 1989).

Thus, although the number of studies being conducted and the number of research reports in nursing journals is expanding, almost exponentially, the incorporation of research findings into the provision of nursing care has, to a great extent, not occurred. Consistent, continued efforts are needed to accomplish this end. The increasing emphasis being placed on cost-effectiveness of care provides an excellent opportunity for nurses to demonstrate that a particular intervention is effective in achieving a patient outcome, and, perhaps, is more cost effective than other treatment modalities. The study by Brooten and colleagues (1988) on the reduction of cost resulting from the use of transitional care for low-birth weight infants is an example of the type of research studies that are needed. When nurses in clinical areas, legislators, and policy makers can see the impact that nursing interventions can make on patient outcomes and costs, nursing will have taken a giant stride forward in being recognized as a practice discipline that uses a scientific knowledge base to make a difference in patient outcomes.

REFERENCES

Broome, M., Lillis, P., & Collette-Smith, M. (1989). Pain interventions with children: A meta-analysis of research. *Nursing Research* 38:154–158.

Brooten, D., Brown, L.P., Munro, B.H., York, R., Cohen, S.M., Roncoli, M., & Hollingsworth, A. (1988). Early discharge and specialist transitional care. *Image: Journal of Nursing Scholarship* 20:64–68.

Cooper, H.M. (1989). *Integrative research: A guide for literature reviews.* Newbury Park, CA: Sage.

Cordray, D.S. (1990). Strengthening causal interpretations of non-experimental data: The role of meta-analysis. Pp. 151–172 in L. Sechrest, E. Perrin, & J. Bunker eds., *Conference proceedings of research methodology: Strengthening causal interpretation of nonexperimental data.* Rockville, MD: Department of Health and Human Services, Agency for Health Care Policy and Research.

Curlette, W.L., & Cannella, K.S. (1985). Going beyond the narrative summarization of research findings: The meta-analysis approach. *Research in Nursing and Health* 8:293–301.

Devine, E., & Cook, T. (1983). A meta-analytic analysis of effects of psychoeducational interventions on length of postsurgical hospital stay. *Nursing Research* 32:267–274.

Fawcett, J. (1982). Utilization of nursing research findings. *Image* 14:57–59.

Friedman, L.M., Furberg, C.D., & DeMets, D.L. (1985). *Fundamentals of clinical trials.* Littleton, MA: PSG.

Gaits, V., Ford, R.N., Kaplow, R., Bru, G., Belcher, A., Brown, M.H., & Bookbinder, M.I. (1989). Unit-based research forums: A model for the clinical nurse specialist to promote clinical research. *Clinical Nurse Specialist* 3:60–65.

Glass, G.V. (1976). Primary, secondary, and meta-analysis of research. *Educational Researcher* 5:3–8.

Goode, C.J., Lovett, M.K., Hayes, J.E., & Butcher, L.A. (1987). Use of research based knowledge in clinical practice. *Journal of Nursing Administration* 17(12):11–18.

Haller, K.B., Reynolds, M.A., & Horsely, J. (1979). Developing research-based innovation protocols: Process, criteria, and issues. *Research in Nursing and Health* 2:45–51.

Hatch, J.P. (1987). Guidelines for controlled clinical trials of biofeedback. Pp. 323–363 in J.P. Hatch, J.G. Fisher, & J.D. Rugh eds., *Biofeedback: Studies in clinical efficacy.* New York: Plenum.

Hathaway, D. (1986). Effect of preoperative instruction on postoperative outcomes: A meta-analysis. *Nursing Research* 35:269–275.

Heater, B., Becker, A., & Olson, R. (1988). Nursing interventions and patient outcomes: A meta-analysis of studies. *Nursing Research* 37:303–307.

Hyman, R., Feldman, H., Harris, R., Levin, R., & Malloy, G. (1989). The effects of relaxation training on clinical symptoms: A meta-analysis. *Nursing Research* 38:216–220.

Jacox, A., & Prescott, P. (1978). Determining a study's relevance for clinical practice. *American Journal of Nursing* 78:1882–1889.

Killien, M.G. (1988). Disseminating and using research findings. Pp. 479–497 in N. Woods & M. Catanzaro eds., *Nursing research—theory and practice.* St. Louis: C.V. Mosby.

Krueger, J.C., Nelson, A.H., & Wolanin, M.O. (1978). *Nursing research: Development, collaboration, and utilization.* Germantown, MD: Aspen.

Lobo, M., & Loveland-Cherry, C. (eds.) (1989). *Individual, family, and community interventions to improve exercise and nutrition behaviors.* Indianapolis: Sigma Theta Tau International.

Moody, L.E. (1990a). Meta-analysis: Qualitative and quantitative methods. Pp. 70–110 in Moody, L.E. ed., *Advancing nursing science through research,* vol. 2. Newbury Park, CA: Sage.

_____. (1990b). Randomized clinical trials. Pp. 15–69 in Moody, L.E. ed., *Advancing nursing science through research,* vol. 2. Newbury Park, CA: Sage.

_____. (1990c). *Advancing nursing science through research,* vol. 2. Newbury Park, CA: Sage.

Moody, L., Wilson, M., Smith, K., Schwartz, R., Tittle, M., & Van Cott, M. (1988). Analysis of a decade of nursing practice research. *Nursing Research* 37:374–379.

Phillips, J.R. (1989). New methods of research; Beyond the shadows of nursing science. *Nursing Science Quarterly* 2:1–2.

Schwartz, R., Moody, L., Yarandi, H., & Anderson, G.C. (1988). A meta-analysis of critical outcome variables in nonnutritive sucking in preterm infants. *Nursing Research* 36:292–295.

Smith, M.C. (1988). *Meta-analysis of nursing intervention research.* Birmingham, AL: University of Alabama-Birmingham.

Stetler, C.B., & Marram, C. (1976). Evaluating research findings for applicability in practice. *Nursing Outlook* 24(9):559–563.

Woods, N.F., & Catanzaro, M. (1988). *Nursing research theory and practice.* St. Louis: C.V. Mosby.

INDEX